AF248944

MRI of the Liver
Imaging Techniques, Contrast Enhancement, Differential Diagnosis

Springer

*Milan
Berlin
Heidelberg
New York
Hong Kong
London
Paris
Tokyo*

Günther Schneider · Luigi Grazioli · Sanjay Saini (Eds.)

MRI of the Liver

Imaging Techniques
Contrast Enhancement
Differential Diagnosis

Contributors

P. Fries
P. Caccia
M.P. Bondioni
K. Altmeyer
M. Harisinghani
R.V. D'Souza
D. Sahani

Foreword by

Pablo R. Ros

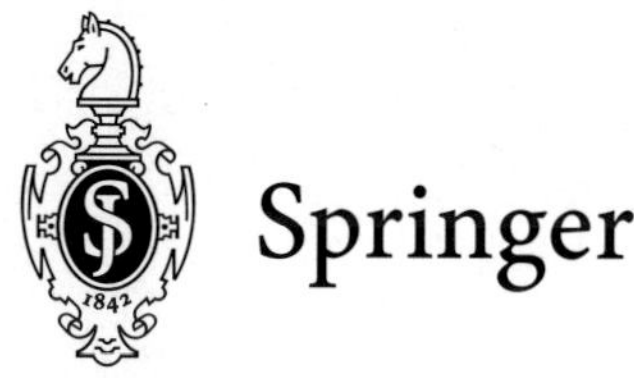

Springer

Editors

GÜNTHER SCHNEIDER, M.D.
Department of Diagnostic Radiology
University Hospital of Saarland
66421 Homburg/Saar, Germany

LUIGI GRAZIOLI, M.D.
Department of Radiology
University of Brescia
Piazale Spedali Civili 1
25023 Brescia, Italy

SANJAY SAINI, M.D.
The Division of Abdominal Imaging
and Intervention
Department of Radiology
and Harvard Medical School
Boston, MA 02114, USA

Contributors

P. FRIES
P. CACCIA
M.P. BONDIONI
K. ALTMEYER
M. HARISINGHANI
R.V. D'SOUZA
D. SAHANI

Springer-Verlag Italia
a member of BertelsmannSpringer Science+Business Media GmbH

© Springer-Verlag Italia, Milano 2003

http://www.springer.de

ISBN 88-470-0209-5

Typesetting: Compostudio, Cernusco sul Naviglio (Milano)
Printing and binding: Staroffset, Cernusco sul Naviglio (Milano)
Cover design: Simona Colombo (Milano)

Printed in Italy

SPIN 10904947

Foreword

It is with pleasure that I am writing the foreword for this textbook entitled "MRI of the Liver: Imaging Techniques, Contrast Enhancement, Differential Diagnosis" by Drs. Schneider, Grazioli and Saini.

If the liver has become the key organ to image in the abdomen, magnetic resonance (MR) imaging has become an indispensable modality for its evaluation. The absence of ionizing radiation, unparalleled soft tissue contrast, inherent multiplanar capability and high temporal resolution in dynamic gadolinium-enhanced imaging are major advantages over other imaging techniques. Furthermore, the introduction of contrast agents with liver specific properties has increased the usefulness of MRI for the detection and characterization of liver lesions.

This book fills a void in the current literature, giving radiologists and other physicians (primarily hepatologists and liver surgeons) interested in liver diseases the opportunity to have an up-to-date, single source of knowledge on MRI applied to the liver. This book is a combination of a manual, a reference textbook and an atlas. The first chapter constitutes a manual of liver MRI including modern imaging techniques and sequences. By including common imaging protocols tailored for the main manufacturers, it offers to practicing radiologists cookbook recipes to obtain superb liver MRI studies like the ones obtained by experts such as the authors. Current approaches to MRI of the liver using phased-array multicoils, enhanced gradients and motion reduction techniques allow us to have images with superb contrast resolution and acceptable spatial and temporal resolution. In chapter two, the authors cover the contrast administration strategy for MRI of the liver, detailing the use of both extracellular and liver specific contrast agents. The reasoning for the intravenous administration of extracellular gadolinium contrast agents as a useful adjunct in liver MRI is discussed. The increase in differences in signal intensity between normal hepatic parenchyma and hypo- or hypervascular neoplastic tissues is discussed, as are the specific enhancement patterns observed in different phases of perfusion following gadolinium administration. In addition, the rationale for using liver specific MR contrast agents is presented, with examples given for both manganese and iron oxide-based agents.

Chapter three presents a detailed overview of the histological classification of focal and diffuse liver pathologies, focusing on the essential needs of radiologists. In addition, possible classifications of focal liver lesions are presented based on their appearance on both unenhanced and contrast-enhanced MRI. Specifically, flow charts and tables for the differential diagnoses of liver lesions are presented, thereby consolidating in a single source the charts and tables found in a multiplicity of books and articles on abdominal and hepatobiliary imaging.

Chapters four and five constitute a reference on liver MRI of focal liver disease, discussing the radiological features of benign and malignant focal lesions in a systematic fashion. All benign and malignant primary liver lesions are presented from the most common such as hemangioma or hepatocellular carcinoma to the rarest such as nodular regenerative hyperplasia or epithelial hemangioendothelioma. Both pediatric and adult liver tumors are included. The sections on secondary liver lesions cover not only metastases and lymphoma, but also inflammatory and parasitic lesions. Where appropriate, the imaging features observed with other techniques (computed tomography and ultrasound) are presented for comparison.

The role of MRI in the characterization and monitoring of diffuse liver disease is recognized with a whole chapter dedicated to cirrhosis, iron overload and vascular pathology. For completion a chapter is included on MRI of the liver post-surgery/post-ablation, an increasing challenge for abdominal radiologists given the increased frequency with which these techniques are performed.

This textbook is very well illustrated with more than 600 figures of high quality, which allow it to be seen as an atlas on liver MRI.

This textbook on MRI of the liver taps on the expertise of three obvious leaders in liver imaging, namely Drs. Günther Schneider, Luigi Grazioli and Sanjay Saini. Their respective institutions, the University Clinic of Homburg-Saar, Germany, the University Hospital of Brescia, Italy, and the Mass. General Hospital in Boston, USA, are well-known for their interest in liver radiology and, specifically, liver MRI. This truly international effort has produced a fully-encompassing source for radiologists anywhere with current and practical information. I predict that this book will influence the way we practice liver imaging: the protocols will be improved, the differential diagnosis charts will be copied and pinned up in reading rooms in many departments and overall it will have a beneficial impact.

I invite you to read the work of Drs. Schneider, Grazioli and Saini with the certainty that you will enjoy their material and information.

November, 2002   **Pablo R. Ros, MD, MPH**

Contents

4 Imaging of Benign Focal Liver Lesions

5 Imaging of Malignant Focal Liver Lesions

6 Imaging of Diffuse Liver Disease

Contributors

Günther Schneider, M.D.
Department of Diagnostic Radiology
University Hospital of Saarland
66421 Homburg/Saar, Germany

Luigi Grazioli, M.D.
Department of Radiology
University of Brescia
Piazale Spedali Civili 1
25023 Brescia, Italy

Sanjay Saini, M.D.
The Division of Abdominal Imaging
and Intervention
Department of Radiology
and Harvard Medical School
Boston, MA 02114, USA

Peter Fries, M.D.
Department of Diagnostic Radiology
University Hospital of Saarland
66421 Homburg/Saar, Germany

Paolo Caccia, M.D.
Department of Radiology
University Hospital of Brescia
Piazzale Spedali Civili no. 1
25030 Brescia, Italy

Maria Pia Bondioni, M.D.
Department of Radiology
University Hospital of Brescia
Piazzale Spedali Civili no. 1
25030 Brescia, Italy

Katrin Altmeyer, M.D.
Department of Diagnostic Radiology
University Hospital of Saarland
66421 Homburg/Saar, Germany

MUKESH HARISINGHANI, M.D.
Division of Abdominal Imaging
Department of Radiology
Massachusetts General Hospital
and Harvard Medical School
White 270, 55 Fruit Street
Boston, MA 02114, USA

ROY V. D'SOUZA, M.D.
Division of Abdominal Imaging
Department of Radiology
Massachusetts General Hospital
and Harvard Medical School
White 270, 55 Fruit Street
Boston, MA 02114, USA

DUSHYANT SAHANI, M.D.
Clinical Instructor
Harvard Medical School
Assistant Radiologist in Abdominal
and Interventional Radiology
Massachusetts General Hospital
White 270, 55 Fruit Street
Boston, MA 02114, USA

Acknowledgements

We are indebted to Miles A. Kirchin, to Diane Wagner-Jochem (University Hospital Homberg-Saar, Germany), to Antonella Cerri (Springer-Verlag Italia, Milan) for their beyond-the-call-of-duty efforts to get this book published in a timely manner.

Our sincere thanks go also to Emma Clarke and Gianni Chiappella for their precious support in the preprint processes of copyediting and type-setting, respectively.

We would also like to thank Mike Bourne (University Hospital of Wales, Cardiff, UK) for his assistance.

November, 2002   **The Editors**

1   Techniques for Liver MR Imaging

Contents

Magnetic resonance imaging (MRI) of the liver has evolved into a powerful imaging modality for the detection and characterization of focal liver pathology. The advent of fast imaging techniques allows rapid breath-hold whole-liver imaging for lesion detection and characterization. This chapter presents an overview of scanning techniques for a comprehensive MR evaluation of the liver.

1.1   Equipment

The liver can be imaged using magnet strengths from 0.5–3.0 Tesla. Since a doubling of the field strength results in a doubling of the signal-to-noise ratio (SNR), the higher field strength units permit higher resolution imaging. However, experience at field strengths above 1.5 Tesla is limited at present, therefore this chapter will focus predominantly on imaging techniques at 1.5 Tesla.

High resolution imaging can also be achieved by using multiple-element phased array surface coils which wrap around the torso. Due to the close proximity to the tissue, surface coils increase the SNR and have been shown to improve liver lesion detection [4]. The disadvantage of phased array coils is that there is a steep signal gradient with the tissues closest to the coil having the highest signal intensity. Newer generation scanners have introduced post-processing algorithms that correct for the signal intensity gradient.

A related problem occurs when there are motion artifacts due to breathing since subcutaneous fat has a very high signal. In order to reduce these artifacts the use of fat saturation, breath-hold imaging/respiratory triggering or saturation bands may be necessary (Fig. 1).

1.2   Imaging Parameters

A combination of T1- and T2-weighted pulse sequences is employed for MR imaging of the liver. The pulse sequence timing parameters (TR, Relaxation Time; TE, Echo Time) of individual T1- and T2-weighted images are based on the relaxation times of normal liver and liver tumors [35]. At 1.5 Tesla, the liver has a T1 relaxation time of approximately 550 ms and a T2 relaxation time of approximately 50 ms. Liver metastases have a T1 relaxation time ranging from 800–1000 ms and a T2 relaxation time of 80–100 ms. Liver hemangiomas and cysts have longer relaxation times, in excess of 1500 ms for T1 and 150 ms for T2. Knowledge of the tissue relaxation times is important for selecting appropriate TR and TE values. The main principle for high quality T1-weighted images is to use the shortest possible TE. This maximizes the T1 contrast, the SNR and the number of slices attainable. T2-weighted images require a TR in excess of 3–4 times the tissue T1 relaxation time and a TE which approximates the tissue T2 relaxation time. The signal intensity of the spleen is often similar to that of malignant liver disease and thus the spleen can act as an internal reference standard on T1- and T2-weighted images.

1.2.1   T1-weighted Imaging

Spin-echo (SE) pulse sequences are less frequently used nowadays as they are not compatible with breath-holding techniques. The prolonged imaging times needed, limit the usefulness of these techniques for imaging during the dynamic phase of contrast enhancement. Hence, breath-hold T1-weighted spoiled gradient-echo (GRE) sequences have now replaced conventional SE T1-weighted sequences in patients capable of suspending respiration [18, 38] (Fig. 2).

GRE techniques do not use a 180° refocusing radio frequency pulse. Since proton dephasing is induced by imaging gradients, the application of a second gradient pulse, equal in direction and magnitude but of opposite polarity, results in a reversal of the dephasing. This produces the gradient-recalled echo. In addition, a spoiling gradient is applied after each TR that eliminates any residual signal in the transverse plane. Absence of the 180° radio frequency pulse allows the slice loop

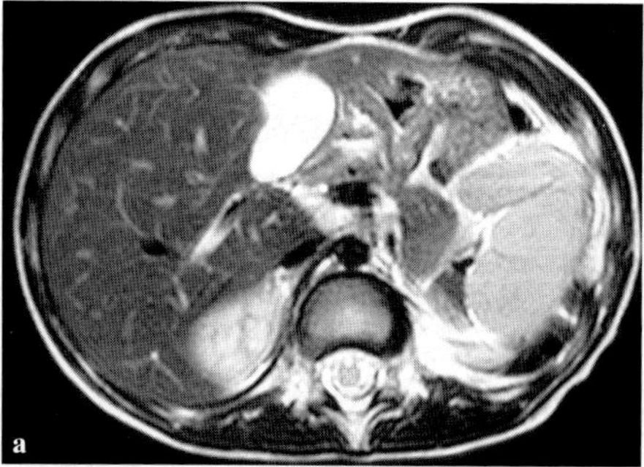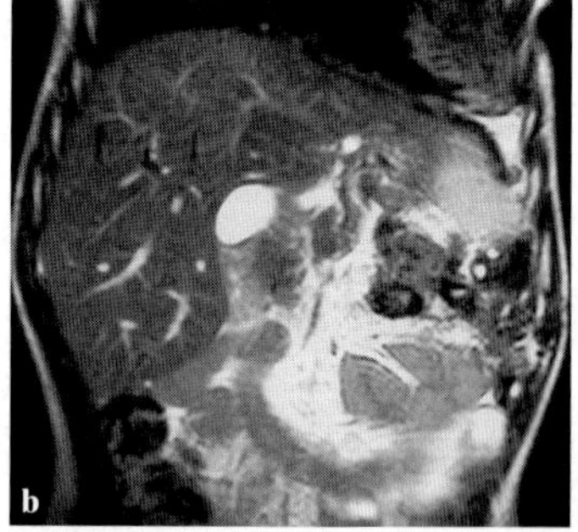

Fig. 1a,b. MR imaging of a spontaneously (free)-breathing 3 year old child with respiratory triggering. Synchronization of image acquisition with the respiratory cycle permits high quality T2-weighted turbo spin echo images to be acquired without artifacts (**a**) axial image, (**b**) coronal image to be shorter, thus enabling more slices to be acquired for the same TR. However, the overall signal level in a GRE image is slightly less than in an SE image.

GRE sequences have various acronyms depending on the vendor. The common acronyms used are SPGR for Spoiled Gradient Echo (General Electric), FLASH for Fast Low Angle Shot (Siemens) and FFE for Fast Field Echo (Philips). 2D GRE sequences use a short TE (< 5 ms), a TR of 100-200 ms and a flip angle of 70–90°. Very short TR and TE values (< 5 ms) with low flip angles are used in 3D GRE imaging. Although this results in a low SNR on unenhanced images, if the signal of the liver is augmented by means of intravenously administered contrast agents, a 3D GRE sequence may be more desirable as this facilitates the reconstruction of thin slices in various planes.

The signal from fat and water protons can affect tissue contrast on GRE images [36]. Hence in-phase and out-of-phase (opposed phase) images are typically acquired with the TE selected such that lipid protons are "in-phase" (4–5 ms at 1.5 Tesla) or "opposed phase" (2–3 ms at 1.5 Tesla). It is important to obtain both in-phase and opposed phase images because hepatic masses may be obscured on opposed phase images in patients with diffuse hepatic steatosis [24] (Fig. 3). Opposed phase imaging can diagnose fatty infiltration of the liver, focal fat sparing and focal

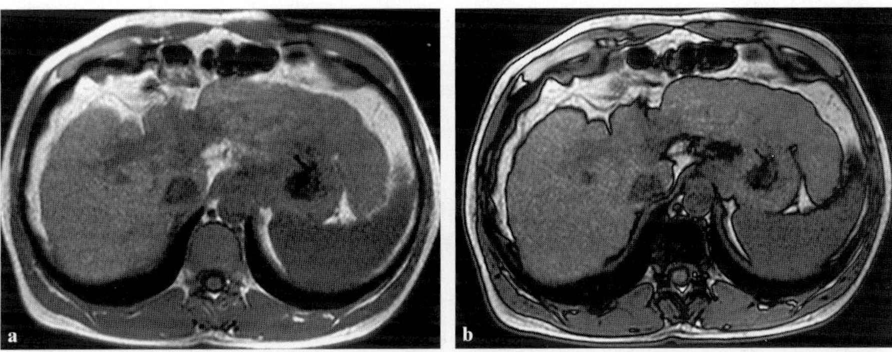

Fig. 2a,b. GRE T1-weighted images in-phase (**a**) and out-of-phase (**b**) in cirrhotic liver. Using this sequence, imaging of the entire liver can be performed in a single breath-hold

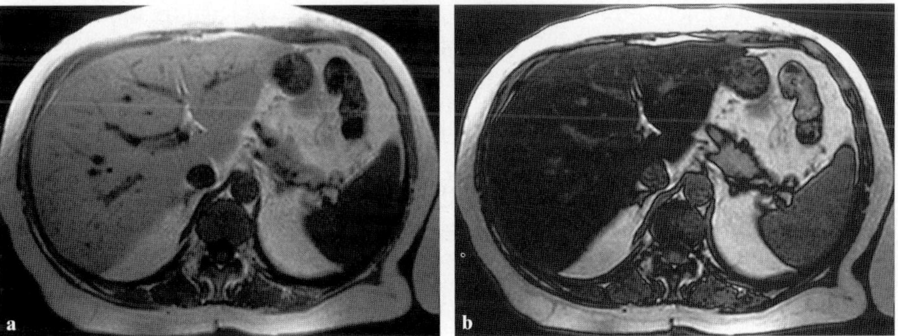

Fig. 3a,b. GRE T1-weighted images in-phase (**a**) and opposed phase (**b**) in a patient with hepatic steatosis. Fat deposition within the hepatocytes determines high signal intensity of the liver on the in-phase acquisition (**a**) and marked signal drop on the opposed phase image (**b**)

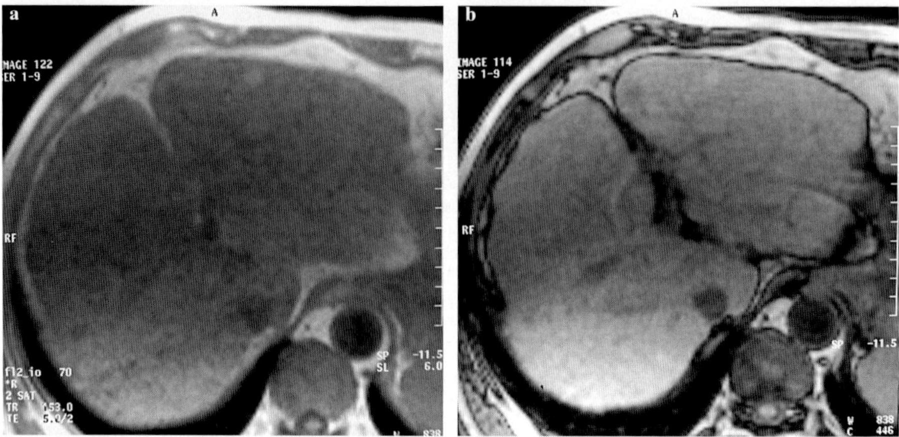

Fig. 4a,b. GRE T1-weighted images in-phase (**a**) and opposed phase (**b**) in a patient suffering from hepatic cirrhosis with concomitant multiple diffuse nodules. On the T1-weighted in-phase image (**a**) numerous nodules are hypointense while others present as hyperintense. On the opposed phase image (**b**) some nodules do not show marked signal drop due to the absence of fat content. Hyperintensity in this case could be due to glycogen or copper deposition within the nodule

fatty infiltration, in addition to demonstrating the presence or absence of lipid in hepatocellular nodules [15, 19] (Fig. 4).

Fat saturation decreases motion artifacts by suppressing subcutaneous and abdominal fat (Fig. 5). In addition, it increases the dynamic range of images and improves the SNR and contrast-to-noise ratio (CNR) of focal liver lesions [17, 27, 29]. For a spoiled GRE T1-weighted sequence, out-of-phase images are preferred for suppressing the signal from fat as the shorter TE for out-of-phase sequences enables a higher number of slices for a given TR.

Several software and hardware options permit the optimization of GRE sequences. Slice zero interpolation (ZIP) [7] techniques allow new slice locations in a 3D volume. This approach changes the slice center but not the slice thickness. The use of slice ZIP smooths reformations and also reduces partial volume artifacts due to the position of the anatomy within the slice. Phase oversampling [1] doubles the field-of-view (FOV), doubles the phase matrix, and halves the number of excitations (NEX) during acquisition and then discards the expanded data during reconstruction to eliminate wrap-around artifacts. Wrap-around artifacts occur when the anatomy extends beyond the FOV. The FOV specifies the area from which the MR signals are sampled. They may be specified separately for the frequency and phase encoding directions (rectangular FOV) or listed as a single number (square FOV). To decrease the FOV, the corresponding gradient amplitude has to be increased. Decreasing the FOV improves the resolution but results in a reduction in SNR. A rectangular FOV requires a more precise placement of anatomy in the center of the FOV. This is accomplished by means of FOV center offsets. Phase wrap-around artifacts occur if anatomy exists outside the new, reduced FOV.

In order to cover the entire liver volume in a single breath-hold on dynamic imaging with gadolinium chelates, the emphasis with T1-weighted GRE imaging is speed (Fig. 6). Options such as rectangular FOV allow for increased speed while maintaining a reasonable pixel size. Although dynamic imaging still remains one of the

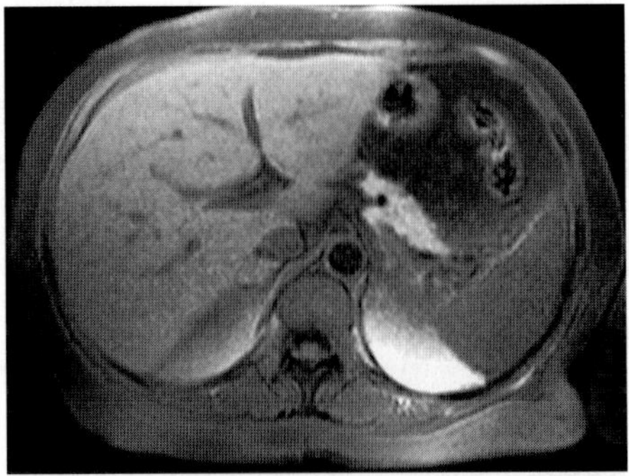

Fig. 5. GRE T1-weighted image with fat saturation. The homogeneous saturation of fat improves the CNR and reduces artifacts

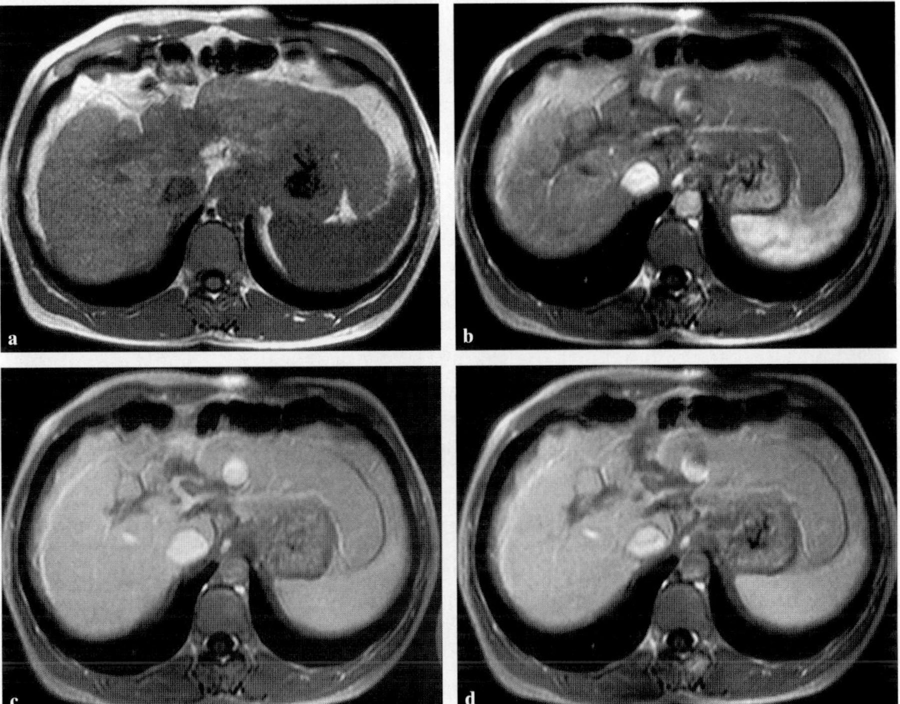

Fig. 6a-d. GRE T1-weighted images before and after the intravenous bolus injection of Gd-BOPTA. Following the acquisition of the unenhanced image (**a**), the sequence permits images to be acquired during the dynamic phase of contrast enhancement at 25–30 sec (arterial phase) (**b**), 70–90 sec (portal-venous phase) (**c**) and 3 – 5 min (equilibrium phase) (**d**)

most important techniques for both the detection and characterization of focal liver lesions, the recent advent of contrast agents that prolong the enhancement of the liver has meant that the limiting temporal factor is no longer present to such an extent (Fig. 7). As a result many techniques are now optimized for increased spatial resolution. As there is considerable liver enhancement, there is ample signal present even on higher resolution images. Spatial resolution can be improved by increasing the matrix size in the phase and frequency directions. This, however, may mean that

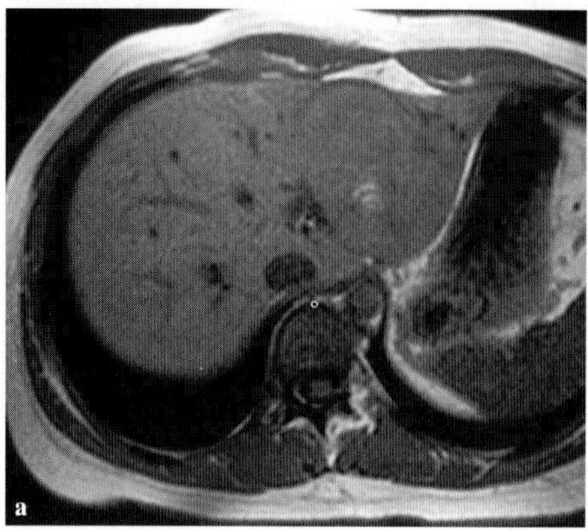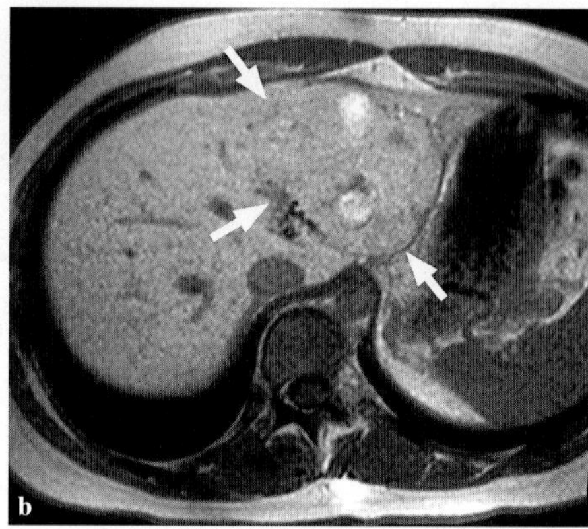

Fig. 7a,b. GRE T1-weighted images acquired before (**a**) and during the hepatobiliary phase at 3h after the administration of Gd-BOPTA (**b**). Liver parenchyma signal intensity at 3 h after Gd-BOPTA is clearly superior to that on the unenhanced image. Similarly, the large FNH (*arrows*) shows increased signal intensity.

two breath-holds instead of one are required to cover the entire liver volume. Using the phase oversampling option and higher excitations, the FOV can also be narrowed with thinner slices to provide higher resolution images and good SNR. Another valid technique for the acquisition of high resolution T1-weighted fat-suppressed images with a slice thickness < 3 mm is the so-called volume interpolated breath-hold examination (VIBE) which is a noved breath-hold 3D spoiled GRE sequence. This technique permits the entire liver to be imaged in one single breath-hold and offers the opportunity for 3D post-processing.

For details on the most common T1-weighted imaging parameters for MR machines from the major manufacturers, see appendix section 1.4, tables 1 and 2.

1.2.2 T2-weighted Imaging

In the 1980s, conventional SE pulse sequences were used to obtain T2-weighted images. Techniques to reduce motion artifacts had to be used with these sequences due to the long acquisition times needed. Subsequently, Hennig et al. developed RARE (rapid acquisition with relaxation enhancement) techniques that permitted the faster acquisition of T2-weighted images [9]. T2-weighted images acquired using RARE sequences are obtained in less time than conventional SE images since more than one phase-encoded signal is obtained for each TR. The echo train length corresponds to the number of echoes obtained per TR. However, RARE sequences provide lower CNR compared to conventional T2-weighted SE sequences and are slightly inferior for focal lesion detection and characterization in the liver [5, 6, 22, 26]. The imaging parameter that affects liver to lesion conspicuity for RARE T2-weighted images is echo train length. The longer the echo train length the poorer the CNR. Typically, an echo train length of 8 or 16 is used.

RARE imaging has been adapted by all vendors and termed fast spin echo (General Electric) or TurboSE (Siemens and Philips). With RARE-based non-breath-hold T2-weighted imaging, the TR is in excess of 5000 ms and saturation of tissues with long T1 relaxation times (e.g. cysts and hemangiomas) is negligible. Imaging is

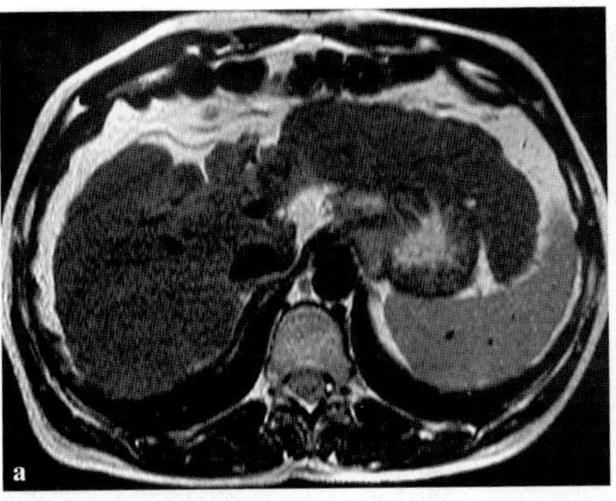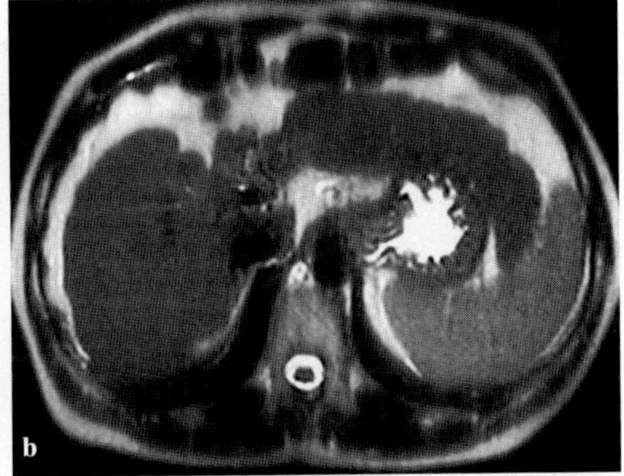

Fig. 8a,b. High resolution T2-weighted images. Turbo SE T2w sequences with high matrix resolution (512) (**a**) improves image quality and CNR. The high resolution matrix reduces the blurring sometimes seen on HASTE sequences (**b**)

performed at two different TEs. An intermediate TE of approximately 75 ms is used for detection of metastases. This TE is selected because it is intermediate between the T2 relaxation times of liver and liver metastases. The longer echo image is obtained at approximately 150 ms, which approximates the T2 relaxation times of cysts and hemangiomas and is optimal for lesion characterization [26].

There are some differences between RARE and conventional SE sequences. Firstly, fat has a higher signal on RARE images than conventional SE images. This results in the need for fat saturation with RARE techniques. Secondly, RARE sequences are less sensitive to magnetic susceptibility effects than conventional spin echo T2-weighted sequences. This is advantageous when imaging patients with embolization coils or orthopedic hardware [33] but is disadvantageous when images are obtained after administration of superparamagnetic iron oxide contrast agents [28]. Magnetization transfer is much greater on RARE images compared with conventional SE images. This effect lowers both the signal intensity and CNR of solid liver tumors. Lastly, tissues with shorter T2 relaxation times may be blurred on a RARE image because of low signal intensity at the end of the echo train. Image blurring can be decreased by reducing the echo spacing in RARE sequences.

A modification of the RARE sequence (HASTE or Half Fourier Acquisition Single-Shot Turbo Spin Echo by Siemens and SSFSE or Single Shot Fast Spin Echo by General Electric) is completed after a single excitation by acquiring only half of k-space in one long echo train [33]. Hence, the TR of these sequences is nearly infinite and images are reconstructed using a half Fourier technique [31]. An advantage of these techniques is that individual slices can be obtained in a few seconds. A disadvantage is that there is significant blurring of tissues within the short TR, resulting from T2 decay during the long echo train. The CNR and SNR are also lower than on RARE images with shorter echo train lengths (Fig. 8).

A recent modification of the RARE sequence, termed Forced Recovery Fast Spin Echo (FRFSE) [13], has been developed for breath-hold T2-weighted imaging. This sequence uses an additional 180° refocusing pulse after the last echo in the RARE echo train. A negative 90° pulse is then used to drive the refocused magnetization back into the longitudinal axis, instead of allowing it to recover via T1 relaxation processes. After several TR intervals a steady state longitudinal magneti-

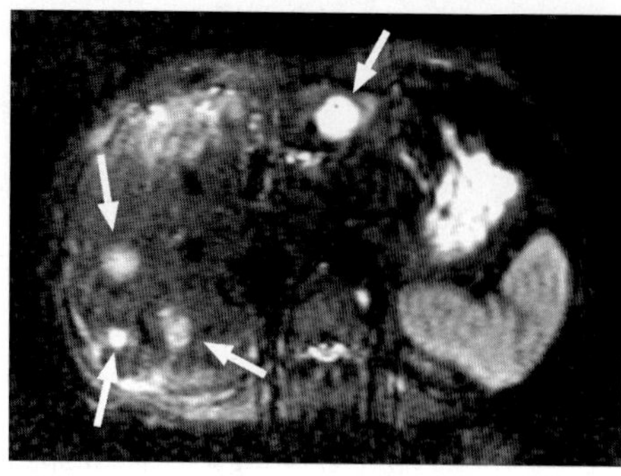

Fig. 9. EPI sequence acquired in a patient with metastatic liver disease. Multiple metastases display with very high signal intensity (*arrows*) as compared with the low signal intensity of the normal liver parenchyma. Note the low signal intensity of abdominal and subcutaneous fat

zation is established with a net enhancement of the long T2 relaxation components. Recovery of the residual transverse magnetization improves the SNR when compared to Single Shot imaging techniques. This sequence permits optimized slice ordering, the cancellation of blurring and fast breath-hold T2 relaxation enhancement. However FRFSE images have a lower CNR for liver lesions of intermediate signal than respiratory-triggered RARE images.

Echo planar imaging (EPI) is another method of obtaining breath-hold T2-weighted images and is currently the fastest MR imaging technique available. This technique does not use 180° refocusing pulses between echoes, but instead uses gradient refocusing which permits fast image acquisition. Specialized gradients are required for the rapid switching necessary. EPI can be performed using single or multishot sequences. Single-shot EPI provides the most rapid ultrafast MR imaging with an acquisition time of under 50 ms [31]. With this technique, the physiologic motion that typically affects abdominal MR images, such as respiration, vascular pulsation, flow, or peristalsis can be frozen. Initial experience has shown that images obtained using T2-weighted SE-EPI sequences offer comparable quality and better lesion-to-liver CNR than images obtained using conventional SE sequences [2, 25] (Fig. 9).

Echo planar images have marked chemical shift artifacts in the phase encoding direction. The major problem of single-shot EPI is severe image distortion due to susceptibility effects. This distortion occurs especially at the liver-air interface. This susceptibility can be reduced using multi-shot acquisitions as the data sampling time at each TR becomes shorter. Unfortunately, the temporal resolution is reduced compared to single-shot EPI and becomes similar to breath-hold T2-weighted RARE imaging which requires breath-holding over a period of 10–20 s. However, the contrast between lesion and liver is superior with multi-shot EPI than with breath-hold RARE T2-weighted imaging [12].

For details on the most common T2-weighted imaging parameters for MR machines from the major manufacturers, see appendix section 1.4, tables 3 and 4.

1.2.3   Contrast Enhanced Imaging

A complete evaluation of the liver requires the injection of an MR contrast agent for lesion detection and characterization. A list of contrast agents available and their method of use is covered in Chapter 2. Breath-hold spoiled GRE images are used for extracellular gadolinium-chelate enhanced T1-weighted imaging of the liver [8, 36]. The minimum possible in-phase TE is usually used to optimize SNR and CNR. Dynamic contrast-enhanced studies of the liver include pre-contrast images and images obtained in the arterial (~30 s), portal venous (~60 s) and equilibrium (~180 s) phases of contrast enhancement [16, 20]. Imaging with hepatocyte-directed gadolinium-based contrast agents is performed with T1-weighted high spatial resolution techniques while imaging with iron-oxide particles targetted to the reticuloendothelial system is performed primarily with T2-weighted techniques.

Breath-hold VIBE sequences are also useful for dynamic evaluation of the liver (Fig. 10). These sequences enable thinner sections (2–3 mm) to be acquired which improve spatial resolution, and also fat saturation, thus permitting increased CNR and 3D reconstruction of both the vasculature and, when hepatobiliary-excreted contrast agents are employed, the biliary tree (Fig. 11).

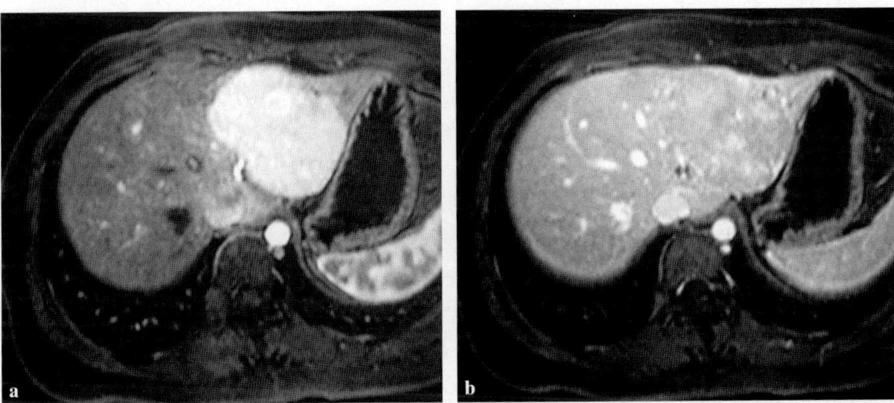

Fig. 10a,b. T1-weighted images acquired with a VIBE sequence. High spatial (slice thickness = 2-3 mm) and contrast (fat saturation) resolution renders the sequence suitable for dynamic evaluation. The arterial phase image (**a**) reveals intense homogenous enhancement of the FNH shown in Fig. 7. The image acquired during the portal-venous phase (**b**) reveals rapid contrast agent washout

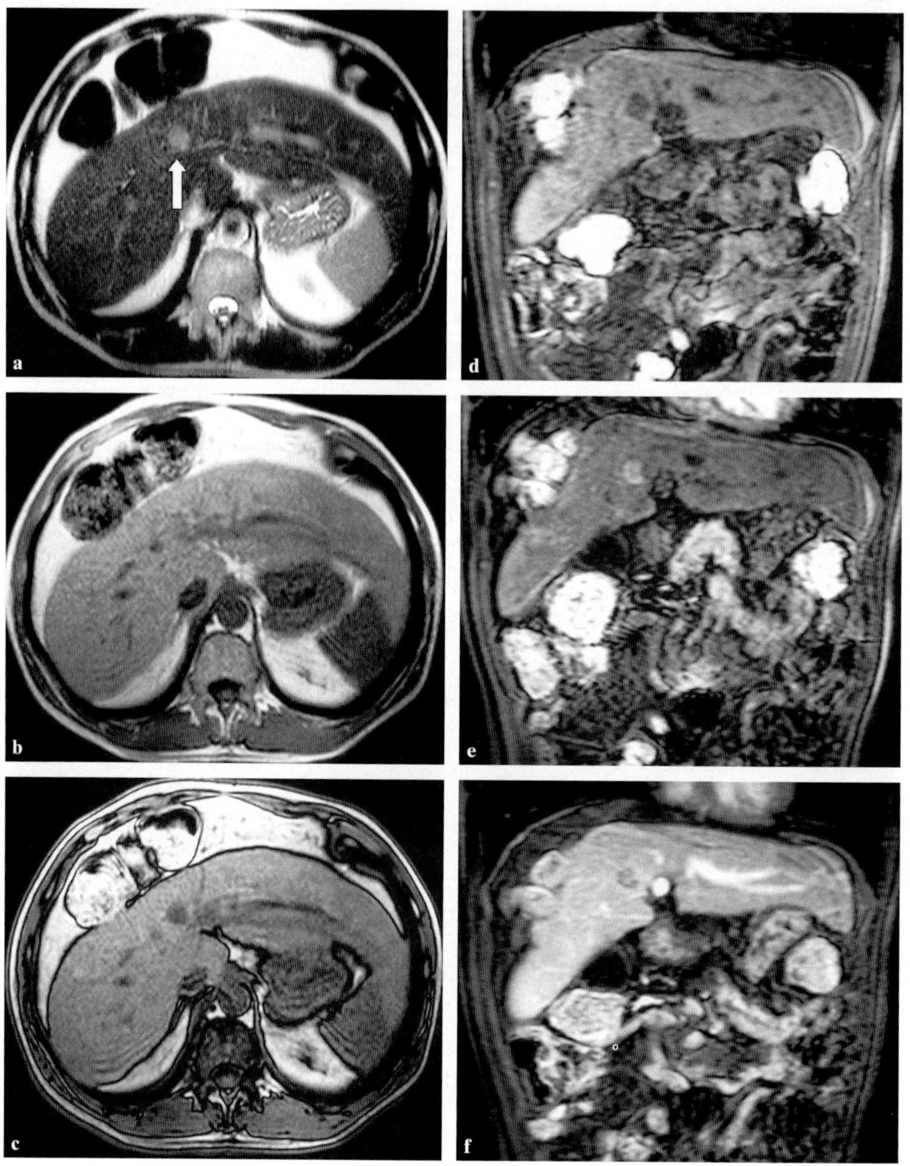

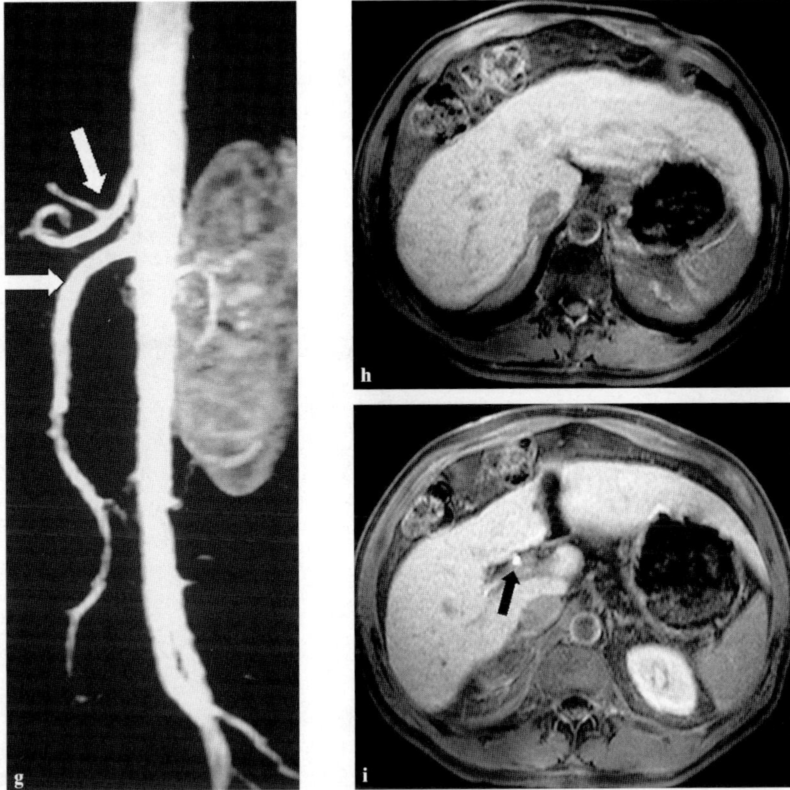

Fig. 11a-i. The unenhanced HASTE T2-weighted image (**a**) reveals a well-defined hyperintense nodule (*arrow*). The lesion is seen as isointense on the unenhanced GE T1-weighted in-phase image (**b**) but as hypointense on the GE T1-weighted opposed-phase image (**c**) because of the presence of fat. The lesion is also seen as hypointense on the unenhanced coronal T1-weighted VIBE image (**d**). Following the bolus administration of Gd-BOPTA, intense enhancement is seen during the arterial phase (**e**) followed by wash-out during the subsequent portal-venous phase (**f**). With the VIBE sequence, MR angiography can be performed: both the celiac tripod and the inferior mesenteric artery (*arrows*) can be visualized with good spatial and contrast resolution (**g**). The GE T1-weighted fs image acquired during the delayed hepatobiliary phase after Gd-BOPTA administration (**h**) indicates that the lesion does not take up the contrast agent and hence appears hypointense against the enhanced background parenchyma. Biliary duct elimination of Gd-BOPTA (*arrow*) can also be seen in this phase (**i**)

1.2.4   Miscellaneous Techniques

An additional use of T2-weighted sequences is for performing magnetic resonance cholangio-pancreatography (MRCP) (Fig. 12). This is usually performed with heavily T2-weighted RARE or single-shot fast spin-echo sequences. RARE MR-CP is performed by using respiratory gating, a long echo train, a long repetition time, an echo time greater than 250 ms, fat saturation and thin collimation. The imaging time is usually 4–6 minutes. Single-shot fast spin-echo is a newer and more rapid MRCP sequence that can be performed in a single breath-hold, thereby significantly reducing motion artifacts and increasing image quality [10, 11, 21, 23]. The imaging time for both single-section and multi-section sequences is less than 30 seconds and typically thick oblique sections are obtained to capture the entire extra hepatic biliary tree in a single plane.

Magnetic Resonance Angiography (MRA) can be performed using a thin slice (< 3 mm) breath-hold 3D spoiled GRE sequence after dynamic intravenous gadolinium chelate injection (Fig. 13) [14]. Zero-fill interpolation with overlapping reconstructions has led to a qualitative improvement in the image quality of reformatted images.

1.3   Normal MR Appearance of the Liver

Normal liver parenchyma has a higher signal intensity than the spleen on T1-weighted images but a lower signal intensity on T2-weighted images (Fig. 14). The higher signal intensity on T1-weighted images is due to the large amount of proteins and rough endoplasmic reticulum within the hepatocytes [3]. On T1-weighted images intrahepatic biliary ducts and vessels generally appear hypointense, although flow-related bright signal can be seen within the vessels. On T2-weighted images the signal intensity of the liver parenchyma appears hypointense against which biliary ducts may appear hyperintense.

In summary, MR imaging is the primary diagnostic examination in many clinical situations and serves as a problem-solving study when other modalities are inconclusive. The emphasis in MR imaging of the liver is on increasing the speed of the examination and at the same time utilizing the different available sequences for improving lesion detection and characterization.

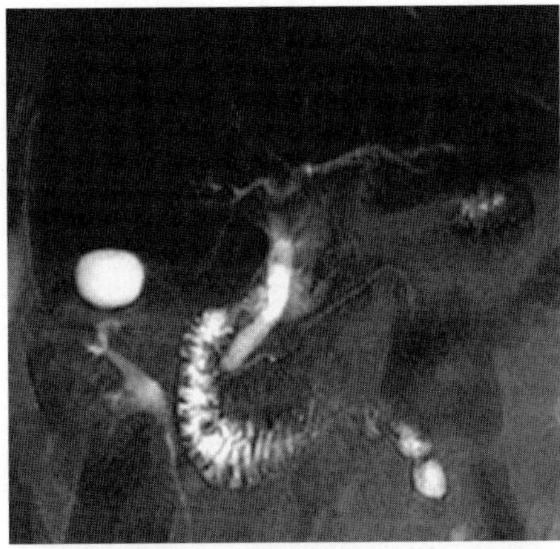

Fig. 12. Coronal Single-Shot Fast Spin-Echo T2-weighted MRCP image shows normal caliber of the bile duct and the pancreatic duct. Also note the bright signal in the duodenum and renal collecting system and an incidental simple cyst in the right kidney

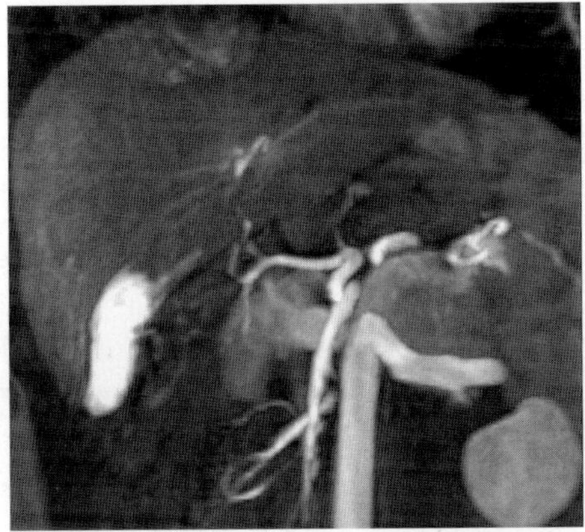

Fig. 13. Coronal MIP image generated from gadolinium enhanced T1-weighted gradient-echo MR sequence shows normal hepatic arterial anatomy

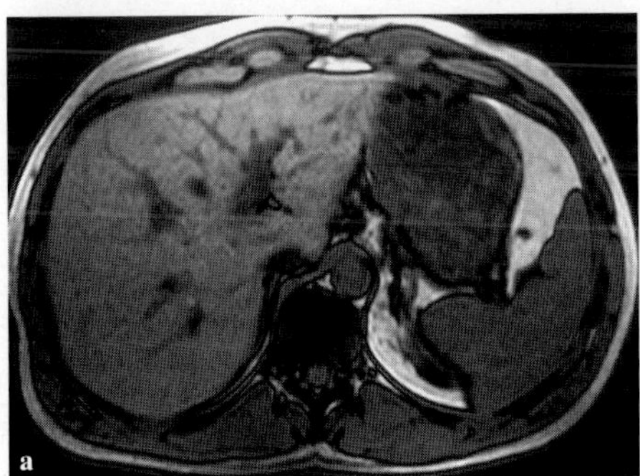
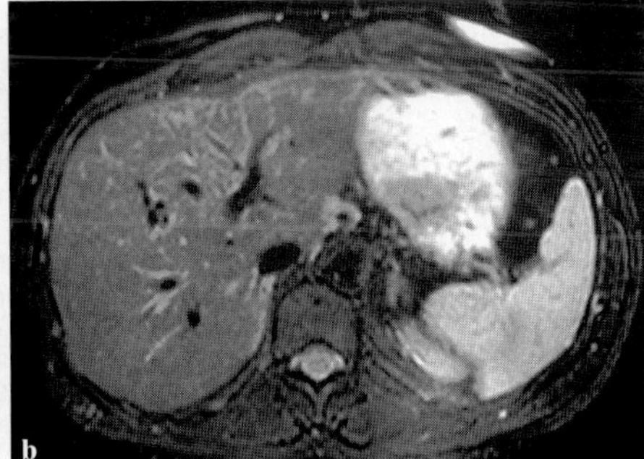

Fig. 14a,b. GRE T1-weighted opposed phase image (**a**) and T2-weighted Turbo SE image with fat saturation (**b**) in a healthy liver. Note that the liver parenchyma has a higher signal intensity than the spleen on the T1-weighted image but a lower signal intensity on the T2-weighted image

References

1. Arena L, Morehouse HT, Safir J. MR imaging artifacts that simulate disease: how to recognize and eliminate them. Radiographics 1995 Nov;15(6):1373-94
2. Butts K, Riederer SJ, Ehman RL, Felmlee JP, Grimm RC. Echo-planar imaging of the liver with a standard MR imaging system. Radiology 1993 Oct;189(1):259-64
3. Cameron IL, Ord VA, Fullerton GD. Characterization of proton NMR relaxation times in normal and pathological tissues by correlation with other tissue parameters. Magn Reson Imaging 1984;2(2):97-106
4. Campeau NG, Johnson CD, Felmlee JP, Rydberg JN, Butts RK, Ehman RL, Riederer SJ. MR imaging of the abdomen with a phased-array multicoil: prospective clinical evaluation. Radiology 1995 Jun;195(3):769-76
5. Carpenter KD, Macaulay SE, Schulte SJ, Obregon RG, Nelson RC, Simon HE, Schmiedl UP. MR of focal liver lesions: comparison of breath-hold and non-breath-hold hybrid RARE and conventional spin-echo T2-weighted pulse sequences. J Magn Reson Imaging 1996 Jul-Aug;6(4):596-602
6. Catasca JV, Mirowitz SA. T2-weighted MR imaging of the abdomen: fast spin-echo vs conventional spin-echo sequences. AJR Am J Roentgenol 1994 Jan;162(1):61-7
7. Du YP, Parker DL, Davis WL, Cao G. Reduction of partial-volume artifacts with zero-filled interpolation in three-dimensional MR angiography. J Magn Reson Imaging 1994 Sep-Oct;4(5):733-41
8. Hamm B, Thoeni RF, Gould RG, Bernardino ME, Luning M, Saini S, Mahfouz AE, Taupitz M, Wolf KJ. Focal liver lesions: characterization with nonenhanced and dynamic contrast material-enhanced MR imaging. Radiology 1994 Feb;190(2):417-23
9. Hennig J, Nauerth A, Friedburg H. RARE imaging: a fast imaging method for clinical MR. Magn Reson Med 1986 Dec;3(6):823-33
10. Ichikawa T, Nitatori T, Hachiya J, Mizutani Y. Breath-held MR cholangiopancreatography with half-averaged single shot hybrid rapid acquisition with relaxation enhancement sequence: comparison of fast GRE and SE sequences. J Comput Assist Tomogr 1996 Sep-Oct;20(5):798-802
11. Irie H, Honda H, Tajima T, Kuroiwa T, Yoshimitsu K, Makisumi K, Masuda K. Optimal MR cholangiopancreatographic sequence and its clinical application. Radiology 1998 Feb;206(2):379-87
12. Kanematsu M, Hoshi H, Itoh K, Murakami T, Hori M, Kondo H, Yokoyama R, Nakamura H. Focal hepatic lesion detection: comparison of four fat-suppressed T2-weighted MR imaging pulse sequences. Radiology 1999 May;211(2):363-71
13. Katayama M, Masui T, Kobayashi S, Ito T, Takahashi M, Sakahara H, Nozaki A, Kabasawa H. Fat-suppressed T2-weighted MRI of the liver: comparison of respiratory-triggered fast spin-echo, breath-hold single-shot fast spin-echo, and breath-hold fast-recovery fast spin-echo sequences. J Magn Reson Imaging 2001 Oct;14(4):439-49
14. Kopka L, Rodenwaldt J, Vosshenrich R, Fischer U, Renner B, Lorf T, Graessner J, Ringe B, Grabbe E. Hepatic blood supply: comparison of optimized dual phase contrast-enhanced three-dimensional MR angiography and digital subtraction angiography. Radiology 1999 Apr;211(1):51-8
15. Kreft BP, Tanimoto A, Baba Y, Zhao L, Chen J, Middleton MS, Compton CC, Finn JP, Stark DD. Diagnosis of fatty liver with MR imaging. J Magn Reson Imaging 1992 Jul-Aug;2(4):463-71
16. Low RN. Contrast agents for MR imaging of the liver. J Magn Reson Imaging 1997 Jan-Feb;7(1):56-67
17. Lu DS, Saini S, Hahn PF, Goldberg M, Lee MJ, Weissleder R, Gerard B, Halpern E, Cats A. T2-weighted MR imaging of the upper part of the abdomen: should fat suppression be used routinely? AJR Am J Roentgenol 1994 May;162(5):1095-100
18. Martin J, Sentis M, Puig J, Rue M, Falco J, Donoso L, Zidan A. Comparison of in-phase and opposed phase GRE and conventional SE MR pulse sequences in T1-weighted imaging of liver lesions. J Comput Assist Tomogr 1996 Nov-Dec;20(6):890-7
19. Mitchell DG. Chemical shift magnetic resonance imaging: applications in the abdomen and pelvis. Top Magn Reson Imaging 1992 Jun;4(3):46-63
20. Mitchell DG. Fast MR imaging techniques: impact in the abdomen. J Magn Reson Imaging 1996 Sep-Oct;6(5):812-21
21. Miyazaki T, Yamashita Y, Tsuchigame T, Yamamoto H, Urata J, Takahashi M. MR cholangiopancreatography using HASTE (half-Fourier acquisition single-shot turbo spin-echo) sequences. AJR Am J Roentgenol 1996 Jun;166(6):1297-303
22. Outwater EK, Mitchell DG, Vinitski S. Abdominal MR imaging: evaluation of a fast spin-echo sequence. Radiology 1994 Feb;190(2):425-9
23. Regan F, Fradin J, Khazan R, Bohlman M, Magnuson T. Choledocholithiasis: evaluation with MR cholangiography. AJR Am J Roentgenol 1996 Dec;167(6):1441-5
24. Rofsky NM, Weinreb JC, Ambrosino MM, Safir J, Krinsky G. Comparison between in-phase and opposed-phase T1-weighted breath-hold FLASH sequences for hepatic imaging. J Comput Assist Tomogr 1996 Mar-Apr;20(2):230-5
25. Saini S, Reimer P, Hahn PF, Cohen MS. Echoplanar MR imaging of the liver in patients with focal hepatic lesions: quantitative analysis of images made with various pulse sequences. AJR Am J Roentgenol 1994 Dec;163(6):1389-93

26. Schima W, Saini S, Echeverri JA, Hahn PF, Harisinghani M, Mueller PR. Focal liver lesions: characterization with conventional spin-echo versus fast spin-echo T2-weighted MR imaging. Radiology 1997 Feb;202(2):389-93

27. Schwartz LH, Seltzer SE, Tempany CM, Silverman SG, Piwnica-Worms DR, Adams DF, Herman L, Herman LT, Hooshmand R. Prospective comparison of T2-weighted fast spin-echo, with and without fat suppression, and conventional spin-echo pulse sequences in the upper abdomen. Radiology 1993 Nov;189(2):411-6

28. Schwartz LH, Seltzer SE, Tempany CM, Silverman SG, Piwnica-Worms DR, Adams DF, Herman L, Herman LA, Hooshmand R. Superparamagnetic iron oxide hepatic MR imaging: efficacy and safety using conventional and fast spin-echo pulse sequences. J Magn Reson Imaging 1995 Sep-Oct;5(5):566-70

29. Semelka RC, Hricak H, Bis KG, Werthmuller WC, Higgins CB. Liver lesion detection: comparison between excitation-spoiling fat suppression and regular spin-echo at 1.5T. Abdom Imaging 1993;18(1):56-60

30. Stehling MK, Charnley RM, Blamire AM, Ordidge RJ, Coxon R, Gibbs P, Hardcastle JD, Mansfield P. Ultrafast magnetic resonance scanning of the liver with echo-planar imaging. Br J Radiol 1990 Jun;63(750):430-7

31. Tang Y, Yamashita Y, Namimoto T, Abe Y, Takahashi M. Liver T2-weighted MR imaging: comparison of fast and conventional half-Fourier single-shot turbo spin-echo, breath-hold turbo spin-echo, and respiratory-triggered turbo spin-echo sequences. Radiology 1997 Jun;203(3):766-72

32. Tartaglino LM, Flanders AE, Vinitski S, Friedman DP. Metallic artifacts on MR images of the postoperative spine: reduction with fast spin-echo techniques. Radiology 1994 Feb;190(2):565-9

33. Van Hoe L, Bosmans H, Aerts P, Baert AL, Fevery J, Kiefer B, Marchal G. Focal liver lesions: fast T2-weighted MR imaging with half-Fourier rapid acquisition with relaxation enhancement. Radiology 1996 Dec;201(3):817-23

34. Van Lom KJ, Brown JJ, Perman WH, Sandstrom JC, Lee JK. Liver imaging at 1.5 tesla: pulse sequence optimization based on improved measurement of tissue relaxation times. Magn Reson Imaging 1991;9(2):165-71

35. Wehrli FW, Perkins TG, Shimakawa A, Roberts F. Chemical shift-induced amplitude modulations in images obtained with gradient refocusing. Magn Reson Imaging 1987;5(2):157-8

36. Yamashita Y, Hatanaka Y, Yamamoto H, Arakawa A, Matsukawa T, Miyazaki T, Takahashi M. Differential diagnosis of focal liver lesions: role of spin-echo and contrast-enhanced dynamic MR imaging. Radiology 1994 Oct;193(1):59-65

37. Yamashita Y, Yamamoto H, Namimoto T, Abe Y, Takahashi M. Phased array breath-hold versus non-breath-hold MR imaging of focal liver lesions: a prospective comparative study. J Magn Reson Imaging 1997 Mar-Apr 7(2):292-7

1.4 Appendices: Common Imaging Parameters of MR Machines from Different Vendors for MRI of the Liver

Table 1. General gradient echo sequences for T1w imaging of the liver

GRE T1w	Magnetom Vision (Siemens)	Magnetom Sonata (Siemens)		ACS NT (Philips)	General Electric (GE)	General Electric (GE)
Field strength (T)	1.5	1.5	1.5	1.5	1.5	1.5
Name	Flash 2D	Flash 2D	VIBE	FFE	SPGR	3D FSPGR
TE (ms)	4.1	4.76	2.27	5.0	4.7	2.8
TR (ms)	174.9	166	4.78	110	175	5.8
Flip angle (°)	80	70	10	70	70	10
Matrix	107×256	166×256	166×256	128×256	128×256	128×256
NSA	1	1	1	1	1	1
Slice thickness (mm)	6	6	2.5	8	7	5
Gap (%)	25	25	–	10	10	–
Breath hold (BH) Respiratory gating (RG)	BH	BH	BH	BH	BH	BH
No. of slices	23	18	64	23	20	30
Acquisition time (s)	18	21	22	18	21	22

Table 2. T1w sequences for dynamic liver imaging

GRE T1w	Magnetom Vision (Siemens)	Magnetom Sonata (Siemens)		ACS NT (Philips)	General Electric (GE)
Field strength (T)	1.5	1.5	1.5	1.5	1.5
Name	Flash 2D	Flash 2D	VIBE	FFE	SPGR
TE (ms)	4.1	4.76	2.27	5.0	4.7
TR (ms)	174.9	166	4.78	110	175
Flip angle (°)	80	70	10	70	70
Matrix	107×256	166×256	128×256	128×256	128×256
NSA	1	1	1	1	1
Slice thickness (mm)	6	6	2.5	8	7
Gap (%)	25	25	–	10	–
Breath hold (BH) Respiratory gating (RG)	BH	BH	BH	BH	BH
No. of slices	23	18	64	3	–
Acquisition time (s)	18	21	22	6	–

Table 3. Turbo spin echo sequences for T2w imaging of the liver

TSE T2w	Magnetom Vision (Siemens)		Magnetom Sonata (Siemens)	ACS NT (Philips)	General Electric (GE)	
Field strength (T)	1.5	1.5	1.5	1.5	1.5	1.5
Name	TSE T2w	TSE T2w	TSE T2w	TSE T2w	FRSE-XL	FRFSE
TE (ms)	138	109	93	100	90	90
TR (ms)	3200	3200	1260	3000	2000	4000
ETL	29	29	27	25	19	16
Matrix	116×256	154×256	256×256 256×512	160×256	224×256	160×256
NSA	1	1	2	5	1	2
Slice thickness (mm)	6	6	6	8	6	6
Gap (%)	25	10	20	10	20	20
Breath hold (BH) Respiratory gating (RG)	BH	BH	RG	RG	BH	RG
No. of slices	2×11	12	20	23	26	25
Acquisition time (s)	2×17	18	>2.08 min	180	2×28	160

Table 4. Additional miscellaneous sequences for T2w imaging of the liver

	Magnetom Vision (Siemens)	Magnetom Sonata (Siemens)	ACS NT (Philips)	General Electric (GE)	
Field strength (T)	1.5	1.5	1.5	1.5	1.5
Name	HASTE (single shot)	HASTE	TSE T2w SPIR	SSFSE Loc-Nom BH	SSFSE Loc BH
TE (ms)	90	57	100	180	90
TR (ms)	4.4	1000	5000	∞	∞
ETL	–	159	18	160	128
Matrix	160×256	212×256	136×256	160×384	128×384
NSA	1	1	5	1	1
Slice thickness (mm)	6	6	8	7	7
Gap (%)	25	15	10	20	20
Breath hold (BH) Respiratory gating (RG)	BH	BH	RG	RG	BH
No. of slices	2×11	2×16	22	15	15
Acquisition time (s)	2×14	2×16	160	140	25

2   Contrast Agents for Liver MR Imaging

Contents

2.1   Introduction

Use of contrast agents in magnetic resonance (MR) imaging of the liver has become an indispensable component of a comprehensive scanning protocol. Several classes of MR contrast agents are currently available for clinical use in MR imaging of the liver [28, 33, 45, 72, 87]. These include non-specific materials that have an extracellular distribution, materials that are taken up specifically by hepatocytes and excreted in part through the biliary system, and materials that are targeted specifically to the Kupffer cells of the reticuloendothelial system (RES) (Table 1).

This chapter describes the properties and indications of each category of contrast agent for liver MR imaging.

2.1.1   Non-specific Gadolinium Chelates

Chelates of the paramagnetic gadolinium ion that have no tissue specific bio-distribution have been commercially available since 1986. Approved gadolinium chelates in the USA and elsewhere include gadopentetate dimeglumine (Magnevist®, Gd-DTPA; Berlex Laboratories/Schering AG), gadoteridol (ProHance®, Gd-HP-DO3A; Bracco Diagnostics), gadodiamide (Omniscan®, Gd-DTPA-BMA; Amersham Health), and gadoversetamide (Optimark®, Gd-DTPA-BMEA; Mallinckrodt). Other non-specific gadolinium agents currently approved in Europe and elsewhere include gadoterate meglumine (Dotarem®, Gd-DOTA; Guerbet) and gadobutrol (Gadovist®, Gd-BT-DO3A; Schering AG) (Table 2). All have an extremely attractive safety profile especially in comparison to iodinated x-ray contrast agents [28, 45, 54, 55, 57, 71, 72, 90, 93].

Table 1. Contrast agents for MR imaging of the liver

Contrast agent type	Manufacturer	Principal mechanism
Extracellular Gd agents		
Gadopentetate dimeglumine; Gd-DTPA (Magnevist®)	Schering[1] / Berlex[2]	T1 shortening
Gadoteridol; Gd-HP-DO3A (ProHance®)	Bracco Imaging[3] / Bracco Diagnostics[4]	T1 shortening
Gadodiamide; Gd-DTPA-BMA (Omniscan®)	Amersham Health[5]	T1 shortening
Gadoversetamide; Gd-DTPA-BMEA (Optimark®)	Mallinckrodt[6]	T1 shortening
Gadoterate meglumine; Gd-DOTA (Dotarem®)	Guerbet[7]	T1 shortening
Gadobutrol; Gd-BT-DO3A (Gadovist®)	Schering[1]	T1 shortening
Hepatobiliary agent		
Mangafodipir trisodium; Mn-DPDP (Teslascan®)	Amersham Health[5]	T1 shortening
Combined extracellular / hepatobiliary agents		
Gadobenate dimeglumine; Gd-BOPTA (MultiHance®)	Bracco Imaging[3] / Bracco Diagnostics[4]	T1 shortening
Gadoxetate; Gd-EOB-DTPA (Eovist®)	Schering[1] / Berlex[2]	T1 shortening
SPIO agent		
AMI-25; Ferumoxides (Feridex®; Endorem®)	Schering[1]-Berlex[8] / Guerbet[7]	T2 shortening
USPIO agents		
SHU 555A (Resovist®)	Schering[1]	T1 and T2 shortening
AMI-227 (Combidex®; Sinerem®)	Advanced Magnetics[8] / Guerbet[7]	T1 and T2 shortening

1 = Berlin, Germany; 2 = Wayne NJ, USA; 3 = Milano, Italy; 4 = Princeton NJ, USA; 5 = Oslo, Norway; 6 = St. Louis MO, USA; 7 = Aulnay-Sous-Bois, France; 8 = Cambridge MA, USA

Table 2. Water proton magnetic relaxivities of various T1-shortening contrast media at 20 MHz

	Relaxivities ($mM^{-1}s^{-1}$)							
	In protein-free aqueous solution				In protein-containing aqueous solution			
Product	r_1	Ref.	r_2	Ref.	r_1	Ref.	r_2	Ref.
Magnevist[®] Gd-DTPA/Dimeg (Gadopentetate dimeglumine)	3.8[b]	[79]	4.3[b]	[79]	~4.3[e] ~5.0[f] ~4.9[g]	[a] [a] [104]	~5.6[e] ~5.4[f] ~6.3[g]	[a] [a] [a]
ProHance[®] Gd-HP-DO3A (Gadoteridol)	3.7[b]	[96]	4.3[b]	[a]	~4.6[f]	[a]	~5.3[f]	[a]
Omniscan[®] Gd-DTPA-BMA (Gadodiamide)	3.9[b]	[10]	4.7[b]	[a]	~4.8[f]	[a]	~5.1[f]	[a]
Doratem[®] Gd-DOTA/Meg (Gadoterate meglumine)	3.5[b]	[96]	4.8[b]	[a]	~4.3[f]	[a]	~5.0[f]	[a]
MultiHance[®] Gd-BOPTA/Dimeg (Gadobenate dimeglumine)	4.4[b]	[a]	5.6[b]	[a]	~8.0[e] ~10.8[f] ~9.7[g]	[a] [a] [a]	~10.8[e] ~12.2[f] ~12.5[g]	[a] [a] [a]
Teslacan[®] Mn-DPDP/Na$_3$ (Mangafodipir trisodium)	1.9[d]	[95]	2.2[d]	[95]	~1.6[h]	[18]	~5.5[h]	[18]

[a] Measurements of Bracco SpA. [b] In 0.15 M NaCl, pH=7.3, at 39°C. [c] In water, at 40°C. [d] In water, at 37°C. [e] In 4% (w/v) bovine serum albumin solution, at 39°C. [f] In Human serum (Seronorm™ Human), at 39°C. [g] In Heparizined human plasma, at 39°C. [h] In blood, at 40°C. These data may be flawed by transmetallation and metabolism.

As paramagnetic compounds, gadolinium chelates shorten tissue relaxation times. At recommended doses of 0.1–0.3 mmol/kg bodyweight their principal effect is to shorten the T1 relaxation time resulting in an increase in tissue signal intensity on T1-weighted images. This effect is best captured on heavily T1-weighted images [42, 46, 86]. Due to rapid redistribution of gadolinium chelates from the intravascular compartment to the extracellular space, the contrast agents must be administered as a rapid bolus, typically at 2 ml/s. Thereafter, imaging of the entire liver is performed in a single breath-hold during the dynamic phases of contrast enhancement. This is most commonly undertaken with a 2D or 3D T1-weighted spoiled gradient echo (GRE) pulse sequence with serial imaging in the arterial dominant phase (25–30 s post-injection), the portal-venous phase (60–80 s post-injection) and the equilibrium phase (3–5 min post-injection).

In the hepatic arterial dominant phase, enhancement occurs principally in the arterial tree and in other arterially-perfused tissues, such as liver tumors [16, 47, 56, 105, 106]. This is important since most focal lesions, especially primary liver tumors and metastases, are supplied primarily by hepatic arteries [30, 47, 105]. Enhancement during the arterial dominant phase is important also for detecting perfusion abnormalities. Typically, transiently increased segmental enhancement may indicate that portal-venous flow is compromised due to compression or thrombosis [80, 108]. This can be of value in patients where findings on unenhanced images are equivocal.

Typically, maximal enhancement of the hepatic parenchyma is seen in the portal-venous phase. In this phase, hypovascular lesions, such as cysts, hypovascular metastases and scar tissue, are most clearly revealed as regions of absent or diminished enhancement. Patency or thrombosis of hepatic vessels is also best shown during this phase [30].

Enhancement of tissues with enlarged extracellular space, such as focal liver lesions and focal nodular hyperplasia (FNH) scar, is usually best seen in the equilibrium phase. Likewise, typical signs of malignancy, such as peripheral washout in colorectal metastases, are best seen during the equilibrium phase. These features frequently contribute towards accurate lesion characterization [48, 49].

Imaging with gadolinium during the arterial phase has been shown to improve the rate of detection of suspected hepatocellular carcinoma (HCC) in cirrhotic patients compared to unenhanced imaging [56, 106, 108]. For lesion characterization, characteristic enhancement patterns have been identified for a variety of benign and malignant masses of both hepatocellular and non-hepatocellular origin [19, 30, 42, 47–49, 105] (Figs. 1, 2).

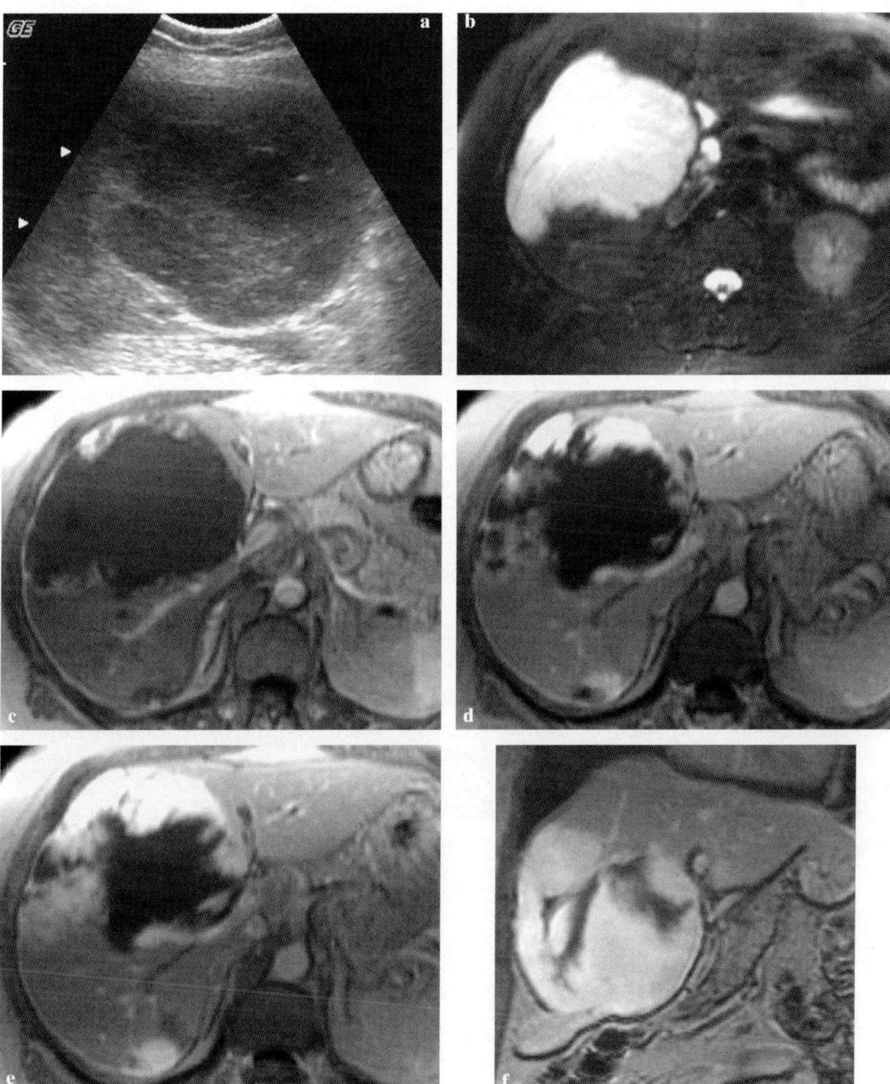

Fig. 1a-f. Hemangioma. A large hypoechoeic mass noted in the liver on ultrasound (**a**) is seen as hyperintense on the T2-weighted MR image (**b**). With dynamic T1-weighted imaging following the bolus administration of Gd-DTPA, the lesion demonstrates intense peripheral nodular enhancement with progressive filling-in on the arterial (**c**), early and late portal-venous (**d** and **e**, respectively) and equilibrium (**f**) phase images. The enhancement pattern is characteristic of a benign hemangioma

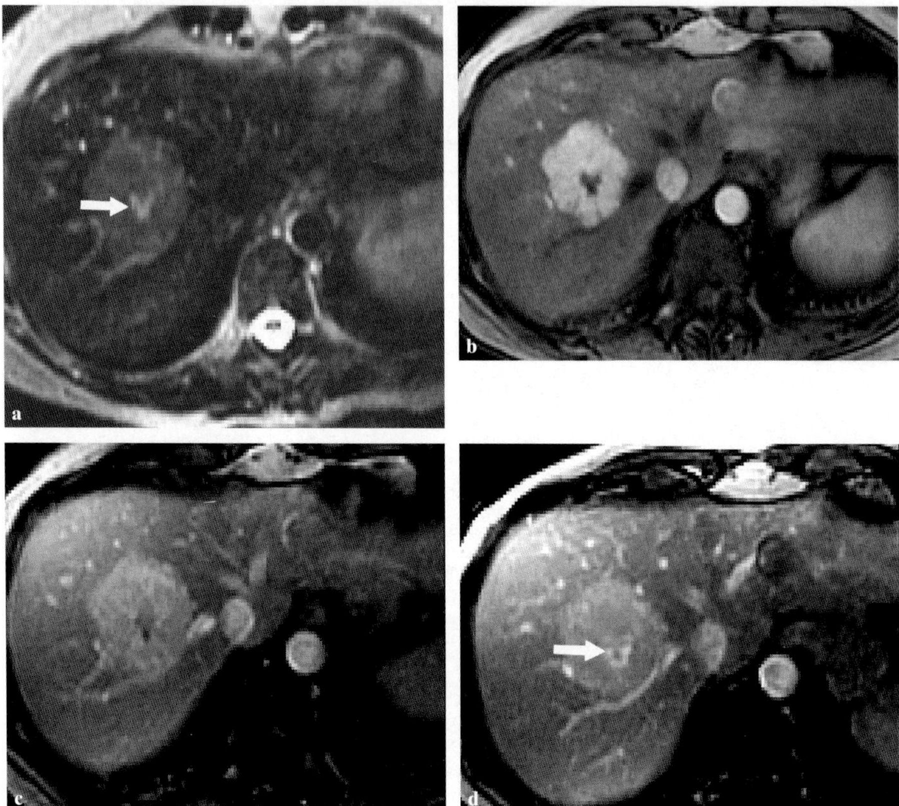

Fig. 2a-d. Focal nodular hyperplasia. A large well-defined mass in the liver is seen as hyperintense in comparison to the normal background parenchyma on the T2-weighted fast spin echo image (**a**). A bright central scar (*arrow*) is also evident. Dynamic T1-weighted imaging following the administration of Gd-DTPA reveals that the lesion shows intense enhancement during the arterial phase (**b**) followed by rapid wash-out during the portal-venous (**c**) phase. The central scar is seen as hypointense on the arterial phase image and as hyperintense on the equilibrium phase image (**d**) (*arrow*)

2.1.2   Hepatocyte-Targeted Contrast Agents

Hepatocyte-selective contrast agents undergo uptake by hepatocytes and are eliminated, at least in part, through the biliary system. A prototypical, dedicated hepatocyte-selective contrast agent is mangafodipir trisodium (Teslascan®, Mn-DPDP; Amersham Health) which was approved for clinical use in 1997 [28, 33, 45, 72, 87, 101]. As with gadolinium chelates, it is considered to have an acceptable safety profile, although injection-related minor adverse events, such as flushing, are relatively common [4, 20]. Moreover, the Mn-DPDP chelate dissociates rapidly following administration to yield free Mn^{++} ion [23] which, in patients with hepatic impairment, may be associated with increased neurological risk [34, 52].

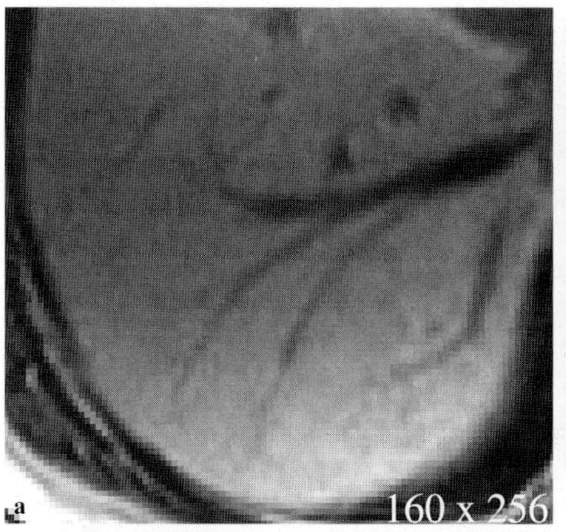
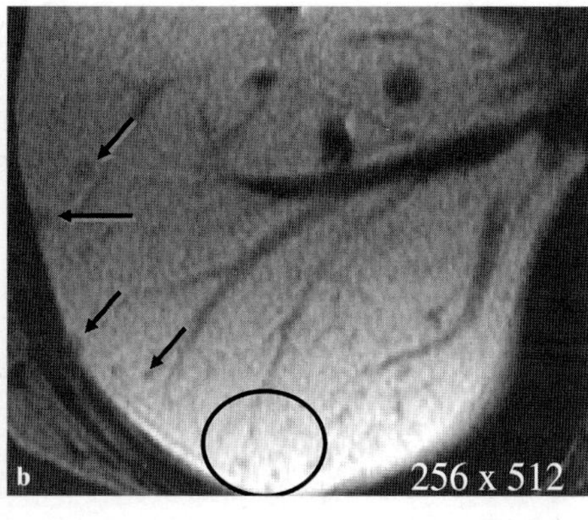

Fig. 3a,b. Detection of liver metastasis with mangafodipir in a young male patient with primary colorectal cancer. Post-mangafodipir-enhanced images obtained with standard (128 × 256) resolution (**a**) and high (256 × 512) resolution (**b**) are shown. Compared to the routine T1-weighted gradient-echo image more lesions (*arrows, circle*) are seen with the high resolution technique

As a paramagnetic contrast agent, mangafodipir trisodium primarily affects T1 relaxation. The increased signal intensity generated in functioning hepatocytes improves the contrast in non-enhancing tissues on T1-weighted images [4, 7, 20, 29, 53, 75]. This agent is administered as a slow intravenous infusion over 1–2 min, which unfortunately precludes the possibility of performing dynamic phase imaging in the manner performed with gadolinium-based agents [4, 35]. Moreover, because the 5–10 mmol/kg dose of mangafodipir is 10% or less than that of the gadolinium agents, imaging with mangafodipir during its distribution phase in the extracellular fluid compartment does not contribute to diagnosis. Doses above 10 mmol/kg do not contribute additional enhancement either [4, 101]. Liver enhancement is maximal within 10 min of mangafodipir trisodium infusion and persists for several hours. Since dynamic images are not acquired with this agent, any T1-weighted sequence can be used. Use of fat saturation has been shown to improve contrast [29, 67, 75]. More importantly, higher spatial resolution imaging can be used effectively even if the entire liver cannot be covered in one data acquisition. A useful sequence is 2D or 3D spoiled GRE with a matrix size of 512/256 x 512 (Fig. 3).

Since liver enhancement in patients with cirrhosis is limited with mangafodipir trisodium [69], liver lesion detection on mangafodipir-enhanced MR imaging is primarily effective in patients with normal liver parenchyma. In these patients, non-hepatocellular focal lesions generally appear hypointense to the normal liver on post-contrast T1-weighted images [5, 102].

Several studies have shown a benefit for liver lesion detection with mangafodipir-enhanced hepatic MR imaging compared with unenhanced MR imaging [4, 5, 20, 29, 101, 102]. Moreover, since hepatocellular lesions, such as FNH, hepatic adenoma and HCC, are generally enhanced with mangafodipir, it is frequently possible to differentiate detected lesions of hepatocellular origin from lesions of non-hepatocellular origin [53, 59, 69]. Unfortunately, because mangafodipir often causes the enhancement of both benign and malignant lesions of hepatocellular origin, it is not

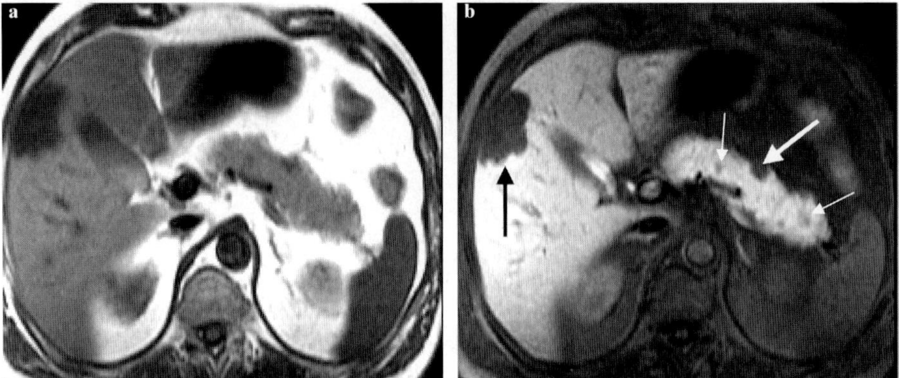

Fig. 4a,b. Mangafodipir-enhanced MRI of the pancreas in a middle-aged man with a history of sarcoma. Compared to the pre-contrast T1-weighted image (**a**) strong enhancement of the pancreas is seen on delayed images after the administration of mangafodipir (**b**). Multiple metastatic deposits in the pancreas (*white arrows*) are much better appreciated on the T1-weighted fat suppressed post-contrast image. Additionally, the conspicuity of the lesions in the liver is improved (*black arrow*)

always possible to differentiate between these lesion-types. In a recent study of 77 patients with histologically-confirmed diagnoses, the sensitivity and specificity of mangafodipir-enhanced MR imaging for the differentiation of histologically-confirmed malignant versus benign lesions was 91% and 67%, respectively, while that for the differentiation of hepatocellular versus non-hepatocellular lesions was 91% and 85%, respectively [59]. Enhancement of both benign and malignant hepatocellular neoplasms [12] limits the usefulness of this agent for the accurate differentiation of hepatocellular lesions, and this, combined with the frequent need for delayed imaging at 4–24 h post-contrast [69], represents a principal shortcoming of this agent [7, 12, 53, 59, 67].

Apart from an inability to differentiate adequately benign from malignant lesions of hepatocellular origin, a further potential limitation of mangafodipir-enhanced liver MR imaging appears to be inadequate characterization of non-hepatocellular lesions. Common benign tumors such as hemangiomas and cysts, as well as non-neoplastic masses such as focal fatty infiltration and focal fat sparing may mimic malignancy in patients with known or suspected cancer. In these settings Gd-chelate-enhanced dynamic multiphase MR imaging is invaluable for satisfactory lesion characterization.

Although mangafodipir trisodium is primarily considered an agent for MR imaging of the liver, a number of early studies demonstrated a potential usefulness for imaging of the pancreas [24, 44, 51] (Fig. 4).

Additionally, since the Mn^{++} ion is excreted in part through the biliary system, mangafodipir trisodium may prove effective for biliary tract imaging on T1-weighted imaging [43].

2.1.3   Agents with Combined Extracellular and Hepatocyte-specific Distribution

In 1998, gadobenate dimeglumine (MultiHance®, Gd-BOPTA; Bracco Imaging SpA) became available in Europe for MR imaging of the liver. Today, gadobenate dimeglumine is approved in Europe and other parts of the world for MR imaging of both the liver and the central nervous system and is under development for other indications including MR Angiography and MR imaging of the breast and heart [1, 11, 13, 38, 40, 74, 78, 81, 97]. Gadobenate dimeglumine differs from the purely extracellular gadolinium agents in combining the properties of a conventional non-specific gadolinium agent with those of an agent targeted specifically to hepatocytes [2, 36]. With this agent, it is possible to perform both dynamic phase imaging as performed with conventional gadolinium-based agents, and delayed phase imaging as performed with mangafodipir trisodium [61, 62]. Thus, arterial, portal-venous and equilibrium phase images are readily attainable using identical sequences to those employed with the conventional non-specific gadolinium agents [82] (Fig. 5a-d). Unlike the conventional agents, however, approximately 3–5% of the injected dose of gadobenate dimeglumine is thereafter taken up by functioning hepatocytes and ultimately excreted into the bile [91]. As with mangafodipir, a result of the hepatocytic uptake is that the normal liver parenchyma shows enhancement on delayed T1-weighted images that is maximal between approximately 1h and 3h after administration [8, 91] (Fig. 5e).

A second feature unique to gadobenate dimeglumine is a capacity for a weak and transient interaction with serum albumin [9, 14]. This feature results in Gd-BOPTA possessing a T1 relaxivity in human serum ($r1=9.7$ mM^{-1}s^{-1}) that is approximately twice that of the conventional gadolinium agents that do not have any capacity for protein interaction [14] (see Table 2). Not only does this increased relaxivity permit lower overall doses to be used to acquire the same information in the dynamic phase as available with conventional agents at a standard dose of 0.1 mmol/kg [82], it also facilitates the improved performance of gadobenate dimeglumine for both intra- and extra-hepatic vascular imaging.

A principal advantage of the selective uptake by functioning hepatocytes is that the normal liver enhances while tumors of non-hepatocytic origin (e.g. metastases, Fig. 6 and cholangiocellular carcinoma, Fig. 7) and non-functioning hepatocytic tumors that are unable to take up Gd-BOPTA (Fig. 8) remain unenhanced, thereby increasing the liver-lesion contrast-to-noise ratio (CNR) and hence the ability to detect lesions [8, 62, 73, 91].

Imaging is typically performed with 2D or 3D T1-weighted GRE sequences while the use of fat saturation has been shown to improve CNR. In the delayed hepatobiliary phase, high-resolution imaging is recommended.

Clinical studies and routine clinical practice have shown that dynamic phase imaging is particularly important for lesion characterization (Fig. 9) while delayed phase imaging in the hepatobiliary phase increases the sensitivity of MRI for liver lesion detection [8, 61, 62]. However, delayed phase imaging also contributes to the improved characterization of lesions, particularly when the results of unenhanced and dynamic imaging are equivocal or when atypicial enhancement patterns are noted on dynamic imaging [25, 26].

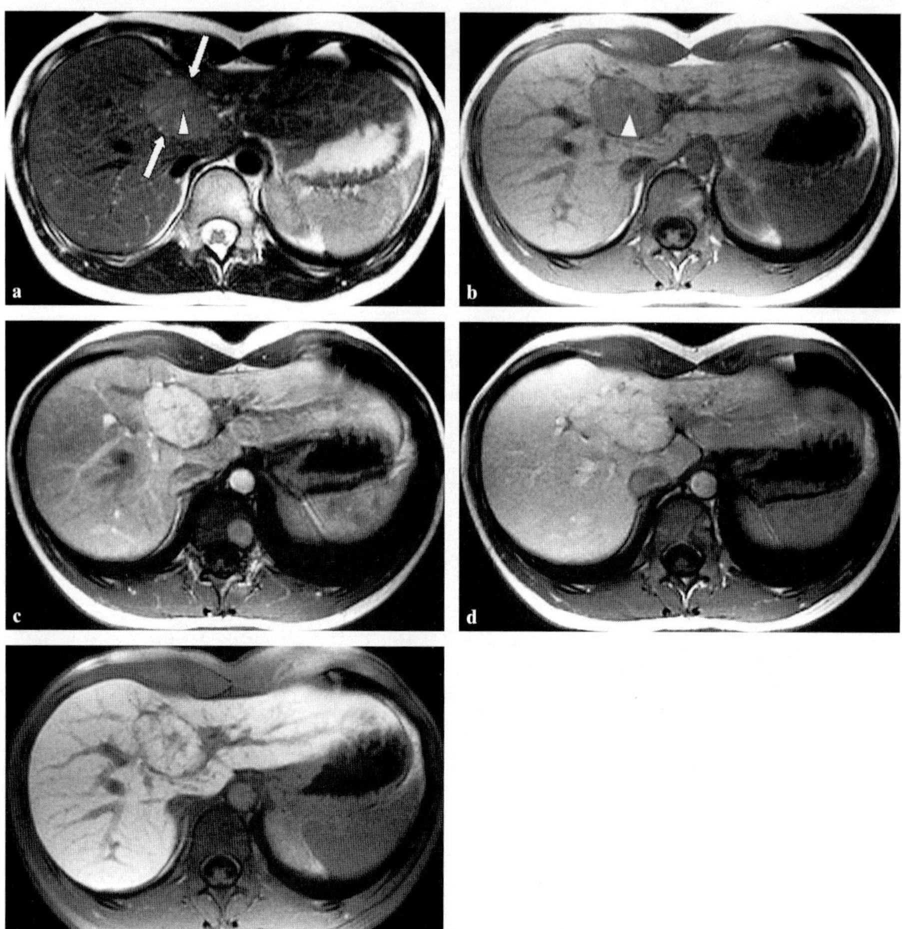

Fig. 5a-e. Characterization of FNH with Gd-BOPTA. On the unenhanced T2w image the lesion (*arrows*) appears slightly hyperintense against the surrounding normal parenchyma. A focus of slight hyperintensity (*arrowhead*) is indicative of a central scar. The corresponding unenhanced T1w image (**b**) reveals a slightly hypointense lesion with a markedly hypointense central area (*arrowhead*) corresponding to the scar. The enhancement pattern observed following the bolus injection of Gd-BOPTA is typical of that observed for FNH after the administration of conventional gadolinium agents i.e., rapid homogenous enhancement during the arterial phase (**c**) followed by rapid washout during the portal-venous phase (**d**). The T1w image acquired during the delayed hepatobiliary phase (**e**) reveals a lesion that is isointense against the surrounding normal parenchyma. This indicates that the lesion contains functioning hepatocytes that are able to take up Gd-BOPTA in the same way as normal hepatocytes. The central scar is seen as hypointense on the delayed image.

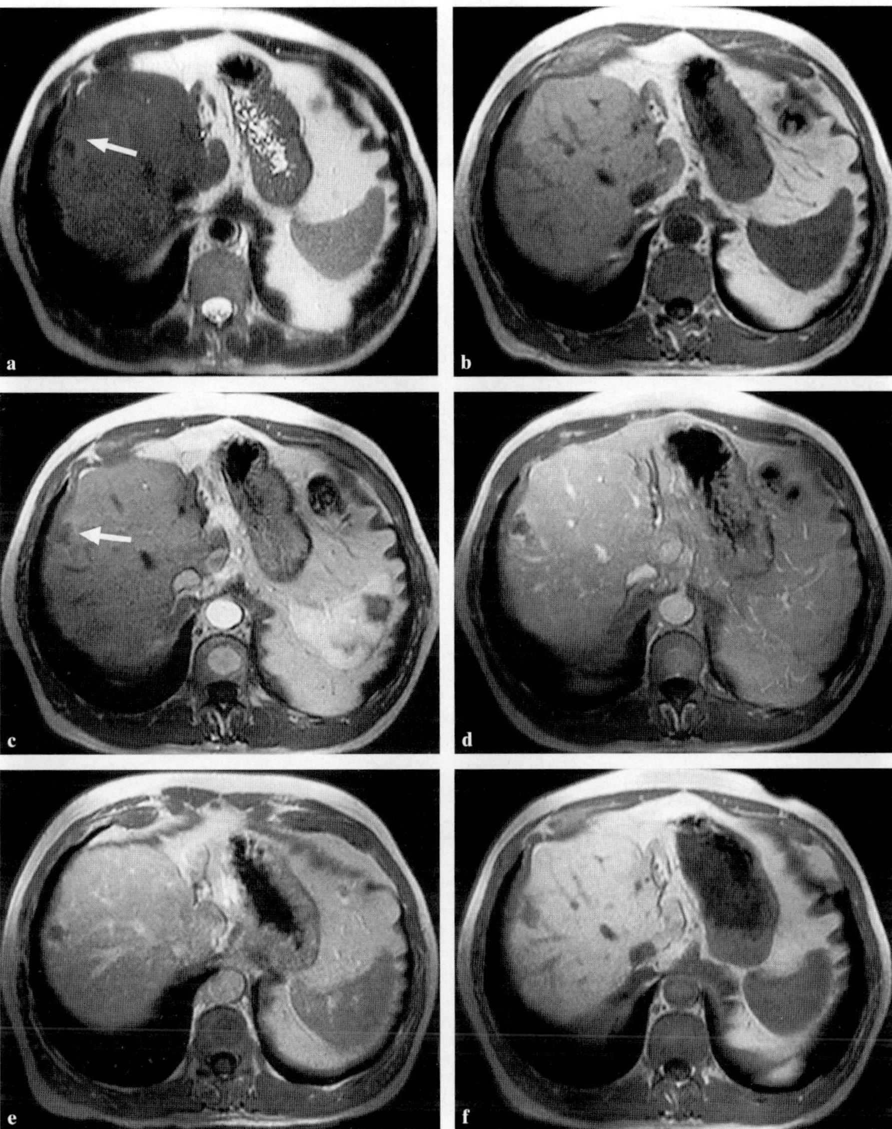

Fig. 6a-f. Characterization of hypovascular metastasis with Gd-BOPTA. Unenhanced T2w and T1w images (**a** and **b**, respectively) both reveal a lesion that is hypointense against the normal liver parenchyma (*arrow in* **a**). The lesion remains hypointense with a hyperintense peripheral rim on arterial (*arrow in* **c**), portal-venous (**d**) and equilibrium (**e**) phase images acquired after the administration of Gd-BOPTA. The hyperintense appearance of the rim is due to the presence of peripheral edema. On the T1w image acquired during the delayed hepatobiliary phase (**f**) the lesion is still hypointense against a strongly enhanced surrounding normal parenchyma. This indicates that the lesion does not take up Gd-BOPTA and is therefore malignant in nature.

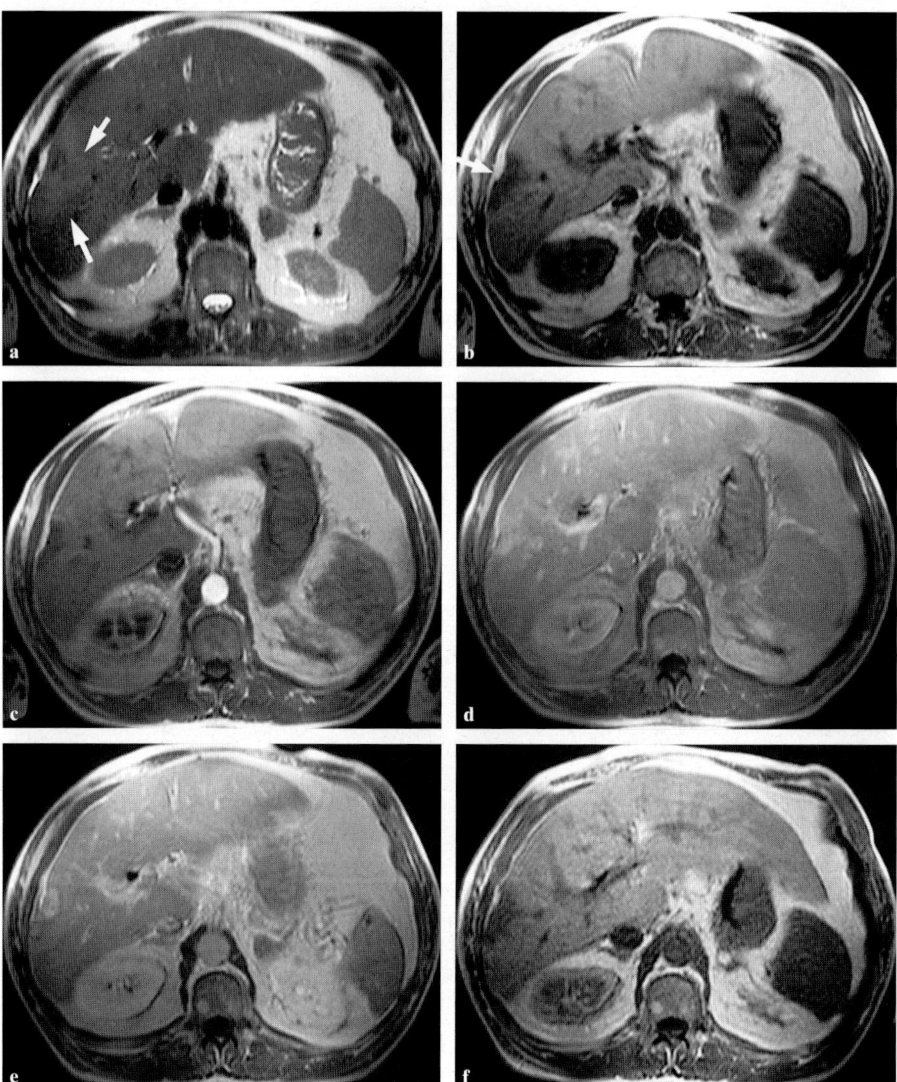

Fig. 7a-f. Characterization of cholangiocellular carcinoma with Gd-BOPTA. The unenhanced T2w image (**a**) reveals a liver of low signal intensity in which a faint area of high signal intensity can be seen in the right lobe (*arrows*). On the unenhanced T1w image (**b**) a marked area of hypointensity is apparent. In addition capsular retraction is evident (*arrow*). The lesion retains an initial hypointense appearance on the T1w arterial phase image acquired after the bolus administration of Gd-BOPTA (**c**), but thereafter demonstrates progressive delayed heterogeneous enhancement during the portal-venous and equilibrium phase images (**d** and **e**, respectively). On the T1w image acquired during the delayed hepatobiliary phase (**f**) the lesion is again hypointense compared to surrounding normal parenchyma indicating that the lesion is malignant in nature

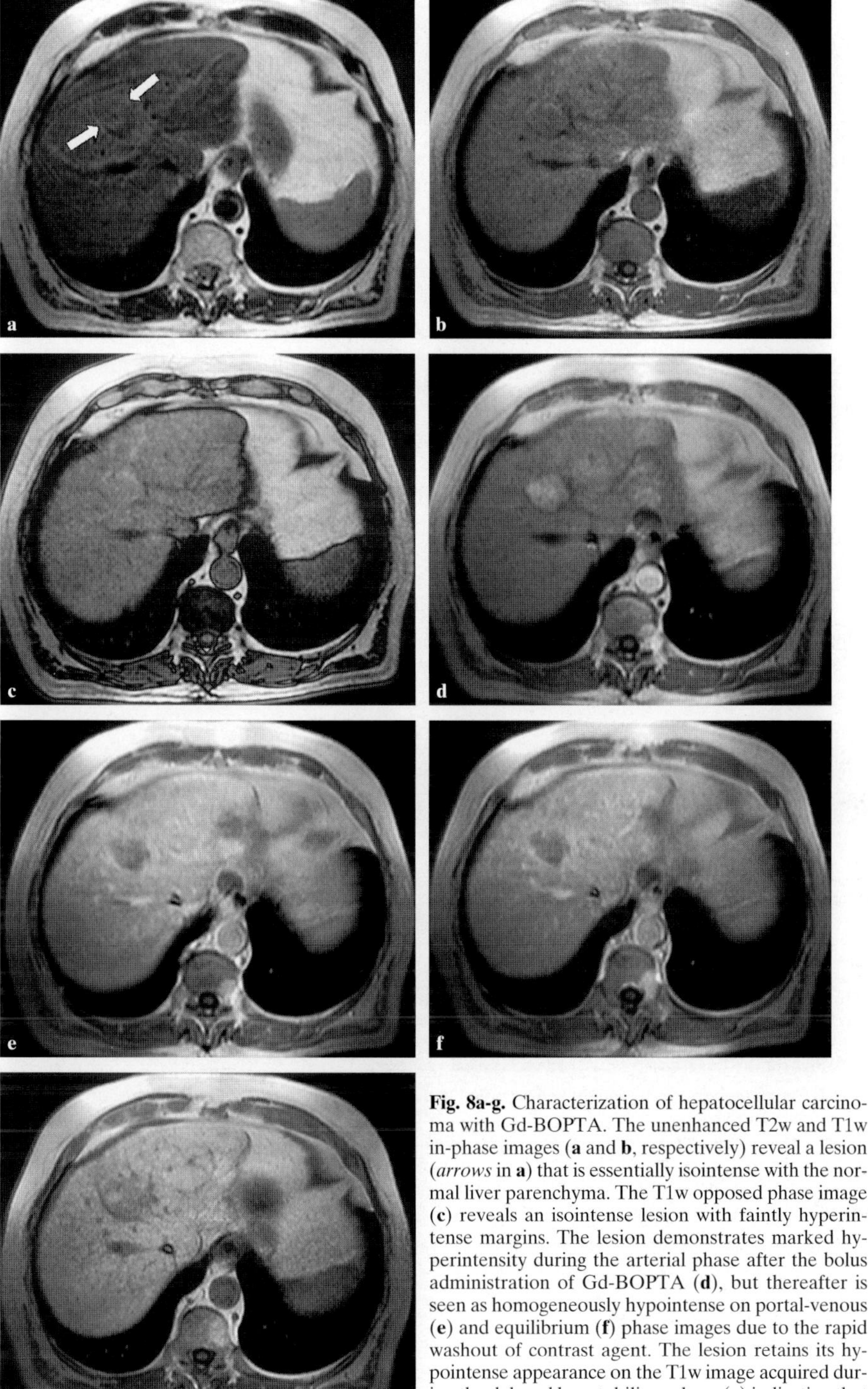

Fig. 8a-g. Characterization of hepatocellular carcinoma with Gd-BOPTA. The unenhanced T2w and T1w in-phase images (**a** and **b**, respectively) reveal a lesion (*arrows* in **a**) that is essentially isointense with the normal liver parenchyma. The T1w opposed phase image (**c**) reveals an isointense lesion with faintly hyperintense margins. The lesion demonstrates marked hyperintensity during the arterial phase after the bolus administration of Gd-BOPTA (**d**), but thereafter is seen as homogeneously hypointense on portal-venous (**e**) and equilibrium (**f**) phase images due to the rapid washout of contrast agent. The lesion retains its hypointense appearance on the T1w image acquired during the delayed hepatobiliary phase (**g**) indicating that the lesion is malignant in nature

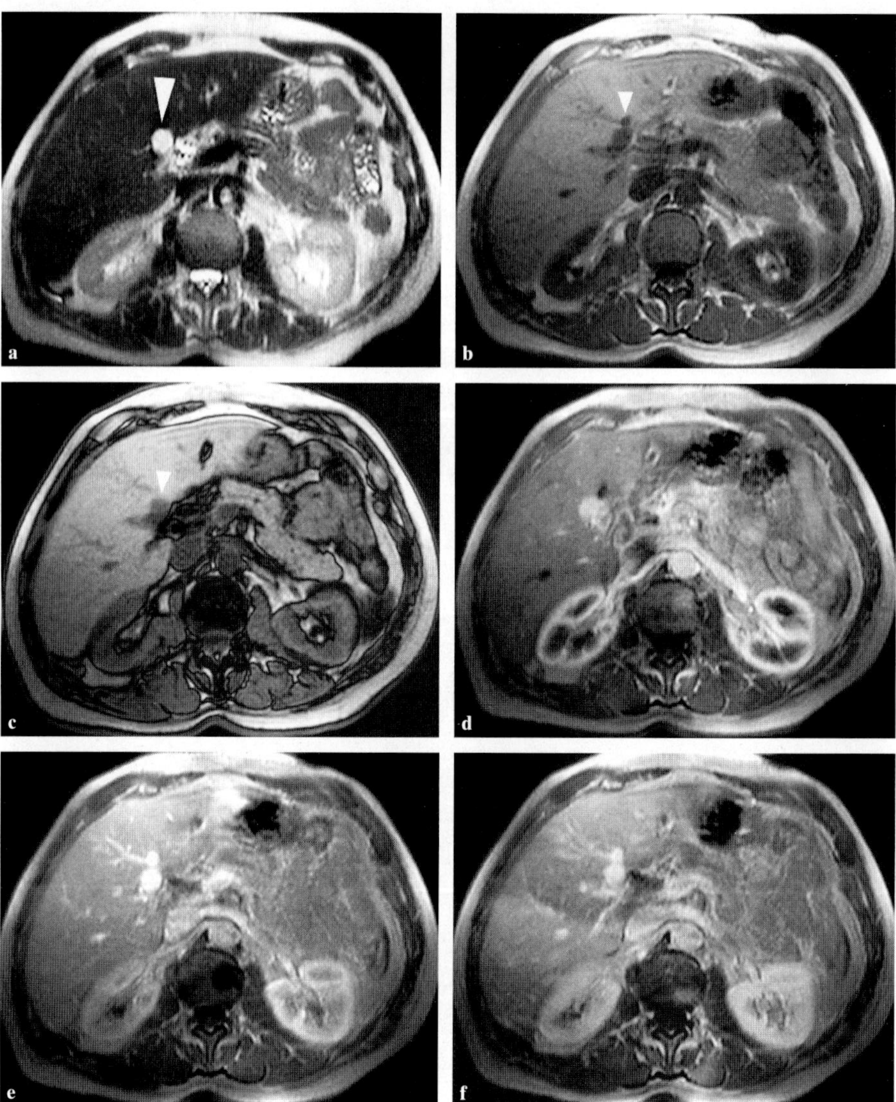

Fig. 9a-f. Characterization of capillary hemangioma with Gd-BOPTA. A markedly hyperintense lesion (*arrowhead*) on the unenhanced T2w image (**a**) is seen as hypointense on the unenhanced T1w in-phase and opposed phase images (**b** and **c**, respectively *arrowheads*). The lesion demonstrates marked hyperintensity during the arterial phase after the bolus administration of Gd-BOPTA (**d**) and retains this hyperintense appearance on the subsequent portal-venous (**e**) and equilibrium (**f**) phase images. The persistent hyperintense appearance on the equilibrium phase image is an indication of the benign nature of the lesion

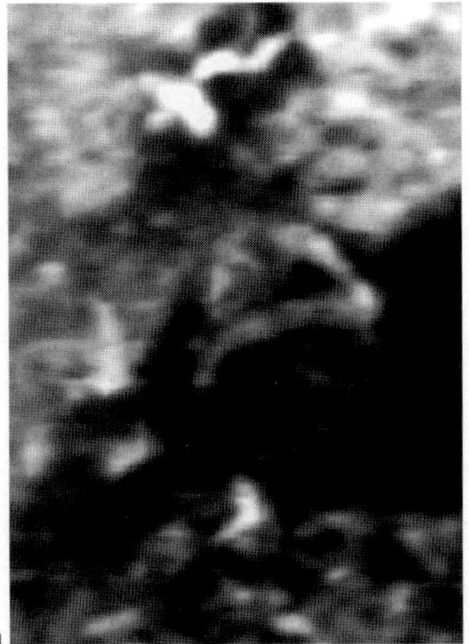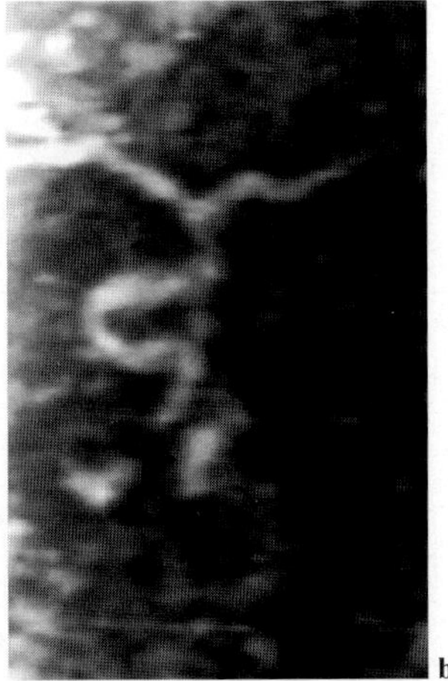

Fig. 10a,b. Unenhanced MRCP (**a**) reveals the common bile duct but gives little additional information regarding functionality. Conversely, the T1-weighted 3D-MIP image (**b**) acquired during the hepatobiliary phase after the administration of Gd-BOPTA reveals the common bile duct and both the left and right hepatic duct. Continuity and normal functionality of the bile duct structures until the papillary region is demonstrated due to excretion of the contrast agent by the bile

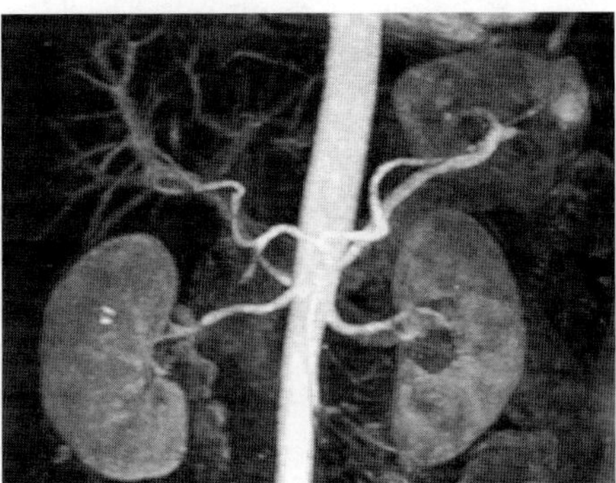

Fig. 11. Contrast-enhanced MR angiography (MRA) after injection of Gd-BOPTA demonstrating normal hepatic vasculature

In addition to the hepatic imaging capability of this agent, its partial biliary excretion should also enable its use for biliary tract imaging (Fig. 10), while the increased relaxivity deriving from weak protein interaction may prove beneficial for intrahepatic MR angiography (Fig. 11). Finally, preliminary studies have already indicated its potential for MR colonography [37].

A second agent with combined extracellular and hepatobiliary properties is gadolinium ethoxybenzyldiethylenetriaminepentaacetic acid (Eovist, Gd-EOB-DTPA, Schering AG), which is currently in the final stages of development [31, 65, 100]. Like Gd-BOPTA, this agent has a higher T1 relaxivity ($r1=8.2$ mM^{-1}s^{-1}) compared to the conventional extracellular agents [65] and distributes initially to the vascular-interstitial compartment after injection. However, whereas only 3–5% of the injected dose of Gd-BOPTA is thereafter taken up by hepatocytes and elimi-

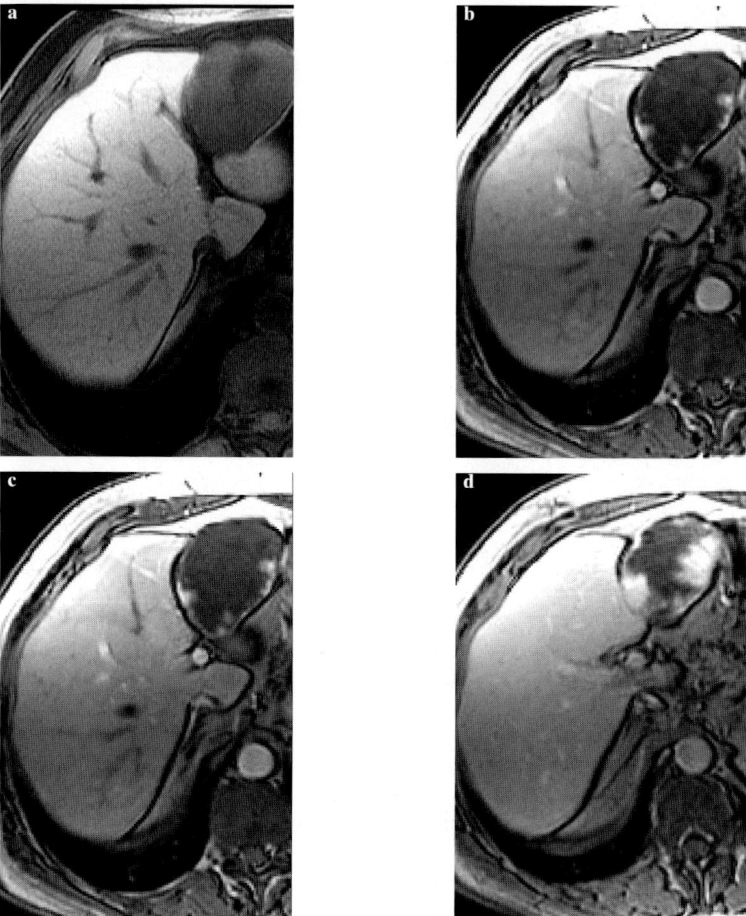

Fig. 12a-d. Hemangioma after Gd-EOB-DTPA. A hypointense lesion on the unenhanced T1-weighted image (**a**) demonstrates the enhancement pattern (peripheral nodular enhancement with progressive filling-in) typical of hemangioma on T1-weighted images acquired during the arterial (**b**), portal-venous (**c**) and equilibrium (**d**) phase after the administration of Gd-EOB-DTPA

nated in the bile, in the case of Gd-EOB-DTPA some 50% of the injected dose is taken up and eliminated via the hepatobiliary pathway after approximately 60 min [31, 84]. The maximum increase of liver parenchyma signal intensity is observed approximately 20 min after injection and lasts for approximately 2 h [31, 70, 83, 84, 100].

As with Gd-BOPTA, the dynamic enhancement patterns seen during the perfusion phase after injection of Gd-EOB-DTPA are similar to those seen with Gd-DTPA (Fig. 12). During the hepatobiliary phase Gd-EOB-DTPA-enhanced im-

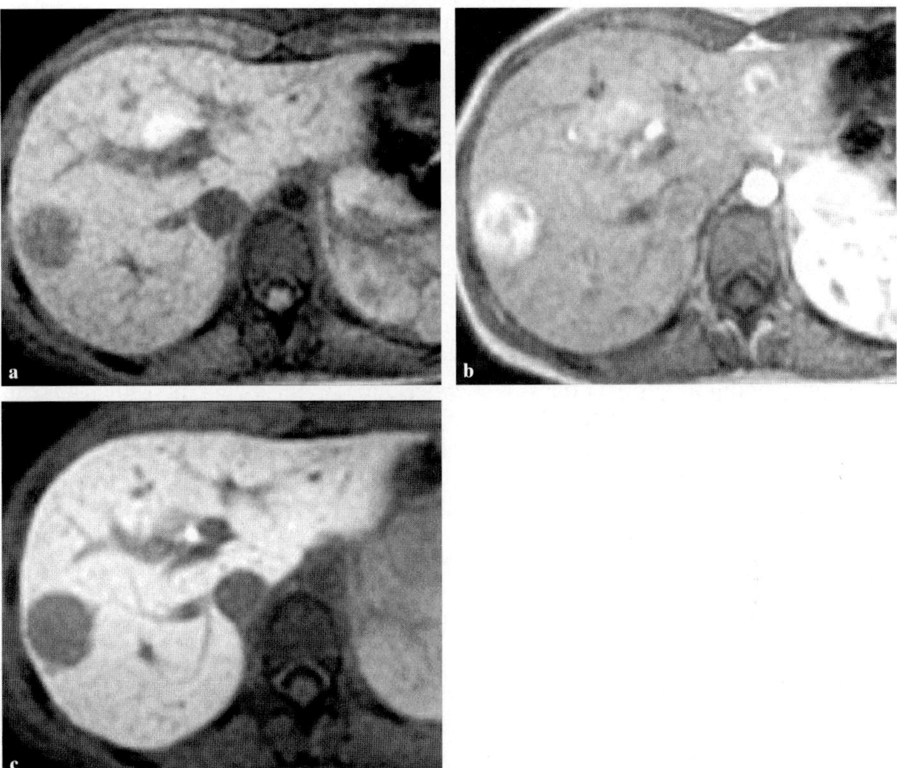

Fig. 13a-c. Lesion detection and characterization with Gd-EOB-DTPA-enhanced MRI in a middle-aged man with carcinoid tumor. Compared to the pre-contrast image (**a**), the early arterial phase image acquired after Gd-EOB-DTPA injection shows uniform arterial phase enhancement of a large liver lesion (**b**). On the delayed phase image acquired 20 min after Gd-EOB-DTPA administration (**c**), the normal liver parenchyma is strongly enhanced due to uptake of the contrast agent by functioning hepatocytes. The lesion-to-liver contrast (conspicuity) is greatly improved due to the inability of the lesion to take up Gd-EOB-DTPA

ages have been shown to improve significantly the detection rate of metastases, HCC, and hemangiomas compared with unenhanced and Gd-DTPA-enhanced images [65, 100] (Fig. 13).

Although Gd-EOB-DTPA is still under development and thus not available for routine clinical practice, it, like Gd-BOPTA [39], is indicated to have a safety profile that is not dissimilar from those of the conventional extracellular gadolinium agents [31, 65].

2.1.4   RES-specific Contrast Agents

Iron oxide particulate agents are selectively taken up by Kupffer cells in the RES, primarily in the liver [28, 85]. Iron oxide particles of different sizes have been developed, which are referred to as superparamagnetic iron oxides (SPIO, mean size > 50 nm) and ultrasmall superparamagnetic iron oxides (USPIO, mean particle size < 50 nm). Of the various formulations, two have so far been developed clinically for MR imaging: ferumoxides (Feridex®, Berlex Laboratories and Endorem®, Laboratoire Guerbet) which has a particle size between 50 and 180 nm and SHU 555 A (Resovist®, Schering AG) which has a particle size ranging between 45 and 60 nm. The safety profiles of these agents are less attractive than those of the paramagnetic contrast agents. With the larger SPIO agents in particular, approximately 3% of patients will experience severe back pain while the contrast agent is being administered [3, 68].

The principal superparamagnetic effect of the larger SPIO particles is on T2 relaxation, and thus MR imaging is usually performed using T2-weighted sequences in which the tissue signal loss is due to the susceptibility effects of iron [21, 22, 63, 64] (Fig. 14). Enhancement on T1-weighted images can also be seen, although this tends to be greater for the smaller SPIO and USPIO formulations [58]. Since there is an overall decrease in liver signal intensity, T2-weighted imaging with SPIO requires excellent imaging techniques that are free of motion artifacts. Typically, moderate T2-weighting echo times of approximately 60–80 ms is adequate for optimizing lesion-liver contrast. Since the larger SPIO agents need to be administered by slow infusion to reduce side effects, imaging is generally performed some 20–30 min after administration (15, 68, 88). Thus, scanning speed is not important and both fast breath-hold and conventional spin echo (SE) imaging can be employed. Pulse sequences that are sensitive to magnetic field heterogeneity tend to be sensitive to the presence of iron oxide. T2*-weighted gradient echo images are very sensitive to SPIO [15, 21, 22, 58, 68]. T2-weighted SE sequences are more sensitive than T2-weighted fast (turbo) SE sequences because the multiple rephasing pulses used in the latter tend to obscure signal losses arising from local variations in the magnetic environment [15]. Administration protocols vary, but typically pre-contrast T1- and T2-weighted imaging is followed by post-contrast T2-weighted imaging.

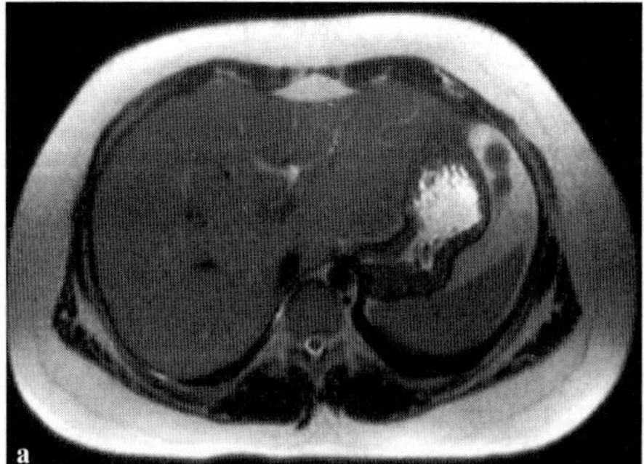
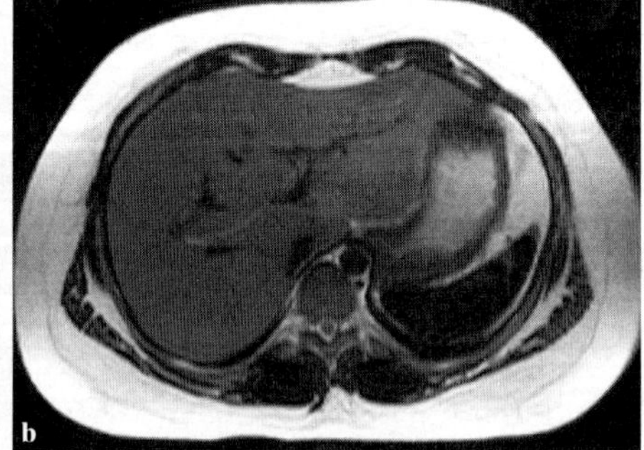

Fig. 14a,b. The signal intensity of the liver is normal on the unenhanced T2-weighted image (**a**). Conversely, a drop of liver and spleen signal intensity is noted on the corresponding T2w image acquired after the administration of SPIO (**b**). This is due to the uptake of iron oxide particles by the Kupffer cells of the RES

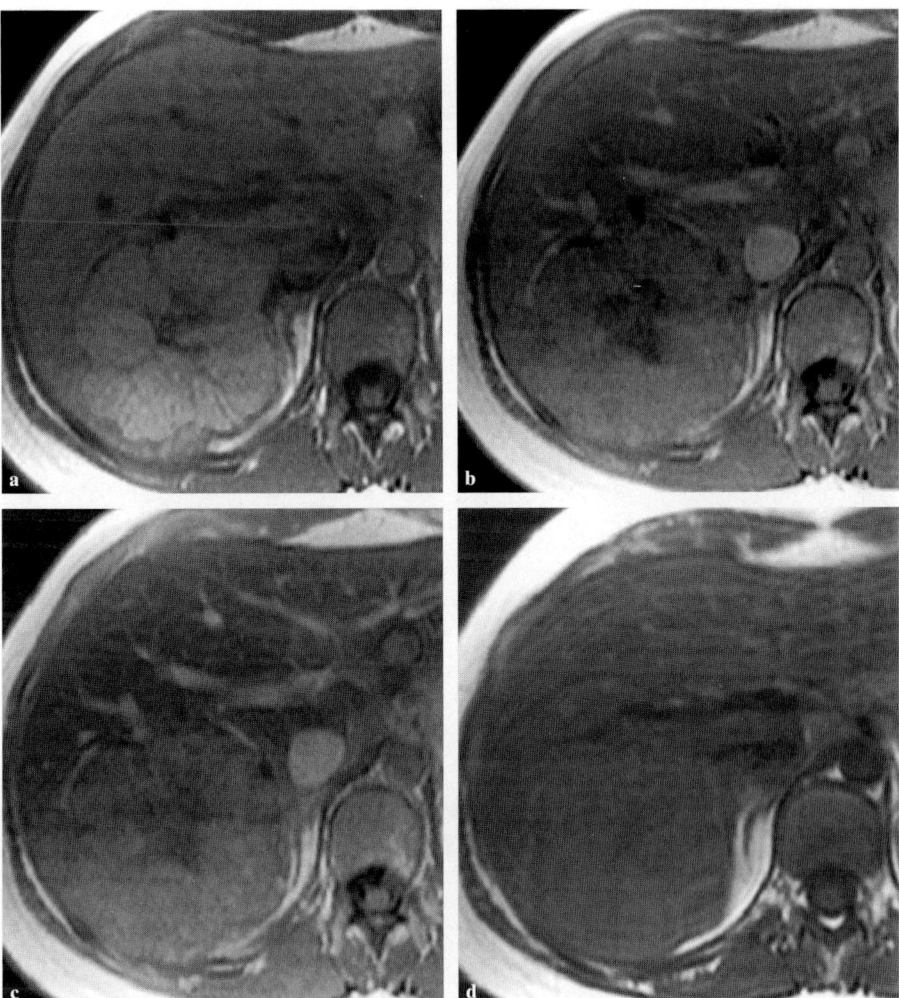

Fig. 15a-d. Dynamic T1w MR imaging of focal nodular hyperplasia with SHU 555 A. A large homogeneously hyperintense lesion can be seen on the arterial phase T1w GRE images acquired at 30 sec after the administration of SHU 555 A (**a**). A central hypointense scar is also apparent on this image. On the portal-venous (**b**) and equilibrium (**c**) phase images acquired after 75 sec and 4 min, respectively, the lesion is seen as slightly hypointense to the surrounding parenchyma. On the delayed phase image acquired after 10 min (**d**) the lesion appears isointense to the surrounding parenchyma while the central scar is seen as slightly hypointense. The isointense appearance on the delayed T1w GRE image indicates that the lesion contains functioning Kupffer cells that are able to take up SHU 555 A. This suggests the lesion is benign in nature

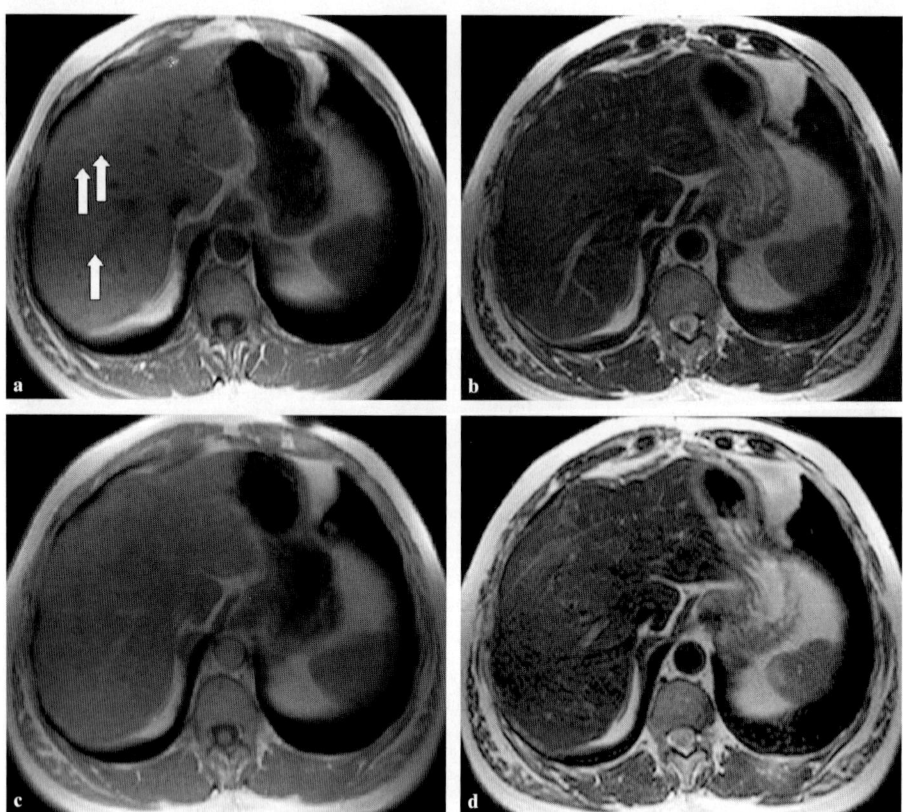

Fig. 16a-d. T2w and T1w MR imaging of nodular regenerative hyperplasia with SHU 555 A. The unenhanced GE T1w image (**a**) reveals several faintly hyperintense nodules (*arrows*) in the right liver lobe. On the corresponding unenhanced TSE T2w image (**b**) these nodules are again seen as slightly hyperintense. On the T1w and T2w images acquired at 10 min after the administration of SHU 555 A (**c** and **d**, respectively) the nodules appear slightly hypointense against the surrounding parenchyma. This indicates that the lesions are able to take up contrast agent and are therefore likely to be benign in nature

Since SPIO particles are removed by the RES, the application of these agents is similar to the use of Tc-sulfur colloid in nuclear scintigraphy. Lesions that contain negligible or no Kupffer cells remain largely unchanged while the signal intensity of the normal liver is reduced on T2-weighted images. As a result, the CNR between liver and lesion is increased [15, 22, 58, 64, 68].

Many well-controlled studies using surgical pathology or intraoperative ultrasound (IOUS) as gold standard, have supported the efficacy of SPIO-enhanced MR imaging [15, 22, 58, 64, 68]. For example, an early multi-center Phase III study showed more lesions in 27% of cases compared to unenhanced MR and in 40% of cases compared to computed tomography (CT) [68]. On the other hand, other early studies were not able to demonstrate a significant benefit over unenhanced imaging for the depiction of hepatic tumors [15]. More recent studies, however, have shown that SPIO-enhanced MR imaging has a significantly greater detection capability for liver malignancies in comparison to spiral CT [88, 103]. Although

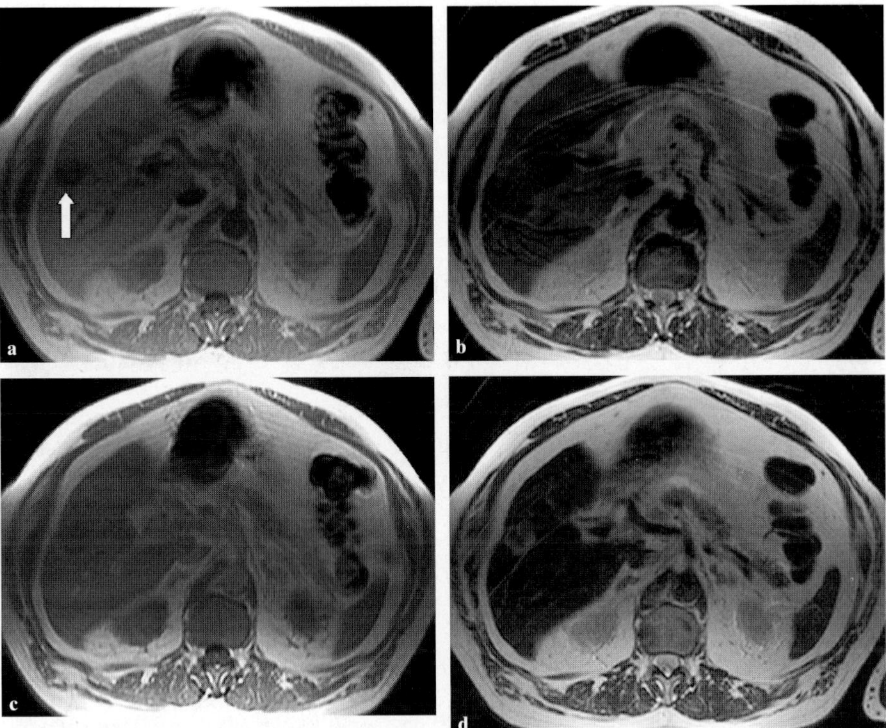

Fig. 17a-d. T2w and T1w MR imaging of peripheral cholangiocellular carcinoma with SHU 555 A. The unenhanced GE T1w image (**a**) reveals a hypointense mass (*arrow*) in the right liver lobe. Slight capsular retraction is also apparent. The lesion is less well seen on the corresponding unenhanced TSE T2w image (**b**). The lesion does not indicate a capacity to take up the contrast agent on the delayed T1w image acquired 10 min after the administration of SHU 555 A (**c**) and remains slight hypointense to the surrounding parenchyma. On the corresponding post-contrast T2w image (**d**) the lesion is clearly delineated with a peripheral hyperintense rim. This enhancement pattern indicates that the lesion is likely to be malignant in nature

comparisons of SPIO-enhanced MR imaging with other gadolinium-enhanced MR techniques have been somewhat limited until recently [6, 27, 60, 94, 98, 99], the general conclusion from the more recent studies is that gadolinium-enhanced imaging is the more valuable approach for the detection of hepatocellular lesions such as HCC and FNH [27, 60, 94].

Limitations of SPIO-enhanced MR imaging include an increased incidence of false positive lesions due to the possibility of vessels mimicking lesions against a background of black liver, and a longer imaging protocol that requires pre- and post-contrast imaging over a period of 30 min or more. Furthermore, the use of SPIO in patients with cirrhosis is also challenging due to the diminished uptake and heterogeneous signal arising from fibrosis [17, 107].

The availability of SHU 555 A may go some way towards overcoming the problems inherent to the larger SPIO agents in that this agent can be administered as a fast bolus in order to observe the early perfusion characteristics of the liver using

T1- or T2*-weighted sequences [64, 66, 89, 99] (Fig. 15). This, combined with the enhancement patterns observed on delayed T1- and T2-weighted images (Figs 16, 17) may prove clinically useful for both the detection and characterization of lesions. Unfortunately, the enhancement during dynamic imaging observed on SHU 555 A–enhanced images is relatively weak due to the small dose that can be injected (1 ml). Thus, it remains to be seen whether this agent will have a widespread clinical impact for liver MRI.

In addition to possessing both T1 and T2 effects, the newer ultrasmall formulations currently under development have a longer intravascular residence time compared to the larger SPIO agents. Hence, they can be considered blood pool agents. As with the larger SPIO particles, the Kupffer cells of the RES take up and eventually clear these USPIO particles over a period of about 24 h. The prolonged imaging window, however, allows for a more favorable image resolution and signal-to-noise ratio because the acquisition parameters are less constrained by time. For liver imaging, the blood-pool effect and combined T1 and T2 effects have shown promise for both the detection and characterization of lesions [32, 77]. A specific advantage is that vessels and lesions show opposite enhancement. On T1-weighted images, vessels are bright while lesions are dark whereas on T2-weighted images the reverse is true. An additional advantage is that MR Angiography may also be performed with these agents. An early study to evaluate the abdominal vasculature on delayed (45 min) images acquired following the infusion of AMI-227, revealed significant enhancement of all vessels [50]. Similarly, time of flight (TOF) MR angiography, prior to and following AMI-227 administration, demonstrated that the renal artery lengths detected increased significantly following contrast administration [92]. Unfortunately, the use of blood-pool agents is flawed, at the present time, by increased background signal and the superimposition of venous structures.

2.2   Summary

Various categories of MR contrast agents are available for clinical use, all of which have been shown to enable the demonstration of more liver lesions than can be depicted on unenhanced imaging alone. The biggest impediment to the more widespread use of contrast agents for liver imaging in the USA in particular is that reimbursement schemes have not yet been established. Thus, these products have so far received only a cautious welcome in the market-place. In addition, the added cost of the extended imaging time needed for the tissue specific (RES and hepatocyte) agents makes their use even less attractive at the current time. On the other hand, it is possible the added value and cost-effectiveness of some of the newer agents will become apparent from clinical use.

In the absence of contrast agents with a combined extracellular and hepatobiliary distribution, at the present time in the USA, one approach to improving both the detection and characterization of liver lesions would be to perform sequential imaging with both a tissue-specific agent and an extracellular gadolinium agent in the same session [41, 76]. The downside of this approach, however, is the need for two injections of two different contrast agents and the associated additional costs involved.

References

1. Baleriaux D, Colosimo C, Ruscalleda J, Korves M, Schneider G, Bohndorf K, Bongartz G, van Buchem MA, Reiser M, Sartor K, Bourne MW, Parizel PM, Cherryman GR, Salerio I, La Noce A, Pirovano G, Kirchin MA, Spinazzi A.. Magnetic resonance imaging of metastatic disease to the brain with gadobenate dimeglumine. Neuroradiol 2002; 44:191-203.
2. Bartolozzi C, Spinazzi A. MultiHance: help or hype? J Comput Assist Tomogr 1999; 23 (Suppl. 1):S151-S159.
3. Bellin MF, Zaim S, Auberton E, Sarfati G, Duron JJ, Khayat D, Grellet J. Liver metastases: Safety and efficacy of detection with superparamagnetic iron oxide in MR imaging. Radiology 1994; 193:657-663.
4. Bernardino ME, Young SW, Lee JK, Weinreb JC. Hepatic MR imaging with Mn-DPDP: Safety image quality and sensitivity. Radiology 1992; 183:53-58.
5. Birnbaum BA, Weinreb JC, Fernandez MP, Brown JJ, Rofsky NM, Young SW. Comparison of contrast enhanced CT and Mn-DPDP enhanced MRI for detection of focal hepatic lesions. Initial findings. Clin Imaging 1994; 18:21-27.
6. Blakeborough A, Ward J, Wilson D, Griffiths M, Kajiya Y, Guthrie JA, Robinson PJ. Hepatic lesion detection at MR imaging: A comparative study with four sequences. Radiology 1997; 203:759-765.
7. Braga HJV, Choti MA, Lee VS, Paulson EK, Siegelman ES, Bluemke DA. Liver lesions: manganese-enhanced MR and dual-phase helical CT for preoperative detection and characterization-comparison with receiver operating characteristic analysis. Radiology 2002: 223:525-531.
8. Caudana R, Morana G, Pirovano GP, Nicoli N, Portuese A, Spinazzi A, Di Rito R, Pistolesi GF. Focal malignant hepatic lesions: MR imaging enhanced with gadolinium benzyloxypropionictetra-acetate (BOPTA) - preliminary results of phase II clinical application. Radiology 1996; 199: 513-520.
9. Cavagna FM, Maggioni F, Castelli PM, Daprà M, Imperatori LG, Lorusso V, Jenkins BG. Gadolinium chelates with weak binding to serum proteins. Invest Radiol 1997; 32:780-796.
10. Chang CA. Magnetic resonance imaging contrast agents. Design and physicochemical properties of gadodiamide. Invest Radiol 1993;28:21-7
11. Cherryman GR, Pirovano G, Kirchin MA. Gadobenate Dimeglumine in MR imaging of Acute Myocardial Infarction: Results of a Phase III study comparing Dynamic and Delayed Contrast Enhanced MR Imaging with EKG, 201Tl SPECT and Echocardiography. Invest Radiol 2002; 37:135-145.
12. Coffin CM, Diche T, Mahfouz A, Alexandre M, Caseiro-Alves F, Rahmouni A, Vasile N, Mathieu D.. Benign and malignant hepatocellular tumors : evaluation of tumoral enhancement after mangafodipir trisodium injection on MR imaging. Eur Radiol 1999; 9:444-449.
13. Colosimo C, Ruscalleda J, Korves M, La Ferla R, Wool C, Pianezzola P, Kirchin MA. Detection of intracranial metastases: a multi-center, intra-patient comparison of gadobenate dimeglumine-enhanced MRI with routinely used contrast agents at equal dose. Invest Radiol 2001; 36:72-81.
14. de Haën C, Cabrini M, Akhnana L, Ratti D, Calabi L, Gozzini L. Gadobenate dimeglumine 0.5M solution for injection (MultiHance"): pharmaceutical formulation and physicochemical properties of a new magnetic resonance imaging contrast medium. J Comput Assist Tomogr 1999; 23 (Suppl. 1):S161-S168.
15. Denys A, Arrive L, Servois V, Dubray B, Najmark D, Sibert A, Menu Y. Hepatic tumors: detection and characterization at 1T MR imaging with AMI-25. Radiology 1994; 193:665-669.
16. Earls JP, Rofsky NM, DeCorato DR, Krinsky GA, Weinreb JC. Hepatic arterial–phase dynamic gadolinium-enhanced MR imaging: optimization with a test examination and a power injector. Radiology 1997; 202:268-273.
17. Elizondo G, Weissleder R, Stark DD, Guerra J, Garza J, Fretz CJ, Todd LE, Ferrucci JT. Hepatic cirrhosis and hepatitis: MR imaging enhanced with superparamagnetic iron oxide. Radiology 1990; 174:797-801.
18. Elizondo G, Fretz CJ, Stark DD, Rocklage SM, Quay SC, Worah D, Tsang YM, Chen MC, Ferrucci JT. Preclinical evaluation of MnDPDP: new paramagnetic hepatobiliary contrast agent for MR imaging. Radiology 1991 Jan;178(1):73-8
19. Fan ZM, Yamashita Y, Harada M, Baba Y, Yamamoto H, Matsukawa T, Arakawa A, Miyazaki T, Takahashi M.. Intrahepatic cholangiocarcinoma : spin echo and contrast-enhanced dynamic MR imaging. Am J Roengenol 1993; 161: 313-317.
20. Federle MP, Chezmar JL, Rubin DL, Weinreb JC, Freeny PC, Semelka RC, Brown JJ, Borello JA, Lee JK, Mattrey R, Dachman AH, Saini S, Harmon B, Fenstermacher M, Pelsang RE, Harms SE, Mitchell DG, Halford HH, Anderson MW, Johnson CD, Francis IR, Bova JG, Kenney PJ, Klippenstein DL, Foster GS, Turner DA.. Safety and efficacy of Mangafodipir Trisodium (Mn-DPDP) Injection for hepatic MRI in adults: results of the U.S. multicenter Phase III clinical trials (safety). J Magn Reson Imaging 2000; 12:186-197.
21. Fretz CJ, Elizondo G, Weissleder R, Hahn PF, Stark DD, Ferrucci JT Jr. Superparamagnetic iron oxide – enhanced MR imaging: Pulse sequence optimization for detection of liver cancer. Radiology 1989; 172:393-397.
22. Fretz CJ, Stark DD, Metz CE, Elizondo G, Weissleder R, Shen JH, Wittenberg J, Simeone J, Ferrucci

JT. Detection of hepatic metastases: Comparison of contrast-enhanced CT, unenhanced MR imaging and iron-oxide-enhanced MR imaging. AM J Roentgenol 1990; 155:763-770.

23. Gallez B, Bacic G, Swartz HM. Evidence for the dissociation of the hepatobiliary MRI contrast agent Mn-DPDP. Magn Reson Med 1996; 35:14-19.

24. Gehl HB, Vorwerk D, Klose KC, Gunther RW. Pancreatic enhancement after low dose infusion of Mn-DPDP: Radiology 1991; 180:337-339.

25. Grazioli L, Morana G, Caudana R, Benetti A, Portolani N, Talamini G, Colombari R, Pirovano G, Kirchin MA, Spinazzi A.. Hepatocellular Carcinoma: Correlation between gadobenate dimeglumine-enhanced MRI and pathologic findings. Invest Radiol 2000; 35:25-34.

26. Grazioli L, Morana G, Federle MP, Brancatelli G, Testoni M, Kirchin MA, Menni K, Olivetti L, Nicoli N, Procacci C. Focal nodular hyperplasia: morphological and functional information from MR imaging with gadobenate dimeglumine. Radiology 2001; 221:731-739.

27. Grazioli L. Morana G, Kirchin MA et al. MR Imaging of focal nodular hyperplasia (FNH) with gadobenate dimeglumine (Gd-BOPTA) and SPIO (Ferumoxides): an intra-individual comparison. J Magn Reson Imaging 2003 In press.

28. Hahn PF, Saini S. Liver-specific MR imaging contrast agents. Radiol Clin North Am 1998; 36:287-97.

29. Vogl TJ, Hamm B, Schnell B, Eibl-Eibesfeldt B, Steiner S, Lissner J. Focal liver lesions: MR imaging with Mn-DPDP – initial clinical results in 40 patients. Radiology 1991; 182:167-174.

30. Hamm B, Thoeni RF, Gould RG, Bernardino ME, Luning M, Saini S, Mahfouz AE, Taupitz M, Wolf KJ.. Focal liver lesions: characterization with nonenhanced and dynamic contrast material–enhanced MR imaging. Radiology 1994; 190:417-423.

31. Hamm B, Staks T, Muhler A, Bollow M, Taupitz M, Frenzel T, Wolf KJ, Weinmann HJ, Lange L.. Phase I clinical evaluation of Gd-EOB-DTPA as a hepatobiliary MR contrast agent: safety, pharmacokinetics and MR imaging. Radiology 1995; 195:785-792.

32. Harisinghani MG, Saini S, Weissleder R, Halpern EF, Schima W, Rubin DL, Stillman AE, Sica GT, Small WC, Hahn PF.. Differentiation of liver hemangiomas from metastases and hepatocellular carcinoma at MR imaging enhanced with blood-pool contrast agent Code-7227. Radiology 1997; 202:687-691.

33. Harisinghani MG, Jhaveri KS, Weissleder R, Schima W, Saini S, Hahn PF, Mueller PR. MRI contrast agents for evaluating focal liver lesions Clin Radiol 2001; 56:714-725.

34. Hauser RA, Zesiewicz TA, Rosemurgy AS, Marinez C, Olanow CW. Manganese intoxication and chronic liver failure. Ann Neurol 1994; 36:871-875.

35. Kettritz U, Schlund JF, Wilbur K, Eisenberg LB, Semelka RC. Comparison of gadolinium chelates with manganese-DPDP for liver lesion detection and characterization: preliminary results. Magn Reson Imaging 1996; 14:1185-1190.

36. Kirchin MA, Pirovano G, Spinazzi A. Gd-BOPTA (Gd-BOPTA): an overview. Invest Radiol 1998; 33:798-809.

37. Knopp MV, Giesel FL, Radeleff J, von Tengg-Kobligk H. Bile-tagged 3D magnetic resonance colonography after exclusive intravenous administration of gadobenate dimeglumine, a contrast agent with partial hepatobiliary excretion. Invest Radiol 2001; 36:619-623.

38. Knopp et al. Assessment of Gadobenate Dimeglumine (Gd-BOPTA) for MR Angiography: Phase I Studies. Invest. Radiol. 2002; In press.

39. Kirchin MA, Pirovano G, Venetianer C, Spinazzi A. Safety assessment of gadobenate dimeglumine (Multihance,): extended clinical experience from phase I studies to post-marketing surveillance. J Magn Reson Imaging 2001; 14: 281-294.

40. Kroencke TJ, Wasser MN, Pattynama PMT et al. Contrast-enhanced magnetic resonance angiography of the abdominal aorta and renal arteries with gadobenate dimeglumine. Am J Roengenol 2002; In press.

41. Kubaska S, Sahani DV, Saini S, Hahn PF, Halpern E. Dual contrast enhanced magnetic resonance imaging of the liver with superparamagnetic iron oxide followed by gadolinium for lesion detection and characterization. Clin Radiol. 2001; 56:410-415.

42. Larson RE, Semelka RC, Bagley AS, Molina PL, Brown ED, Lee JK. Hypervascular malignant liver lesions: comparison of various MR imaging pulse sequences and dynamic CT. Radiology 1994; 192:393-399.

43. Lee VS, Rofsky NM, Morgan GR, Teperman LW, Krinsky GA, Berman P, Weinreb JC. Volumetric mangafodipir trisodium-enhanced cholangiography to define intrahepatic biliary anatomy. Am J Roentgenol 2001; 176: 906-8.

44. Liou J, Lee JK, Borrello JA, Brown JJ. Differentiation of hepatomas from nonhepatomatous masses: use of Mn-DPDP-enhanced MR images. Magn Reson Imaging 1994; 12:71-79.

45. Low RN. Contrast agents for MR imaging of the liver. J Magn Reson Imaging 1997; 7:56-67.

46. Low RN, Francis IR, Sigeti JS, Foo TK. Abdominal MR imaging: comparison of T2-weighted fast conventional spin-echo, and contrast-enhanced fast multiplanar spoiled gradient-recalled imaging. Radiology 1993; 186:803-811.

47. Mahfouz AD, Hamm B, Taupitz M, Wold KJ. Hypervascular liver lesions: differentiation of focal nodular hyperplasia from malignant tumors with dynamic gadolinium-enhanced MR imaging. Radiol-

ogy 1993; 186:133-138.

48. Mahfouz AE, Hamm B, Wolf KJ. Peripheral washout: a sign of malignancy on dynamic gadolinium-enhanced MR images of focal liver lesions. Radiology 1994; 190:49-52.

49. Mathieu D, Rahmouni A, Anglade MC, Falise B, Beges C, Gheung P, Mollet JJ, Vasile N. Focal nodular hyperplasia of the liver: assessment with contrast-enhanced Turbo-FLASH MR imaging. Radiology 1991; 180:25-30.

50. Mayo-Smith WW, Saini S, Slater G, Kaufman JA, Sharma P, Hahn PF. MR contrast material for vascular enhancement: value of supermagnetic iron oxide. Am J Roentgenol 1996; 166:73-77.

51. Mayo-Smith WW, Schima W, Saini S, Slater GJ, McFarland EG. Pancreatic enhancement and pulse sequence analysis using low dose mangafodipir trisodium. Am J Roentgenol 1998; 170: 649-652.

52. Misselwitz B, Muhler A, Weinmann HJ. A toxicological risk for using manganese complexes? A literature survey of existing data through several medical specialities. Invest Radiol 1995; 30:611-620.

53. Murakami T, Baron RL, Peterson MS, Oliver III, JH, Davis PL, Confer SR, Federle MP. Hepatocellular carcinoma: MR imaging with mangafodipir trisodium (Mn-DPDP). Radiology 1996; 200:69-77.

54. Nelson KL, Gifford LM, Lauber-Huber C, Gross CA, Lasser TA. Clinical safety of Gd-DTPA. Radiology 1995; 196: 439-443.

55. Niendorf HP, Kallend D. Gadolinium chelates: adverse reactions. In: Textbook of contrast media (Dawson P, Cosgrove DO. Grainger RG. Eds.). ISIS Medical Media, Oxford, UK; 1999, pp. 323-332.

56. Oi H, Murakami T, Kim T, Matsushita M, Kishimoto H, Nakamura H. Dynamic MR imaging and early-phase helical CT for detection small of intrahepatic metastases of hepatocellular carcinoma. Am J Roentgenol 1996; 366:36-374.

57. Olukotun AY, Parker JR, Meeks MJ, Lucas MA, Fowler DR, Lucas TR. Safety of gadoteridol injection: U.S. clinical trial experience. J Magn Reson Imaging 1995; 5:17-25.

58. Oudkerk M, van den Heuvel AG, Wielopolski PA, Schmitz PIM, Borel Rinke IHM, Wiggers T. Hepatic lesions: detection with ferumoxide-enhanced T1-weighted MR imaging. Radiology 1997; 203:449-456.

59. Oudkerk M, Torres CG, Song B, Konig M, Grimm J, Fernandez-Cuadrado J, Op de Beeck B, Marquardt M, van Dijk P, Cees de Groot J.. Characterization of liver lesions with mangafodipir trisodium-enhanced MR imaging : multicenter study comparing MR and dual-phase spiral CT. Radiology 2002; 223:517-524.

60. Pauleit D, Textor J, Bachmann R, Conrad R, Flacke S, Layer G, Kreft S, Schild H. Hepatocellular carcinoma: detection with gadolinium- and ferumoxides-enhanced MR imaging of the liver. Radiology 2002; 222:73-80.

61. Petersein J, Spinazzi A, Giovagnoni A, Soyer P, Terrier F, Lencioni R, Bartolozzi C, Grazioli L, Chiesa A, Manfredi R, Marano P, Van Persijn Van Meerten EL, Bloem JL, Petre C, Marchal G, Greco A, McNamara MT, Heuck A, Reiser M, Laniado M, Claussen C, Daldrup HE, Rummeny E, Kirchin MA, Pirovano G, Hamm B. Evaluation of the Efficacy of Gadobenate Dimeglumine in MR Imaging of Focal Liver Lesions: a Multicenter Phase III Clinical Study. Radiology 2000; 215:727-736.

62. Pirovano G, Vanzulli A, Marti-Bonmati L, Grazioli L, Manfredi R, Greco A, Holzknecht N, Daldrup-Link HE, Rummeny E, Hamm B, Arneson V, Imperatori L, Kirchin MA, Spinazzi A. Evaluation of the accuracy of gadobenate dimeglumine-enhanced MR imaging in the detection and characterization of focal liver lesions. Am J Roentgenol 2000; 175:1111-1120.

63. Reimer P, Kwong KK, Weisskoff R, Cohen MS, Brady TJ, Weissleder R. Dynamic signal intensity changes in liver with superparamagnetic MR contrast agents. J Magn Reson Imaging 1992; 2:177-181.

64. Reimer P, Rummeny EJ, Daldrup HE, Balzer T, Tombach B, Berns T, Peters PE. Clinical results with Resovist: A phase II clinical trial. Radiology 1995; 195:489-496.

65. Reimer P, Rummeny EJ, Shamsi K, Balzer T, Daldrup HE, Tombach B, Hesse T, Berns T, Peters PE.. Phase II clinical evaluation of Gd-EOB-DTPA: dose, safety aspects, and pulse sequences. Radiology 1996; 199:177-183.

66. Reimer P, Muller M, Marx C, Wiedermann D, Muller R, Rummeny EJ, Ebert W, Shamsi K, Peters PE. T1 effects of a bolus-injectable superparamagnetic iron oxide, SH U 555 A: dependence on field strength and plasma concentration – preliminary clinical experience with dynamic T1-weighted MR imaging. Radiology 1998; 209:831-836.

67. Rofsky NM, Earls JP. Mangafodipir trisodium injection. A contrast agent for abdominal MR imaging. Magn Reson Imaging Clin North Am 1996; 4:73-85.

68. Ros PR, Freeny PC, Harms SE, Seltzer SE, Davis PL, Chan TW, Stillman AE, Muroff LR, Runge VM, Nissenbaum MA, et al. Hepatic MR imaging with ferumoxides: a multicenter clinical trial of the safety and efficacy in the detection of focal hepatic lesions. Radiology 1995; 196:481-488.

69. Rummeny EJ, Torres CG, Kurdziel JC, Nilsen G, Op de Beeck B, Lundby B. Mn-DPDP for MR imaging of the liver. Results of an independent image evaluation of the European Phase III studies. Acta Radiol 1997; 38:638-642.

70. Runge VM. A comparison of two MR hepatobiliary gadolinium chelates: Gd-BOPTA and Gd-EOB-DTPA. J comput Assist Tomogr 1998; 22:643-650.

71. Runge VM. Safety of approved MR contrast media for intravenous injection. J Magn Reson Imaging 2000; 12:205-213.
72. Runge VM, Pels Rijcken TH, Davidoff A, Wells JW, Stark DD. Contrast-enhanced MR imaging of the liver. J Magn Reson Imaging 1994; 4:281-9.
73. Runge VM, Lee C, Williams NM. Detectability of small liver metastases with gadolinium BOPTA. Invest Radiol 1997; 32:557-565
74. Runge VM, Armstrong MR, Barr RG, Berger BL, Czervionke LF, Gonzalez CF, Halford HH, Kanal E, Kuhn MJ, Levin JM, Low RN, Tanenbaum LN, Wang AM, Wong W, Yuh WT, Zoarski GH.. A clinical comparison of the safety and efficacy of MultiHance (gadobenate dimeglumine) and Omniscan (gadodiamide) in magnetic resonance imaging in patients with central nervous system pathology. Invest Radiol 2001; 36:65-71.
75. Sahani DV, O'Malley ME, Bhat S, Hahn PF, Saini S. Contrast-enhanced MRI of the liver with mangafodipir trisodium: imaging technique and results. J Comput Assist Tomogr 2002; 26:216-22.
76. Sahani DV, Saini S, Kalra MK, Michael M, Hahn PF. Liver lesion detection and characterization with sequential use of hepatobiliary contrast agent mangafodipir trisodium and gadolinium-DTPA in a single imaging protocol. Acad Radiol 2002; 9 (Suppl 2):S460-2.
77. Saini S, Edelman RR, Sharma P, Li W, Mayo-Smith W, Slater GJ, Eisenberg PJ, Hahn PF. Blood–pool MR contrast agent material for detection and characterization of focal hepatic lesions. Initial clinical experience with superparamagnetic iron oxide (AMI-227). Am J Roentgenol 1995; 164:1447-1152.
78. Sandstede JJW, Beer M, Lipke C, Pabst T, Kenn W, Harre K, Neubauer S, Hahn D. Time course of contrast enhancement patterns after Gd-BOPTA in correlation to myocardial infarction and viability: a feasibility study. JMRI 2001; 14:789-794.
79. Schering AG, Berlin. Magnevist,. Nierengängiges paramagnetisches Kontrastmittel für die magnetische Resonanztomographie (MRT). 1987.
80. Schlund JF, Semelka RC, Kettritz U, Eisenberg LB, Lee JKT. Transient increased segmental hepatic enhancement distal to portal vein obstruction on dynamic gadolinium-enhanced gradient echo MR images. J Magn Reson Imaging 1995; 4:375-377.
81. Schneider G, Kirchin MA, Pirovano G, Colosimo C, Ruscalleda J, Korves M, Salerio I, La Noce A, Spinazzi A.. Gadobenate dimeglumine-enhanced magnetic resonance imaging of intracranial metastases: effect of dose on lesion detection and delineation. J Magn Reson Imaging 2001; 14:525-539.
82. Schneider G, Maas R, Schultze Kool L et al. Low-dose gadobenate dimeglumine versus standard dose gadopentetate dimeglumine for contrast-enhanced MR imaging of the liver: an intra-individual crossover comparison. Invest Radiol 2003; In press
83. Schuhmann-Giampieri G. Liver contrast media for magnetic resonance imaging. Interrelations between pharmacokinetics and imaging. Invest Radiol 1993; 28:753-761.
84. Schuhmann-Giampieri G, Mahler M, Röll G, Maibauer R, Schmitz S. Pharmacokinetics of the liver-specific contrast agent Gd-EOB-DTPA in relation to contrast enhanced liver imaging in humans. J Clin Pharmacol 1997; 37:587-596.
85. Schwartz LH, Seltzer SE, Tempany CM, Silverman SG, Piwnica-Worms DR, Adams DF, Herman L, Herman LA, Hooshmand R.. Superparamagnetic iron oxide hepatic MR imaging: efficacy and safety using conventional and fast spin-echo pulse sequences. J Magn Reson Imaging 1995; 5:566-570.
86. Semelka RC, Worawattanakul S, Kelekis NL, John G, Woosley JT, Graham M, Cance WG. Liver lesion detection, characterization, and effect on patient management: comparison of single-phase spiral CT and current MR techniques. J Magn Reson Imaging 1997; 7:1040-1047.
87. Semelka RC, Helmberger TKG. Contrast agents for MR imaging of the liver. Radiology 2001; 218:27-38.
88. Seneterre E, Taourel P, Bouvier Y, Pradel J, Van Beers B, Daures JP, Pringot J, Mathieu D, Bruel JM.. Detection of hepatic metastases: ferumoxides-enhanced MR imaging versus unenhanced MR imaging and CT during arterial portography. Radiology 1996; 200:785-792.
89. Shamsi K, Balzer T, Saini S, Ros PR, Nelson RC, Carter EC, Tollerfield S, Niendorf H-P. Superparamagnetic iron oxide particles (SH U 555 A): evaluation of efficacy in three doses for hepatic MR imaging. Radiology 1998; 206:365-371.
90. Shellock FG, Kanal E. Safety of magnetic resonance imaging contrast agents. J Magn Reson Imaging 1999; 10:477-484.
91. Spinazzi A, Lorusso V, Pirovano G, Kirchin M. Safety, tolerance, biodistribution and MR imaging enhancement of the liver with gadobenate dimeglumine. Acad Radiol 1999; 6:282-291.
92. Stillman AE, Wilke N, Li D, Haacke M, McLachlan S. Ultrasmall superparamagnetic iron oxide to enhance MRA of the renal and coronary arteries: Studies in human patients. J Comput Assist Tomog 1996; 20:51-55.
93. Swan SK, Baker JF, Free R, Tucker RM, Barron B, Barr R, Seltzer S, Gazelle GS, Maravilla KR, Barr W, Stevens GR, Lambrecht LJ, Pierro JA.. Pharmacokinetics, safety and tolerability of gadoversetamide injection (Optimark) in subjects with central nervous system or liver pathology and varying degrees of renal function. J Magn Reson Imaging 1999; 9:317-321.
94. Tang Y, Yamashita Y, Arakawa A, Namimoto T, Mitsuzaki K, Abe Y, Katahira K, Takahashi M.. De-

tection of hepatocellular carcinoma arising in cirrhotic livers : comparison of gadolinium- and ferumoxides-enhanced MR imaging. Am J Roentgenol 1999; 172:1547-1554.

95. Tirkkonen B, Aukrust A, Couture E, Grace D, Haile Y, Holm KM, Hope H, Larsen A, Lunde HS, Sjogren CE. Physicochemical characterization of mangafodipir trisodium. Acta Radiol 1997;38:780-9

96. Tweedle MF. Physicochemical properties of gadoteridol and other magnetic resonance contrast agents. Invest Radiol 1992;27:1-6

97. Völk M, Strotzer M, Lenhart M, Seitz J, Manke C, Feuerbach S, Link J. Renal time-resolved MR angiography: quantitative comparison of gadobenate dimeglumine and gadopentetate dimeglumine with different doses. Radiology 2001; 220:484-488.

98. Vogl TJ, Hammerstingl R, Schwarz W, Mack MG, Muller PK, Pegios W, Keck H, Eibl-Eibesfeldt A, Hoelzl J, Woessmer B, Bergman C, Felix R.. Superparamagnetic iron oxide-enhanced versus gadolinium-enhanced MR imaging for differential diagnosis of focal liver lesions. Radiology 1996; 198:881-887.

99. Vogl TJ, Hammerstingl R, Schwarz W, Kummel S, Muller PK, Balzer T, Lauten MJ, Balzer JO, Mack MG, Schimpfky C, Schrem H, Bechstein WO, Neuhaus P, Felix R.. Magnetic resonance imaging of focal liver lesions: comparison of the superparamagnetic iron oxide Resovist versus gadolinium in the same patient. Invest Radiol. 1996; 31:696-708.

100. Vogl TJ, Kummel S, Hammerstingl R, Schellenbeck M, Schumacher G, Balzer T, Schwarz W, Muller PK, Bechstein WO, Mack MG, Sollner O, Felix R.. Liver tumors: comparison of MR imaging with Gd-EOB-DTPA and Gd-DTPA. Radiology 1996; 200:59-67.

101. Wang C, Ahlstrom H, Ekholm S, Fagertun H, Hellstrom M, Hemmingsson A, Holtas S, Isberg B, Jonnson E, Lonnemark-Magnusson M, McGill S, Wallengren NO, Westman L.. Diagnostic efficiency of Mn-DPDP in MR imaging of the liver: a phase III multicenter study. Acta Radiol 1997; 38:643-649.

102. Wang C, Ahlstrom H, Eriksson B, Lonnemark M, McGill S, Hemmingsson A. Uptake of mangafodipir trisodium in liver metastases from neuroendocrine tumors. J Magn Reson Imaging 1998; 8:682-686.

103. Ward J, Niak KS, Gurthrie JA, Wilson D, Robinson PJ. Hepatic lesion detection: comparison of MR imaging after the administration of superparamagnetic iron oxide with dual-phase CT by using alternative–free response receiver operating characteristic analysis. Radiology 1999; 210:459-466.

104. Weinmann HJ, Bauer H, Gries H, Radüchel B, Platzek J, Press WR. New contrast agents for MRI. In: Rinck PA, ed. Contrast and contrast agents in magnetic resonance imaging. Mons, Belgium: European Workshop on Magnetic Resonance in Medecine, State University, 1989:135-48.

105. Whitney WS, Herfkens RJ, Jeffrey RB, McDonnell CH, Li KC, Van Dalsem WJ, Low RN, Francis IR, Dabatin JF, Glazer GM.. Dynamic breath-hold multiplanar spoiled gradient-recalled MR imaging with gadolinium enhancement for differentiating hepatic hemangiomas from malignancies at 1.5 T. Radiology 1993; 189:863-870.

106. Yamashita Y, Mitsuzaki K, Yi T, Ogata I, Nishiharu T, Urata J, Takahashi M. Small hepatocellular carcinoma in patients with chronic liver damage: prospective comparison of detection with dynamic MR imaging and helical CT of the whole liver. Radiology 1996; 200:79-84.

107. Yamashita Y, Yamamoto H, Hirai A, Yoshimatsu S, Baba Y, Takahashi M. MR imaging enhancement with superparamagnetic iron oxide in chronic liver disease: Influence of liver dysfunction and parenchymal pathology. Abdom Imaging 1996; 21:318-323.

108. Yoshida H, Itai Y, Ohtomo K, Kokubo T, Minami M, Yashiro N. Small hepatocellular carcinoma and cavernous hemangioma; differentiation with dynamic FLASH MR imaging with Gd-DTPA. Radiology 1989; 171:339-342.

3 Histopathologic and Radiologic Classification of Liver Pathologies

Contents

Section 1

3.1 Benign and Malignant Nodular Hepatocellular Lesions

3.1.1 Regenerative Lesions

3.1.1.1 Monoacinar Regenerative Nodule

Generally, a regenerative nodule is a well circumscribed area of parenchyma showing enlargement as a response to necrosis, altered circulation or other stimuli.

A monoacinar regenerative nodule is a regenerative nodule limited to one portal tract. Usually, multiple nodules are found involving most of the liver. This is referred to as diffuse nodular hyperplasia [185].

Diffuse nodular hyperplasia can be subdivided into nodular regenerative hyperplasia in which no fibrous septa can be found or diffuse nodular hyperplasia containing fibrous septa or which occurs in coexisting cirrhosis.

3.1.1.1.1 *Diffuse Nodular Hyperplasia without Fibrous Septa (Nodular Regenerative Hyperplasia, NRH)*

Nodular hyperplasia is defined by the presence of non-neoplastic nodules that are not limited by fibrous septa. The cells of the surrounding parenchyma are atrophic. Nodular hyperplasia is usually a regenerative response occurring after circulatory stress. Portal vein obstruction may be responsible for widespread hepatocellular atrophy and secondary hepatic arterial dilatation. Increased arterial flow and possible hepatotropic factors cause hepatocellular hyperplasia with the formation of nodules.

Monoacinar regenerative nodules may also occur in other cases of disturbed circulation, such as hepatic vein obstruction and circulation disorders of the sinusoids. However, the resulting nodules are less uniformly distributed and are accompanied by more congestion and fibrous septa.

The term nodular regenerative hyperplasia was originally applied to livers with minimal or no parenchymal fibrosis. Nodular regenerative hyperplasia can be found in up to 5% of the older population. A higher prevalence occurs in patients with concomitant systemic diseases associated with vasculopathy, such as polycythemia, rheumatoid arthritis and polyarteritis nodosa.

Clinical symptoms which aid the diagnosis in affected patients include oesophageal varices, splenomegaly, moderate increased alkaline phosphatase and ascites [176, 118] (Fig. 1, 2).

3.1.1.1.2 *Diffuse Nodular Hyperplasia with Fibrous Septa or in Cirrhosis*

As described above, this lesion corresponds to nodular regenerative hyperplasia with concomitant fibrous septa or which is superimposed on a previous hepatic cirrhosis [177, 184].

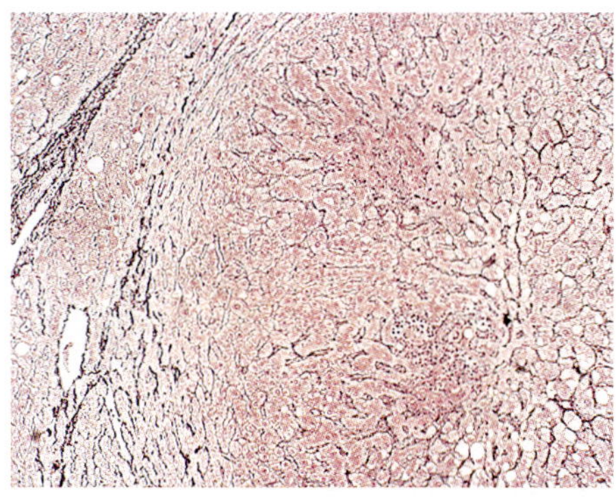

Fig. 1. Nodular regenerative hyperplasia demonstrating a non-neoplastic nodule with hyperplastic liver cells surrounded by atrophic parenchyma

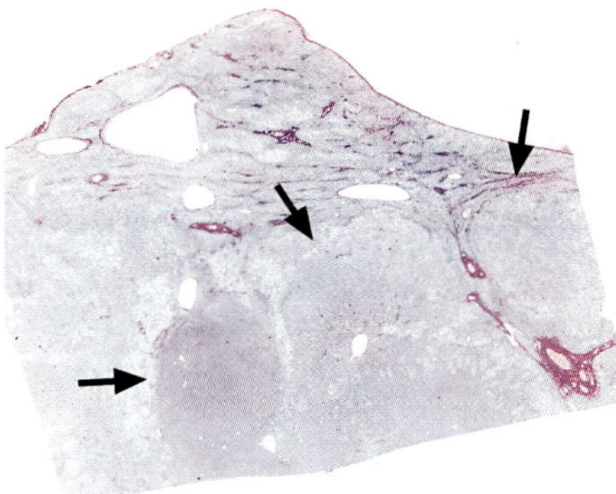

Fig. 2. Histology of diffuse nodular regenerative hyperplasia with demonstration of multiple nodules (*arrows*) surrounded by atrophy in adjacent liver tissue caused by Budd-Chiari syndrome

3.1.1.2 Multiacinar Regenerative Nodule

A regenerative nodule involving more than one solitary portal tract is called a multiacinar regenerative nodule. Normally, it presents in livers with preexisting pathology such as cirrhosis, or in cases of severe disease of the portal veins, hepatic veins, or sinusoids. Usually, multiple nodules occur within the liver and these can correspond to cirrhotic nodules if they are surrounded by fibrous septa. Being larger than most cirrhotic nodules of the same liver or measuring at least 5 mm in diameter, multiacinar regenerative nodules are also called large regenerative nodules or macroregenerative nodules [172] (Fig. 3).

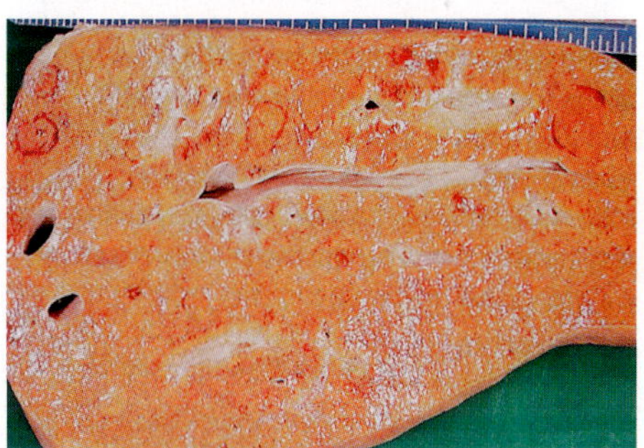

Fig. 3. Nodular regenerative hyperplasia with a diffuse micronodular pattern

3.1.1.3 Lobar or Segmental Hyperplasia

Lobar or segmental hyperplasia is defined as the enlargement of an entire lobe or the major part of a lobe in one or several liver segments, while other parts of the liver show atrophy, necrosis or fibrosis. This pathologic pattern has also been described as atrophy-hypertrophy complex [71].

Lobar or segmental hyperplasia may occur in Budd-Chiari syndrome or in primary sclerosing cholangitis involving the hepatic veins or bile ducts. It introduces both a hyperplasia and an atrophy or fibrosis in the liver parenchyma. As hyperplasia typically arises in regions with increased blood flow in cases of Budd-Chiari syndrome, the caudate lobe often presents as hyperplastic because the drainage of this part of the liver is usually independent of the main hepatic veins. Normally lobar or segmental hyperplasia measures at least several centimeters in diameter but consists of histologically normal liver cells [164].

3.1.1.4 Cirrhotic Nodule (Monoacinar Cirrhotic Nodule / Multiacinar Cirrhotic Nodule)

Generally, a cirrhotic nodule is defined as a regenerative nodule in which hepatocytes are partially or completely surrounded by fibrous septa. It can be subdivided according to its expansion. Thus, a monoacinar cirrhotic nodule contains no more than one terminal portal tract whereas a multiacinar cirrhotic nodule is composed of two or more portal tracts. However, this definition is not in accordance with the classification *micronodule* and *macronodule* in cirrhosis. This is usually defined by size with a division point at 3 mm in diameter [14].

3.1.1.5 Focal Nodular Hyperplasia (FNH)

Focal nodular hyperplasia (FNH) is defined as a nodule that consists of benign-appearing hepatocytes which are accompanied by fibrous stroma and which may contain ductules that form a characteristic central stellate scar. It usually occurs in an otherwise histologically normal or nearly normal liver.

Similar to adenoma (3.1.2.1), FNH is predominantly found in female patients. However, although oral contraception does not seem to be causal, continuous enlargement of lesions has been reported concomitant with the taking of birth-control pills and during pregnancy [182].

Multiple FNH occur in 10–20% of all cases while an association with hemangioma occurs in 5–10% of cases [78, 107].

Macroscopically, FNH shows septations and, in classical cases, a central scar. In contrast to fibrolamellar carcinoma (3.1.2.5) it is not a true scar but rather congeries of blood vessels and bile ducts and sometimes a focal area of cirrhosis. However, in up to 30% of all cases a central scar is not present. An elevated fat- and glycogen-content can often be demonstrated. FNH is thought to derive from an initial regional vascular arterio-venous (AV) malformation which undergoes consecutive localized overgrowth of all liver constitutents. Thus, histologically, FNH consists of normal liver cells abnormally arranged (Fig. 4). In contrast to adenoma, small bile

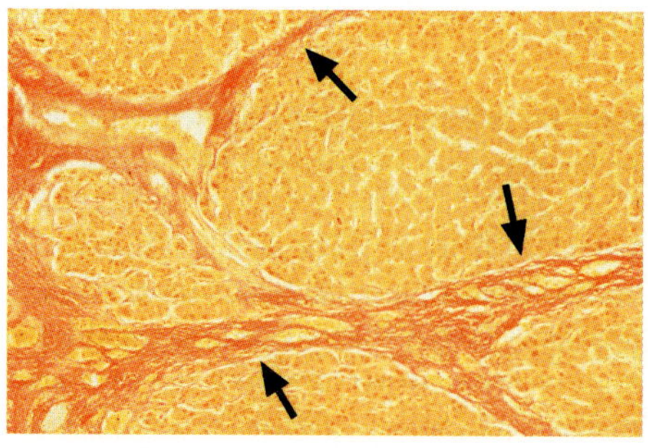

Fig. 4. Focal nodular hyperplasia consists of liver nodules which are separated by fibrous septa (*arrows*). Bile ducts, sometimes numerous, are always present at the interface between liver nodules and septa

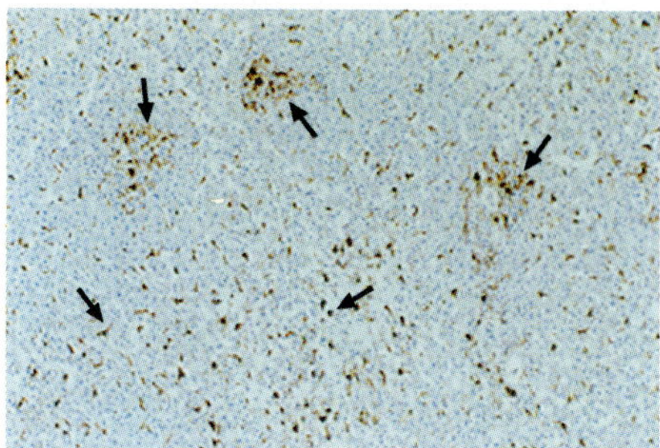

Fig. 5. Histology of focal nodular hyperplasia demonstrating Kupffer cells (*arrows*)

ductules are found which do not communicate with larger bile ducts. Kupffer cells are also present although these are frequently deficient in function (Fig. 5).

A so-called FNH syndrome is present if the coexistence of more than two FNH, intracerebral vascular malformations and meningioma or astrocytoma is observed. If any of the associated lesions are found in the presence of a solitary FNH the syndrome is probably present with incomplete expression. Since the risk of rupture is quite low and patients usually do not present relevant symptoms (90% of all FNH are discovered by chance), surgical intervention is not mandatory [88].

Control of lesion size by means of ultrasound or MRI should be undertaken in order to rule out the possibility of fibrolamellar carcinoma, especially in cases of intralesional calcification.

In general, FNH lesions may be solid or teleangietatic in type, with both types often present in the same liver [178].

3.1.1.5.1 *Focal Nodular Hyperplasia, Solid Type*

This represents the most common type of FNH. Solitary lesions are observed in two thirds of individuals, while two or more lesions may be present in the remaining one third of individuals.

On cut sections most solid FNH have a central fibrous stalk region (Fig. 6, 7). However, this is often absent in lesions smaller than one centimeter in diameter. The stalk region contains an artery that typically is larger than expected for the localization. Degenerative changes such as post-thrombotic arterial fibrosis and cholestasis may be observed in larger lesions.

3.1.1.5.2 *Focal Nodular Hyperplasia, Teleangiectatic Type*

This type of FNH shows multiple dilated blood spaces near the center of the lesion, thus large lesions may resemble hemangioma or peliosis. Compared with solid FNH, the arteries in the central region are small and numerous. The teleangiectatic type of FNH is usually observed in cases of multiple FNH syndrome.

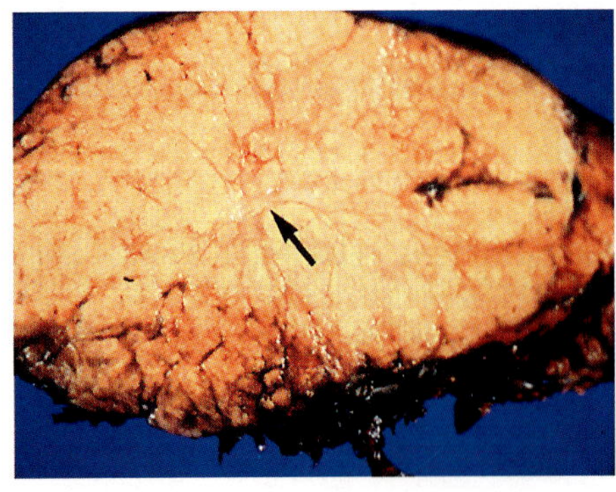

Fig. 6. Focal nodular hyperplasia with characteristic central fibrous region (*arrow*) and radiating fibrous cords

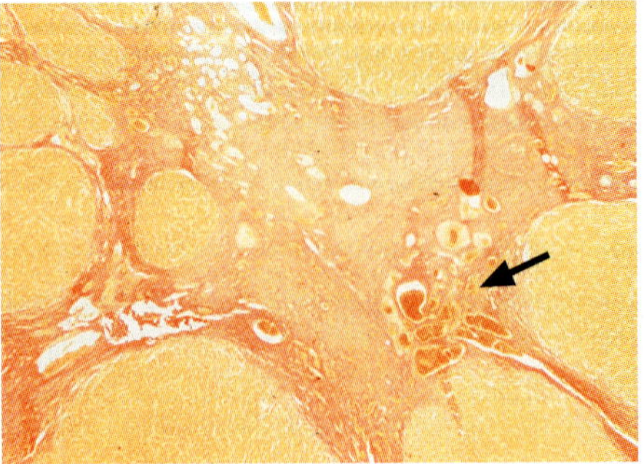

Fig. 7. Histology of a central stellate scar in FNH demonstrating thick-walled vessels (*arrow*) of a large arterial malformation surrounded by fibrous tissue

3.1.2 Dysplastic or Neoplastic Lesions

3.1.2.1 Hepatocellular Adenoma

Liver cell adenoma has an incidence of 1/1,000,000 and is mainly found in women of child-bearing age [65].

In contrast to the situation with FNH, oral contraceptives seem to lead to an increased incidence of hepatocellular adenoma [16]. Moreover, both lesion size and complication rate seem to correlate positively with the duration of oral contraception [26]. Some authors have noted tumor regression after discontinuation of oral contraception [43].

Androgen therapy, familial insulin-dependent diabetes, fanconi anemia and some glycogen storage diseases tend to predispose subjects to adenoma [61].

A so-called adenomatosis is present in subjects observed to have more than 10 hepatic adenoma. This entity is independent of gender or hormone therapy and seems to be associated with an elevated complication rate.

Biopsy of adenoma reveals enlarged and glycogen-rich hepatocytes, sometimes surrounded by a capsule (Fig. 8). Portal tracts and bile ducts are characteristically absent and, in contrast to FNH, there is a substantially increased risk of spontaneous bleeding [121] (Fig. 9).

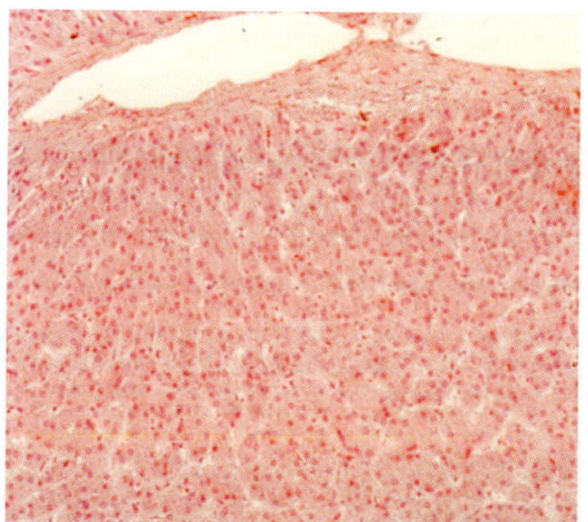

Fig. 8. Histology of hepatic adenoma arranged in plates that are two to three cells thick, separated by sinusoids

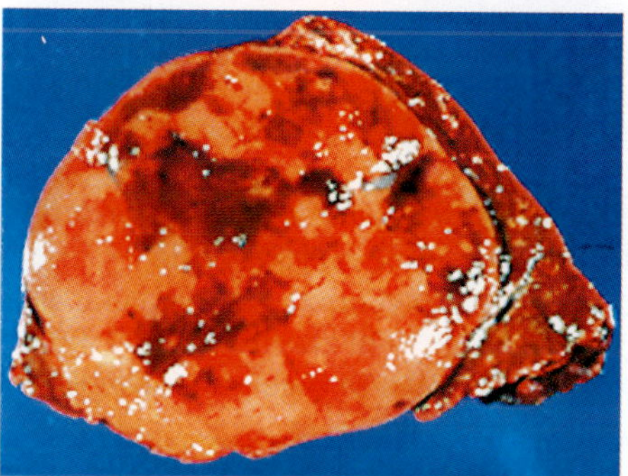

Fig. 9. Macroscopic aspect of liver adenoma with large intralesional hemorrhage

The missing bile ducts enable the differential diagnosis of adenoma from FNH on hepatobiliary sequence scintigraphy. Around 80% of patients with liver cell adenoma complain of abdominal symptoms, which are typically caused by compression, intratumoural bleeding or even rupture and hemoperitoneum [154].

Patients with liver cell adenoma should undergo resection to avoid these complications, and female patients should discontinue oral contraception. Some authors report on individual cases of malignancy developing in liver cell adenoma, however, as yet, there is no valid proof of malignant transformation [60].

On rare occasions it may be impossible to distinguish adenoma from well-differentiated hepatocellular carcinoma (HCC) on biopsy.

3.1.2.2 Dysplastic Focus

Dysplastic focus is defined as congeries of hepatocytes, measuring less than 1 mm in diameter, which show dysplasia but no histological signs of malignancy. Dysplastic foci generally occur in cirrhosis of any origin and are extremely rare in non-cirrhotic livers. In addition, patients suffering from α1-antitrypsin deficiency, tyrosinemia or chronic viral hepatitis B or C demonstrate a comparatively high prevalence of dysplastic foci. Usually, serum α-fetoprotein is normal or minimally increased. However, in patients with tyrosinemia high level serum α-fetoprotein can be found even before nodules are macroscopically visible [12, 181].

3.1.2.3 Dysplastic Nodule

Dysplastic nodule is defined as a nodular region of hepatocytes, measuring at least 1 mm in diameter which show signs of dysplasia but no definite histological signs of malignancy. These nodules are usually found in cirrhotic livers. Dysplastic nodules may be differentiated into two subgroups on the basis of the degree of cellular dysplasia [59, 165].

3.1.2.3.1 *Dysplastic Nodule, Low-grade*

A low-grade dysplastic nodule is a lesion in which the degree of atypia is mild.

3.1.2.3.2 *Dysplastic Nodule, High-grade*

High-grade dysplastic nodules are lesions with at least a moderate degree of atypia which is insufficient for the diagnosis of malignancy. However, this type of lesion can be considered a precursor of HCC and thus resection has to be considered. These lesions may be of any size within the grossly visible range (Fig. 10), however, as the size of the lesion increases, so too does the likelihood that high grade or malignant lesions are present: benign lesions are usually not greater than 20 mm in diameter. Necrosis and hemorrhage are not usually seen in high-grade dysplastic nodules.

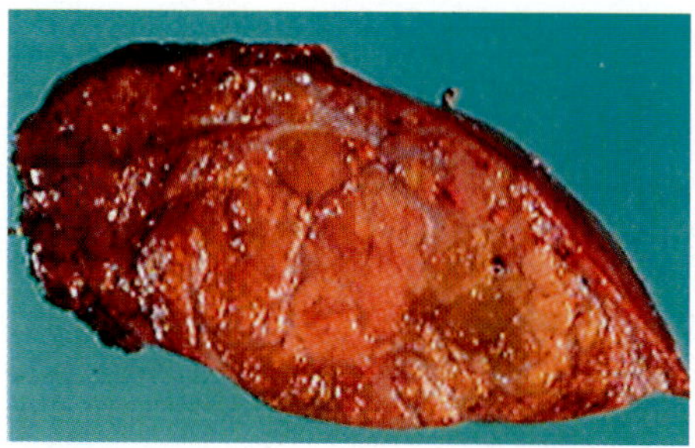

Fig. 10. Cross section of a large high-grade dysplastic nodule in a cirrhotic liver which can only be differentiated microscopically from a HCC

3.1.2.4 Hepatocellular Carcinoma (HCC)

Whereas in Europe and North America the incidence of HCC is generally below 3/100,000 inhabitants, in parts of Asia and Africa it is about thirty times higher. The endemic occurrence of chronic hepatitis B and exposure to Aflatoxin B1 seem to be primary reasons for this [8]. In Europe and Japan the leading cause of HCC is chronic hepatitis C with consecutive cirrhosis [53].

Patients with chronic hepatitis, as in hemochromatosis, have the highest risk of developing HCC. On the other hand, alcohol-induced cirrhosis, autoimmune hepatitis and α_1-antitrypsin-deficiency do not seem to increase the risk significantly. Similarly, primary biliary cirrhosis and Wilson's disease do not predispose subjects to an increased incidence of HCC [135].

Generally, the prognosis for patients with HCC is poor, and is largely dependent upon the extent of surgical intervention, the size of tumor growth, the functionality of the remaining liver parenchyma and the possibility of infiltration of the portal vein [199] (Fig. 11).

Whereas the ultimate procedure for the potential cure of patients with HCC remains liver transplantation [153], possibilities for palliative treatment include the intraarterial injection of [131]Iod-Lipiodol or alcohol [55].

The macropathological division of HCC, which dates from the beginning of the 20th century, correlates relatively well with imaging findings. Three main types can be distinguished:
- the multinodular type with multiple sharply demarcated tumor nodules
- the massive type with one single tumor node and smaller satellite nodules
- the diffuse type with interspersed tumor areas throughout the liver

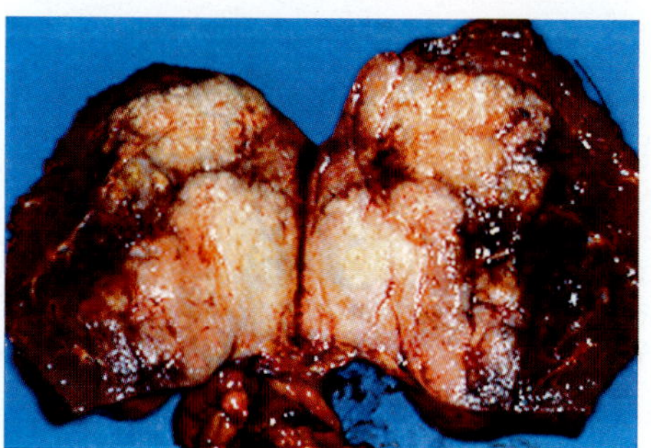

Fig. 11. Cut surface of a hepatocellular carcinoma without capsule infiltrating the liver parenchyma

Additionally, an encapsulated tumor type can be distinguished, which seems to be an early phase of the other histological types. Unfortunately, there doesn't seem to be a correlation between these morphological criteria and epidemiological findings or prognosis. The new World Health Organisation (WHO) classification presents a much more differentiated system of criteria for characterizing HCC [81].

Apart from the above-mentioned pathologies, it is evident that almost any chronic liver disease leading to cirrhosis may be complicated by HCC. Neoplastic development in the liver can be seen as a multistep process that is triggered by a variety of events. Normal liver is mitotically inactive, but, when cells are stimulated to divide, which takes place in a variety of conditions, including liver cirrhosis, it becomes sensitive to carcinogenesis. However, HCC also occurs in the absence of cirrhosis in a small but significant (about 7%) proportion of cases [100].

A proposal as to how the multistep development of HCC can be interpreted is presented in Table 1. However, it is important to realize that reliable differentiation between pre-cancerous developments, such as high-grade dysplastic nodules, and well-differentiated HCC is not always possible [58, 142].

Microscopically, HCC has several patterns. HCCs are composed of malignant hepatocytes that differentiate into normal liver structures and mimic normal hepatocyte growth, but without forming normal hepatic acini (Fig. 12). Cells in well-differentiated HCCs are difficult to distinguish from normal hepatocytes or hepatocellular adenoma cells. Malignant hepatocytes may even produce bile (Fig. 13). In other cases, there are microscopic variations, with HCCs containing fat (Fig. 14), tumoural secretions (large amounts of watery material), fibrosis, necrosis and

Table 1. HCC development and liver cirrhosis

Macro-regenerative nodule

⇓

Low grade dysplastic nodule

⇓

High grade dysplastic nodule

⇓

Well-differentiated HCC

⇓

Dedifferentiated HCC

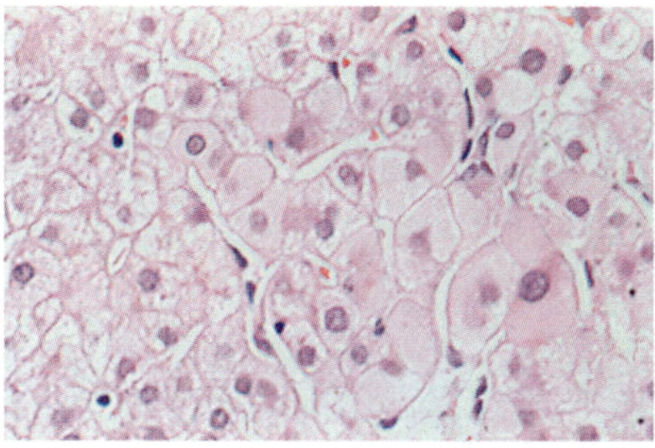

Fig. 12. Grade 1 HCC consisting of small liver-like tumor cells arranged in thin trabecular layers, which may be difficult to distinguish from liver-cell adenomas and atypical hyperplastic nodules

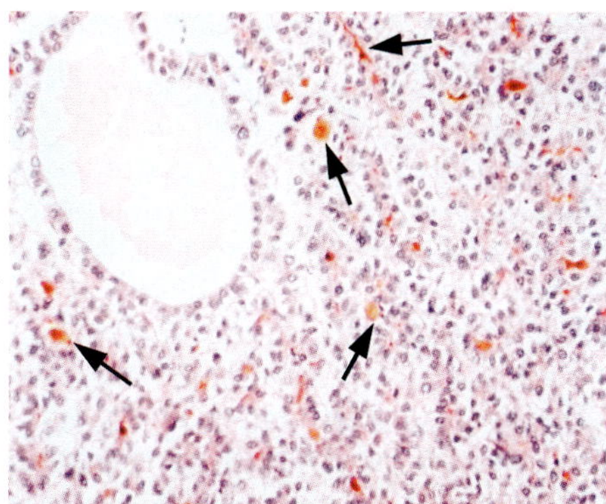

Fig. 13. Histological aspect of a well-differentiated HCC showing bile production (*arrows*)

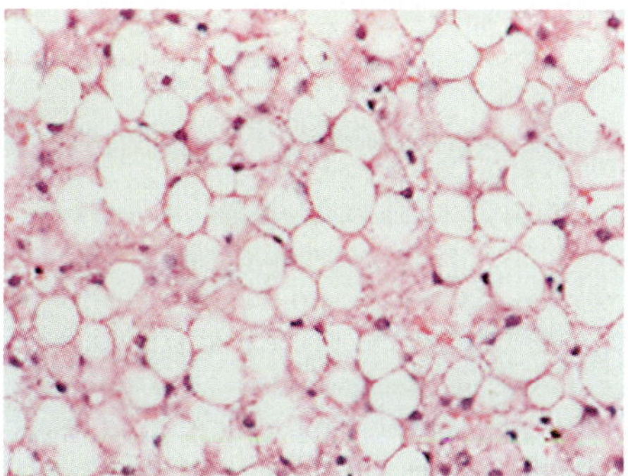

Fig. 14. HCC with fatty metamorphosis

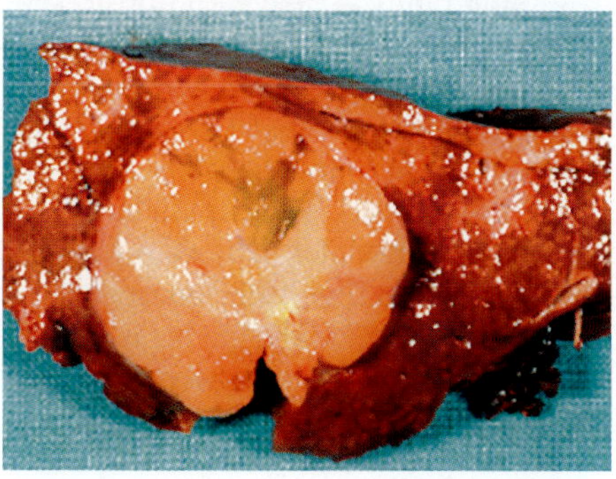

Fig. 15. Cut section of an HCC with a mosaic pattern containing fat, solid nodules, necroses, fibrosis and cystic areas

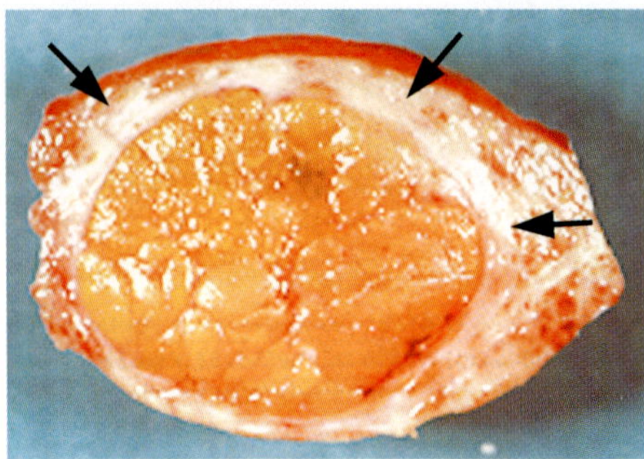

Fig. 16. Cut section of an HCC with a nodular pattern and fibrous capsule (*arrows*)

amorphous calcifications (Fig. 15). This variable microscopic presentation gives rise to different appearances according to the imaging techniques employed.

Macroscopically, there are also several patterns of growth. HCC is referred to as single or massive when there is either a solitary small or a large mass, with or without a capsule (Fig. 16). Multifocal HCC, the second most common pattern, is characterized by multiple separate nodules. The least common pattern of diffuse or cirrhotomimetic growth is composed of multiple small tumoral foci distributed throughout the liver, mimicking nodules of cirrhosis. HCC is said to be encapsulated when it is completely surrounded by a fibrous capsule. Patients with encapsulated HCC have a better prognosis due to increased possibilities for resection. However, vascular invasion of intrahepatic (portal hepatic vein branches) and perihepatic vessels (inferior vena cava and portal vein) is common.

3.1.2.5 Fibrolamellar Carcinoma (FLC)

This type of hepatocellular carcinoma occurs both in male and female patients typically under the age of 25 years. In contrast to HCC, underlying cirrhosis is not usually present in FLC. Pain in the right upper quadrant, nausea and weight loss are the leading symptoms, while jaundice is quite rare. Often the tumors are relatively large (> 15 cm) at the time of detection. If resected early, the 5-year survival rates are about 50%. Metastases from FLC are mostly located in the lymph nodes and lungs, and, in roughly half of the cases, metastatic lymph nodes are present at the time of diagnosis. Macroscopically, the tumors have a lobular appearance with fibrous septa and a central scar, which, in contrast to the scar in FNH, is a true scar.

FLC lesions have a distinctive microscopic pattern and are composed of eosinophilic, malignant hepatocytes containing prominent nuclei. FLCs express hepatic as well as biliary keratin. The fibrous component accounts for 50% of the tumoral mass and is distributed in multilamellar strands (Fig. 17), except in larger tumors containing large central scars (Fig. 18). Satellite nodules are often present. The appearance of FLC can be similar to that of FNH in that both tumors have a central scar and multiple fibrous septa (Fig. 19). In FLC, hemorrhage is rare, while necrosis and coarse calcifications are often present, especially in the central scar (approx. 30%). The origin of FLC is still to be clearly defined, although mixed FLC / HCC types seem to exist [38].

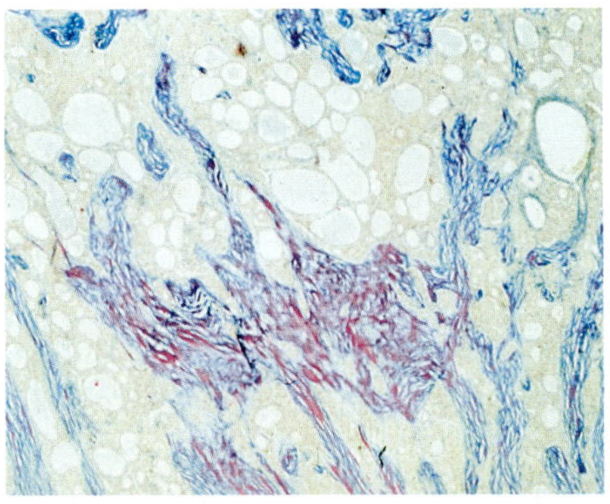

Fig. 17. Histology of a fibrolamellar carcinoma demonstrating tumor cells separated by characteristic parallel lamellae of coarse, ropy collagen

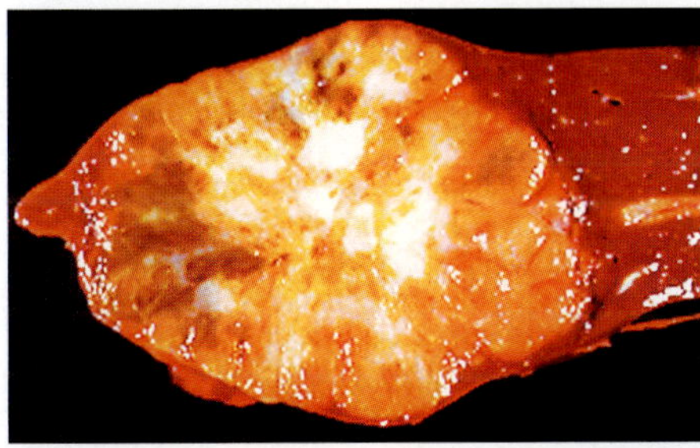

Fig. 18. Cut section of a fibrolamellar carcinoma with a lobular arrangement with interconnecting fibrous septa and a central stellate scar

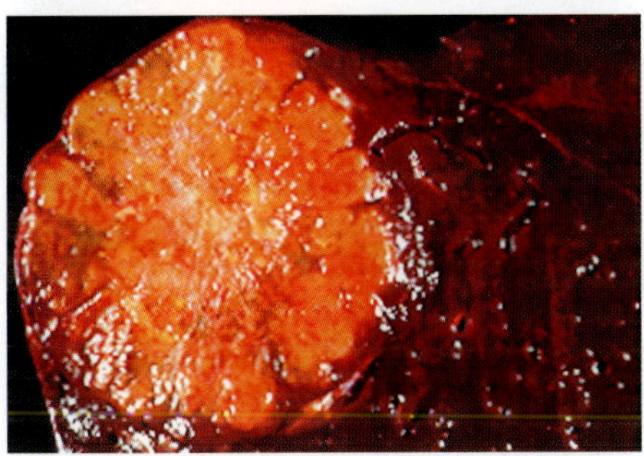

Fig. 19. Cut section of a fibrolamellar carcinoma with a nodular appearance but with minimal demonstration of a central stellate scar

3.2   Benign and Malignant Tumors of the Biliary Tract

3.2.1   Bile-duct Adenoma

This tumor is found mainly by chance and its maximal size often does not exceed 2 cm. Microscopically small bile ducts lined by mucine-producing cells are embedded in a fibrous stroma. A malignant transformation has not yet been reported [3].

3.2.2 Bile-duct Cystadenoma

Hepatic cystadenoma is a very rare tumor, although analogous forms are quite common in the pancreas or ovaries. Most of the patients are women in the fifth decade, and the major symptoms include pain and jaundice. Infection, rupture and malignant transformation of these slowly growing tumors may occur. Surgical resection is the therapy of choice [98] (Fig. 20).

Microscopically, cystic spaces, filled with viscous yellowish or reddish fluid can be seen. The most common mucinous type needs to be distinguished from the serous and papillary cystic types. The tumoral stroma may only comprise a thin hyaline rim, but alternatively it may appear as a compact layer [79].

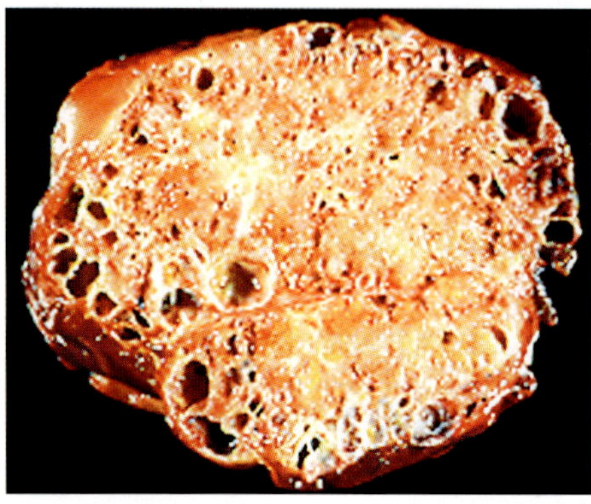

Fig. 20. Macroscopic aspect of a biliary cystadenoma which in contrast to congenital simple cysts, demonstrates a multilocular appearence. Cysts may show hemorrhage and fluid-fluid levels

3.2.3 Biliary Papillomatosis

About 50 cases of multiple small papillomas of the intra- and extrahepatic bile ducts have been described. Jaundice may be the only presenting symptom, although sepsis and hemobilia with a subsequent fatal outcome may result. A temporary biliary stoma may bring about some relief, although the only curative method to date involves liver transplantation. The presence of biliary papillomas seems to coincide with ulcerative colitis, Caroli's syndrome and polyposis coli [124].

3.2.4 Bile-duct Carcinoma (Cholangiocarcinoma, CCC)

Bile duct carcinomas are divided according to their location into intrahepatic cholangiocarcinoma [9], hilar adenocarcinoma (Klatskin-tumor) [91] and carcinoma of the extrahepatic bile ducts [5].

On cut sections, CCC is characterized by the presence of large amounts of whitish fibrous tissue (Fig. 21). Inside the tumor, especially in large examples, a variable amount of central necrosis may be present, while hemorrhage is rare. Histologically, the tumor is an adenocarcinoma with a glandular appearance and cells that resemble biliary epithelium with fibrous stroma (Fig. 22). Mucin production and calcification can sometimes be demonstrated. At autopsy there is often a layer of atypical cells surrounding the main tumor, which probably propa-

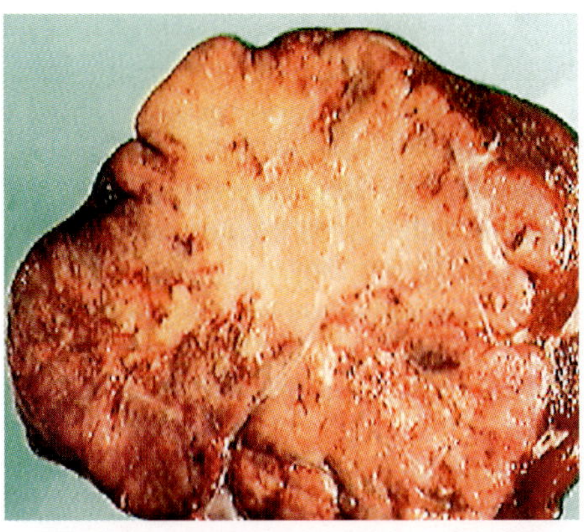

Fig. 21. Cut section of a intrahepatic cholangiocellular carcinoma diffusely infiltrating the liver with finger-like extensions and central sclerosis

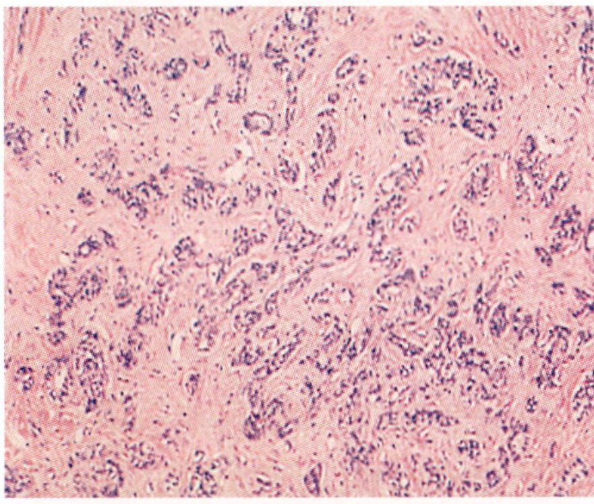

Fig. 22. Histology of the periphery of a CCC which demonstrates tumor cells in a tubular pattern in an abundant fibrous stroma entrapping normal liver cells

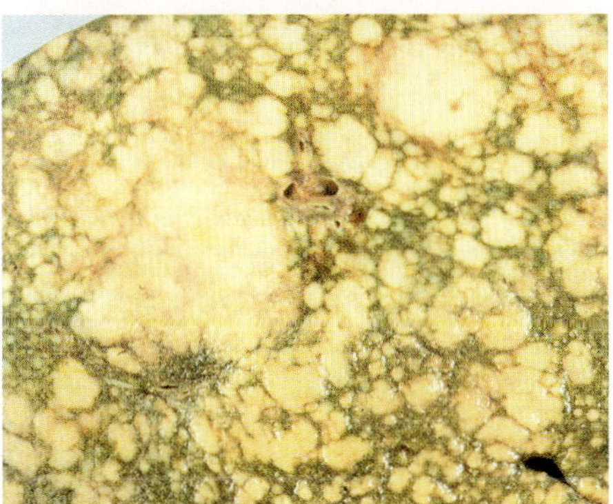

Fig. 23. Macroscopic distribution of diffuse hepatic metastases of a CCC

gates relapsing tumor growth after an initial curative resection. Overall the prognosis is poor.

A large desmoplastic reaction is typical of CCC. Diagnostic studies often reveal lymph node metastases and hematogeneous spread to the lungs, bones, adrenals, spleen and pancreas. Intrahepatic carcinomas often arise in the Fifth or sixth decade, usually in patients that are older than those with HCC. Non-specific signs such as pain and weight loss are typical, while jaundice is generally atypical. The tumor is usually hypovascular but it may show late enhancement in cases of desmo-plastic changes. Early signs of metastases include finger-like extensions along lymphatic channels and these represent another reason for the poor prognosis of intrahepatic CCC (Fig. 23). Infections with *Clonorchis sinensis* and *Opisthorchis viverrini*, hepatolithiasis and congenital anomalies of the bile ducts predispose subjects to bile duct carcinoma. Other risk factors include Caroli's syndrome, sclerosing cholangitis and congenital hepatic fibrosis [18, 93, 94, 136].

The most common extrahepatic locations of CCC are along the common hepatic duct and the cystic duct. In these cases, painless jaundice is the leading symptom. Associations with choledochal cysts, congenital malformations of the bile ducts and ulcerative colitis have been reported. CCC with a high cuboid epithelium located in the liver hilum is typically referred to as Klatskin tumor.

3.2.5 Bile-duct Cystadenocarcinoma

In contrast to bile duct carcinoma, the prognosis for patients with this tumor is somewhat better. Bile duct cystadenocarcinoma is quite rare and metastases are only seldom found. It is usually diagnosed by histologic analysis of a resected cystic mass lesion.

The majority of bile duct cystadenocarcinomas occur in middle-aged women and cause no symptoms until they are quite large in size. Since local or metastatic spread is quite rare, patients are usually referred for surgery [79, 108].

3.2.6 Gallbladder Carcinoma

This tumor is mainly found in female patients predominantly in the sixth decade of life. The main symptoms include right upper quadrant pain, nausea and jaundice. Patients frequently have gallstones or, on occasion, a so-called "porcelain" gallbladder caused by recurrent inflammation [84].

Whereas adenocarcinoma growth usually involves just the bladder, squamous cell carcinoma and undifferentiated carcinoma often infiltrate neighboring structures. Local complications involving fistula, perforation or empyema may arise. Distant metastases typically occur in advanced cases [87, 70].

Other quite rare tumor types in the gallbladder are sarcoma, primary malignant melanoma, carcinoid and lymphoma [111, 193, 198].

3.3 Benign non-Epithelial Tumors

3.3.1 Hemangioma

The most common liver lesions are hemangiomas which are found with a prevalence of 0.4–7.3% and only rarely cause any clinically relevant symptoms [78]. Thus, they are most often detected by chance. Small capillary hemangiomas need to be distinguished from larger cavernous hemangiomas, which are frequently categorized as benign congenital hamartomas. Macroscopically, cystic blood-filled

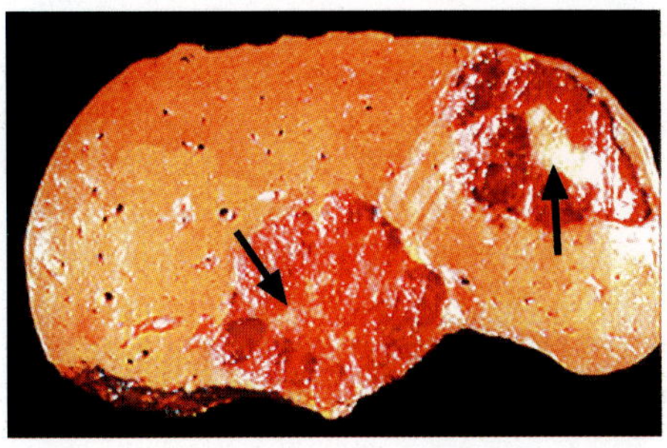

Fig. 24. Cut section of two large hepatic hemangiomas showing central fibrosis and hyalin changes (*arrows*)

spaces can be visualized. When detected intraoperatively, these lesions can be diagnosed as hemangiomas by simple palpation. The lining of these spaces consists of endothelial cells and thin fibrous walls. With increasing tumor size, central thrombosis with consecutive fibrosis, myxoid changes or calcification may occur.

Therapeutic intervention should only be considered in cases of symptomatic or giant hemangioma (larger than 10 cm) [192].

Complications such as rupture, thrombocytopenia or disseminated introvascular coagulation (DIC), caused by stasis of blood flow in the dilated vessels, may occur on rare occasions. Multiple hemangiomas are considered part of the syndrome of systemic hemangiomatosis. Diagnostic fine needle biopsy should be avoided because of possible bleeding and because in many cases only blood is aspirated leading to poor diagnostic results. The diagnosis can usually be established by means of blood pool scintigraphy [166] or MRI.

On cut sections, larger hemangiomas almost always present a heterogeneous composition with areas of fibrosis, necrosis and cystic changes and intratumoral coarse calcifications (Fig. 24). In some cases abundant fibrous tissue completely replaces the lesion.

3.3.2 Infantile Hemangioendothelioma (IHE)

Most of these infantile mesenchymal tumors are found during the first six months of life, and there seems to be a slight female predominance [157].

Common symptoms include hepatomegaly or a palpable mass, sometimes together with diminished growth or high output cardiac failure caused by shunting. Rupture, thrombocytopenia and hypofibrinogenemia may occur on rare occasions. Surgical intervention may be avoided if no life-threatening complications appear as the tumor tends to regress gradually. Therapeutic strategies may consist of steroids, chemo- or radiotherapy, embolization or resection. Macroscopically, IHEs are usually multiple and diffuse. A solitary lesion is an uncommon variant. The nodules vary from a few millimeters to 15 cm or more in size, and are round, reddish-brown and spongy, or white-yellow with fibrotic predominance in mature cases.
Microscopically, two types can be distinguished:
Type 1 has intercommunicating vascular channels with a single-layered endothelial lining. Thrombosis and infarction in cavernous spaces is quite frequent as well as extramedullary hematopoesis.

Type 2 demonstrates nuclear atypia and a multi-layered endothelial lining. There seems to be some resemblance to angiosarcoma, but the finding of a metastasizing IHE has not yet been reported [46].

3.3.3 Lymphangioma

Hepatic lymphangioma are congeries of dilated lymphatic channels containing proteinaceous fluid or blood. Lymphangiomas in the liver occur most frequently as multiple masses, although solitary lesions are found on occasions. In some cases concomitant hemangiomas can be found. When diagnosing hepatic lymphangioma, whole body cross-sectional imaging is indicated because multiple organs and tissues, (i.e. spleen, kidneys, lungs, gastrointestinal tract and skeleton), are usually involved, particularly in children. Thus, the condition is often referred to as lymphangiomatosis [72, 170].

3.3.4 Angiomyolipoma

Angiomyolipomas are rare soft tissue tumors found most frequently in the kidneys but occasionally also in the liver. There is an increased incidence of these tumors in association with tuberous sclerosis [24, 67, 122].

Angiomyolipomas consist of blood vessels, fat and smooth muscle [66] (Fig. 25).

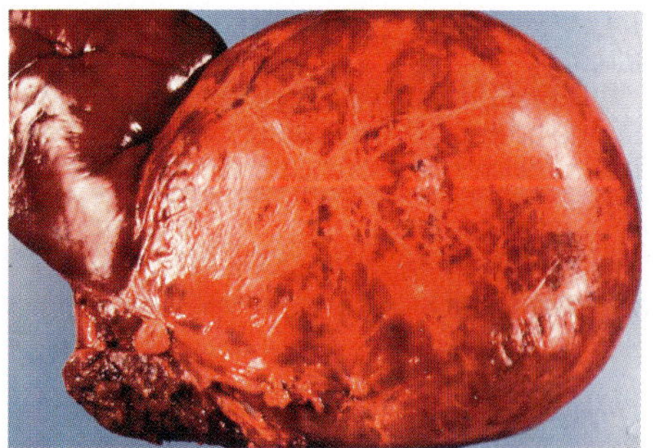

Fig. 25. Macroscopic aspect of an angiomyolipoma of the liver

3.4 Malignant non-Epithelial Tumors

3.4.1 Angiosarcoma

These tumors are the most frequent sarcomas of the liver and arise typically in the sixth and seventh decades, predominantly in male subjects. Thorotrast, monomers of vinyl chloride and chronic arsenic intoxication are known to be associated with angiosarcoma. Liver cell hyperplasia with dilatation of the sinusoids and increased fibrosis leading to portal hypertension are typical early stages of tumor growth. Macroscopically, angiosarcomas are ill-defined sponge-like hemorrhagic tumors

(Fig. 26). They are composed of malignant endothelial cells lining vascular channels of variable size, from cavernous to capillary, which attempt to form sinusoids. Metastases to lymph nodes, spleen, lung, bone and adrenals are rarely found.

Thorotrast particles can be found within the malignant endothelial cells in cases of Thorotrast-induced angiosarcoma. The majority of angiosarcomas present as multiple nodules, often with areas of internal hemorrhage. When angiosarcoma appears as a single, large mass, it does not have a capsule and frequently contains large cystic areas filled with blood debris [125, 152, 163, 194].

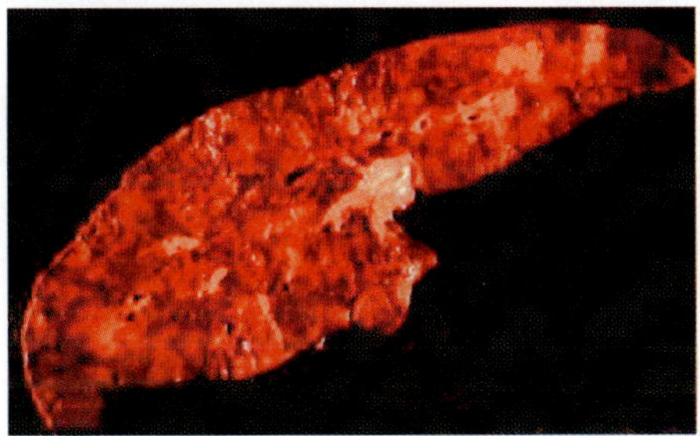

Fig. 26. Cut section of a diffuse infiltrating hepatic angiosarcoma

3.4.2 Malignant Epithelioid Hemangioendothelioma

This tumor most often arises in female patients in the fifth decade. Patients complain of weight loss and right upper quadrant pain, sometimes in combination with jaundice. An association with oral contraceptives may exist. The tumor is located most frequently at subcapsular sites (50–65%) and macroscopically, it is a solid, fibrous mass, sometimes with calcifications and an encasement of vessels. In contrast to angiosarcoma, the prognosis seems to be better; increasingly patients are undergoing hepatectomy and consecutive liver transplantation. Typically, in malignant epithelioid hemangioendothelioma a retraction of the liver surface can be noted (Fig. 27). The only other primary liver lesion in which this sign is observed is CCC. Microscopically, epithelioid hemangioendotheliomas are composed of epithelioid and dentritic cells within a tumor matrix that may become sclerotic, hyalinized and calcified. Intratumoral necrosis and hemorrhage are common findings [54, 80].

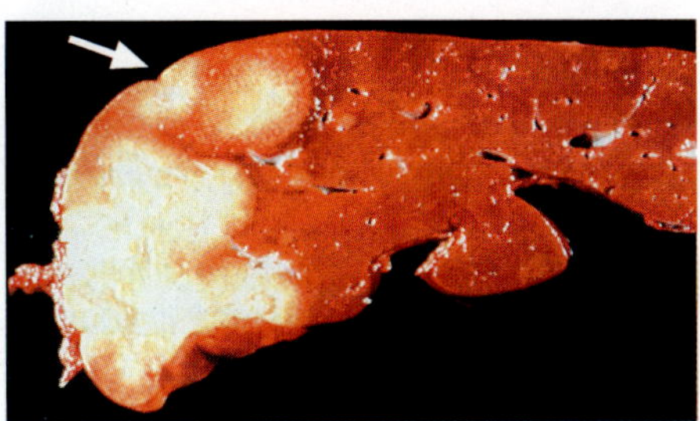

Fig. 27. Cut section of a subcapsular located malignant epithelioid hemangioendothelioma showing a characteristic retraction of the liver surface (*arrow*)

3.4.3 Undifferentiated (Embryonal) Sarcoma

Along with hepatoblastoma and IHE this is one of the most frequent primary malignant hepatic tumors in children, arising typically between the ages of six and ten years. Increased girth and weight loss are common signs while a newly discovered heart murmur induced by a tumor thrombus may be present on rare occasions. Macroscopically, sarcomas have solid and cystic areas, hemorrhage or necroses, and are sometimes surrounded by a pseudocapsule. In 50% of all cases, extramedullary hematopoesis can be demonstrated. Complete tumor resection followed by chemotherapy and radiation can increase the 5-year survival rate to about 15% [160, 173].

3.4.4 Rhabdomyosarcoma (Sarcoma Botryoides)

Hepatic rhabdomyosarcoma is a tumor typically found in children below the age of five. Only on very rare occasions do they arise in adults. Typically, the tumor has a grape-like appearance and grows in the lumina of larger bile ducts. Its presence leads to intermittent icteric episodes, fever and weight loss.

The prognosis and treatment modalities are similar to those of undifferentiated embryonal sarcoma [76].

3.4.5 Other Primary Sarcomas

Almost every type of sarcoma of the liver has been reported. They usually occur in middle and old age, in either sex and are typically large and at an advanced stage when discovered. Although most of the tumors are slow-growing, in most cases prognosis is poor as complete excision is seldom possible due to the size and degree of advancement. Leiomyosarcomas may arise from the ligamentum teres, the portal and hepatic veins, as well as from the liver capsule. Other rare malignant soft-tissue tumors of the liver include fibrosarcoma, malignant fibrous histiocytoma, liposarcoma, osteosarcoma, malignant hemangiopericytoma and sarcomas with divergent cell lines (malignant mesenchymoma).

3.4.6 Primary Lymphoma of the Liver

Hodgkin's lymphoma, non-Hodgkin's lymphoma and leukaemia, as well as histiocytosis and mastocytosis, may affect the liver secondarily. Nevertheless, an increasing number of primary lymphomas of the liver are being described [139, 150]. The recognition of primary hepatic lymphoma is important since these conditions frequently have a favorable outcome. The tumor may occur at any age, from childhood to adolescence, and is around four times more likely to occur in males. Patients present with abdominal pain, hepatomegaly or a mass. Additional B-symptoms (fever, weight loss) are found in 50% of cases. On rare occasions the tumor may be associated with autoimmune disorders, chronic hepatitis, cirrhosis, HBV infection and HIV. Although the tumors most frequently present as solitary (Fig.

28) or multiple masses, diffuse infiltration can also be found on occasions. Upon histology, most non-Hodgkin lymphomas are described as high-grade. Possible misdiagnoses include metastatic carcinoma, chronic hepatitis and inflammatory pseudotumor.

Surgical resection gives the best prognosis although multi-agent chemotherapy and/or radiation therapy are also worthwhile [83].

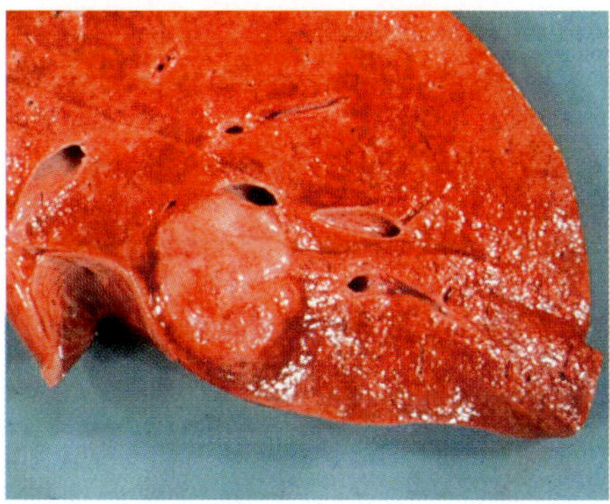

Fig. 28. Macroscopic presentation of a solid solitary primary hepatic manifestation of Hodgkin's disease

3.5   Hepatoblastoma

Hepatoblastoma is typically found in young children. Up to one third of patients have concomitant anomalies such as hemihypertrophy, cleft palate, Beckwith-Wiedemann or Down's syndrome. The tumors are often palpable, While failure to thrive and weight loss, together with extremely elevated α-fetoprotein (AFP)-levels, are typical symptoms. Cystic, necrotic and/or hemorrhagic areas as well as fibrosis and calcifications are common while the tumor may also be partially encapsulated. In 20% of cases the tumors are multifocal.

Most tumors are of the epithelial, mixed or mesenchymal type. In very rare cases of teratoid or even chondroid hepatoblastoma, muscle or neuronal cells may be found. Epithelial hepatoblastoma is composed of fetal and/or embryonal malignant hepatocytes. A mixed hepatoblastoma has both an epithelial (hepatocyte) and a mesenchymal component consisting of primitive mesenchymal tissue. Amorphous calcifications are seen in about 30% of cases. This histological classification has prognostic implications: the epithelial type has a better prognosis than the other forms, especially when there is a predominant hepatocyte presence. Embryonal epithelial cells are more primitive than fetal epithelial and mesenchymal cells and tumors with the former histological type carry a poorer prognosis.

Surgical resection is the primary treatment although operative mortality is high (about 25%). Accurate tumor staging is essential to determine the need for additional chemo- or radiotherapy. The long term survival rate is about 15–35%. Factors that contribute to a worse prognosis are age under one year, large tumor size, involvement of vital structures and the predominance of anaplastic cells [77, 95, 183].

3.6 Tumor-like Lesions

3.6.1 Cysts

Non-parasitic Cysts

The etiology and pathogenesis of solitary liver cysts have not yet been totally clarified. Moreover, it is equivocal as to whether they are developmental or neoplastic in origin. Primary, non-parasitic liver cysts are subdivided into unilocular and multilocular varieties. Whereas unilocular cysts are more likely to be developmental in origin, multilocular cysts may be neoplastic with an increased, but nevertheless very low potential for malignant change (Fig. 29). Primary, non-parasitic liver cysts may occur at any age although the peak incidence is between the fourth and sixth decades of life with a male to female ratio of 4–5:1. Liver cysts smaller than 8–10 cm seldom cause symptoms and are therefore most often diagnosed by chance. In cases of symptomatic cysts, patients present with an upper abdominal mass and fullness, nausea and occasional vomiting. An acute abdominal crisis may be due to torsion, strangulation, hemorrhage into the cyst or rupture [143].

Symptomatic large solitary cysts are twice as likely to be found in the right lobe as opposed to the left. Jaundice is a frequent complication. Whereas excision has often been the treatment of choice, aspiration and injection of sclerosing agents such as alcohol, polidocanol or minocyclin chloride represent an accurate therapeutic option in many cases [52, 63].

Malignant tumors arising from either type of solitary cyst may occur on very rare occasions. Although these tumors are usually adenocarcinomas, squamous cell carcinomas and even carcinoid have been reported [20, 167].

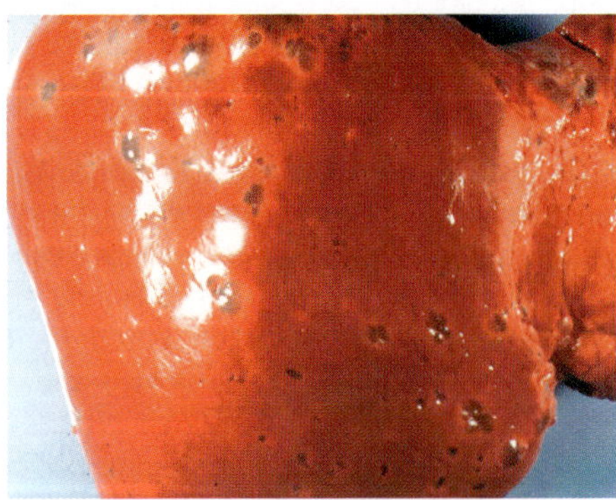

Fig. 29. Liver surface with diffuse distribution of non-parasitic uncomplicated liver cysts

3.6.2 Mesenchymal Hamartoma

Mesenchymal hamartoma most likely represents a localized abnormality of ductal plate development that precedes birth. They occur almost exclusively in young children with an average age of 15 months and the male to female ratio is 2:1. Association with polycystic kidney disease, congenital hepatic fibrosis and biliary hamartoma has been described. Children typically present with progressive abdominal enlargement and imaging techniques show a cystic mass which is usually large. Microscopically, a variable mixture of tissue is seen from which the liver is normally made up. Extramedullary hematopoiesis is commonly present. Surgical excision is curative and malignant transformation has not yet been reported [49, 161].

3.6.3 Biliary Hamartoma

Biliary hamartoma often occur as small lesions, found by chance on fine needle biopsies. They contain irregularly formed dilated bile ducts in a fibrous stroma and may occur together with cystic kidneys. It is still a matter of discussion as to whether cholangiocarcinomas arise from these lesions [50].

3.6.4 Inflammatory Pseudotumor

A rare differential diagnosis among solid liver tumors is the so-called inflammatory pseudotumor (IPT). This lesion may appear in almost every tissue and anatomic location and on diagnostic imaging mimics other common histological and imaging findings. Despite numerous reports, the pathogenesis of IPTs remains unclear. Recent publications have explained the etiology of this lesion as either a post-inflammatory regenerative process or a primary neoplastic process [11, 34, 47].

The suspicion of neoplasm is based on histologic findings in which an IPT is shown to consist of myofibroblasts, fibroblasts, lymphocytes and plasma cells. In such cases the pathologist may be persuaded to diagnose a sarcoma with primary benign clinical behaviour. The suspicion that the lesion is of true neoplastic origin may be reinforced by the presence of histiocytes and spindel cells and when immunohistochemical and ultrastructural examinations reveal signs of benign as well as malignant growth [36].

However, examination of IPTs of the ileo-caecum have shown that it may be infection-associated. The histology of this lesion was shown to be comparable with results on mycobacterial pseudotumors of the lymph nodes, spleen and lung in a patient with HIV-infection [101].

From this observation it was concluded that the immune system plays an important role in the pathogenesis of this kind of mass lesion. Additionally, electron microscopy may demonstrate intracellular bacilliform organisms. Molecular analysis of DNA fragments was able to identify Pseudomonas sub-populations that were not known to be infectious in humans. In this regard, pathogenic organisms such as Eppstein-Barr virus, actinomyces and nocardia, especially in hepatic lesions, are suspected to contribute to the development of IPT [187].

3.6.5 Other Tumor-like Lesions: Peliosis Hepatis

The microscopic type is characterized by an area of absent reticuline fibers, thus resulting in a dilation of the sinusoids, which normally are lined by endothelium [196].

There seems to be an increased incidence of peliosis with thiopurine, anabolic steroids, vitamin A and Thorotrast. The macroscopic type of peliosis shows cystic blood-filled spaces, which occur in malnutrition, leukemias, tuberculosis, some forms of vasculitis, lepra and HIV. Due to the large cystic blood-filled areas imaging studies may misinterpret the lesion as hemangioma [48, 149, 155, 195].

These lesions typically have no clinical relevance, but may cause some irritation for the differential diagnosis of focal liver lesions.

3.7 Infectious Diseases of the Liver

3.7.1 Liver Abscess

A liver abscess generally develops by one of three different routes:
- ascending infection of the bile ducts
- hematogeneous spread in endocarditis, pneumonia and pulmonary AV-malformations
- purulent infections draining to the portal vein, e.g. in diverticulitis

Mostly, the origins of pyogenic abscesses within the liver are not obvious. Contributory factors include diabetes mellitus, perforated duodenal ulcer or diverticulosis. The most common pathogenic germs are *E. coli*, other coliforms, and *Streptococcus milleri*. Anaerobes are being reported with increasing frequency. However, amebiasis and several worm infections (ascariasis, clonorchiasis, fascioliasis) of the biliary tree, which predispose subjects to bacterial cholangitis, should be considered as possible pathogenic agents in the differential diagnosis of pyogenic liver abscesses [68].

Infection spread via the biliary tree may be due to an acute ascending cholangitis complicating a large bile duct obstruction by stones. In addition, suppurative cholecystitis, postoperative biliary stricture, acute or chronic pancreatitis and tumors in the biliary tree and pancreas may cause focal inflammation which spreads to the liver.

Today, bacterial infection via the portal vein is less common among industrialized nations. Hepatic spread arises from inflammatory processes in the appendix, the colon (as in diverticulitis) and the pancreas, leading to septic portal thrombophlebitis and thereafter to liver abscesses. In developing countries umbilical sepsis plays a leading role and is the source of portal pyemia which may also induce splenic vein occlusion leading to splenomegaly.

An arterial spread of infection to the liver is common. Patients usually develop clinical symptoms before a visible abscess can be depicted. Pathogenic germs include *staphylococcus, Neisseria gonorrhoeae* and *Chlamydia trachomatis* which may induce complicated pelvic infections. Chronic granulomatosis disease facilitates arterial septic spread to the liver [119].

On rare occasions acute cholecystitis or liver trauma may be the cause of a liver abscess. In Europe amebic abscesses are not very frequent. Whereas abscesses might not have a fibrous capsule initially, they tend to form coagulative necrosis and subsequently liquifaction (Figs. 30, 31). Thereafter, abscesses may rupture and induce a peritonitis, which usually has a bad prognosis.

Hepatic *Aspergillus* infection typically demonstrates multiple small hemorrhagic necrosis. Hyphae may also obstruct vessels and lead to infarction.

Multiple portal or periportal abscesses with granuloma formation are typical of candida. In *cryptococcus* infection large abscesses are absent, but small foci of necrosis may be observed which sometimes follow the bile ducts in a manner similar to sclerosing cholangitis [10].

Patients under immunosuppression or with hematologic disease are particularly at risk of developing hepatic abscesses.

Abscess Formation in Bile Ducts

Usually a cholangitis is induced by biliary obstruction caused by lithiasis or strictures, and more rarely by a malignant neoplasm. Ascension from the gastrointestinal tract is the typical route of spread.

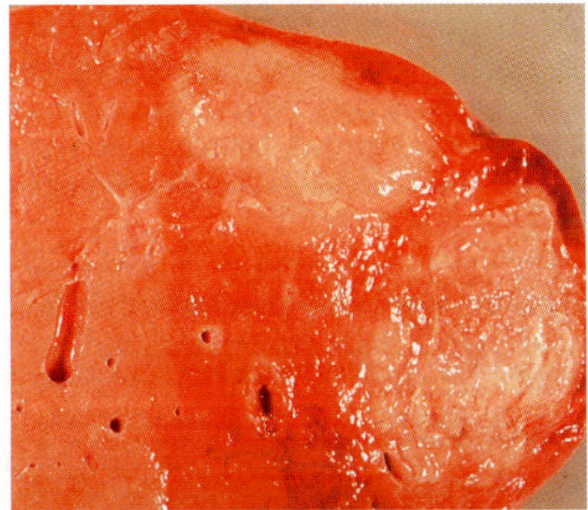

Fig. 30. Macroscopic aspect of an early-stage intrahepatic abscess formation with beginning central necrosis, in a patient with immune deficiency

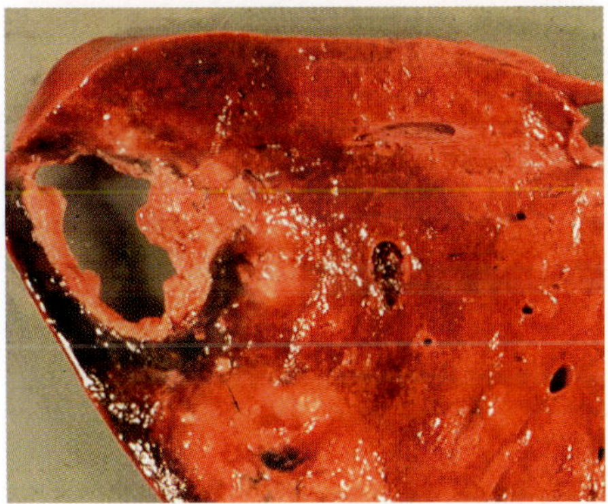

Fig. 31. Abscess formation with central liquified necrosis caused by septic emboli in a patient with AV-malformations of the pulmonary vasculature

3.7.2 Helmintic Infections

3.7.2.1 Nematodes (Ascariasis)

Transmission of helminths is usually by the fecal-oral route. Hepatomegaly with an eosinophilic granulomatous reaction may be present during migration of the larvae. This may lead to mechanical obstruction of the bile or pancreatic ducts and subsequent cholecystitis, hepatic abscesses and septicemia [89].

3.7.2.2 Cestodes (Echinococcus)

Echinococcus granulosus, which is the cause of the unilocular hydatosis, is found throughout Europe and is mainly transmitted by contact with dogs. The larval oncospheres reach the hepatic parenchyma via the portal vein. There they form slowly growing cysts, which may lead to compression or bacterial infection of the bile ducts. The cysts may grow to a size of 30 cm, and are typically surrounded by a fibrous rim which may calcify. Daughter cysts may also occur. A liver biopsy should be avoided because of the potential risk of peritoneal spread, anaphylactic reactions and dissemination of disease. Partial liver resection or sucking of the cysts and treatment with Albendazole may bring about remission.

Unlike the situation with *E. granulosus* infection, patients with *E. multilocularis* infection typically complain of jaundice and ascites. Untreated alveolar hydatidosis is frequently fatal. Cysts may rupture spontaneously. There are typically multiple irregularly formed cysts with a malignant-like tendency to invade surrounding parenchyma [2, 25] (Fig. 32).

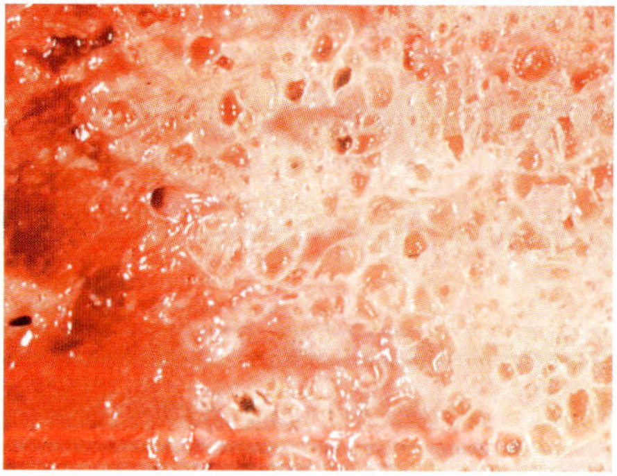

Fig. 32. Cut section of a hepatic infection with *Echinococcus alveolaris*. Congeries of small hepatic cysts are presented which infiltrate the liver parenchyma

3.7.2.3 Trematodes (Schistosomiasis)

Worldwide, schistosomiasis is the leading cause of portal hypertension. Typically, there is a latency between infection and the phase when trematodes (*S. mansoni, S. japonicum, S. mekongi*) are found in the portal vein. Here the female schistosoma begins egg-laying. This may lead to the so-called Katayama fever and transient hepato-splenomegaly. In advanced schistosomiasis microscopic examination reveals a periportal fibrosis (Symmers'clay-pipe stem fibrosis), which follows the periportal tracts. Concomitant granulomatous inflammation occurs with scarring. This leads to the typical portal hypertension of the presinusoidal type. The length and intensity of infection correlates positively with the degree of portal hypertension [42, 171].

3.8 Parenchymal Disease

3.8.1 Hemochromatosis

In hemochromatosis there is typically an increased uptake of iron in the small intestine despite already adequate iron storage. This leads to iron deposition in the liver, pancreas, joints, myocardium and hypophysis. There is an inherited type of hemochromatosis and a transfusion-induced type. Typical symptoms include diabetes, arthralgias, cardiac insufficiency and hypogonadism. To avoid permanent organic deficiency it is important to diagnose the inherited type. Whereas blood examination is able to hint at the possibility of hemochromatosis, a liver biopsy with increased iron storage in hepatocytes establishes the diagnosis [56, 144] (Fig. 33).

In MRI the increased iron content can be demonstrated by calculation of the T2-relaxation time. Therefore diagnosis as well as follow-up under therapy can be assessed. Patients suffering from untreated hemochromatosis typically develop liver cirrhosis and are at high risk to develop HCC. Consequently, regular imaging studies should be initiated.

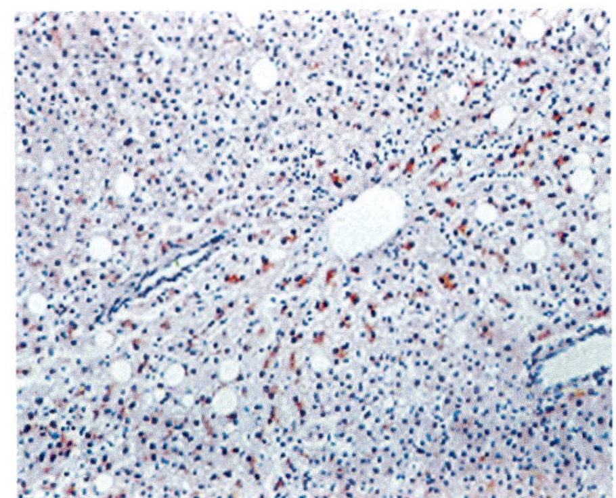

Fig. 33. Histology of hepatic parenchyma affected by hemochromatosis. Hemosiderin is predominantly accumulated in periportal parenchymal cells, which is in contrast to siderosis of the liver in which iron is stored predominantly in Kupffer cells

3.8.2 Transfusional Iron Overload (Hemosiderosis)

In some aplastic or hemolytic anemias frequent transfusions are necessary, which lead to increased iron storage in the spleen, liver, lymph nodes and bone marrow. This induces fibrosis of the hepatic parenchyma. If there is additional iron uptake in the intestine, such as in thalassemia, there is the possibility of liver cirrhosis even in young patients [99].

3.8.3 Fatty Liver

In pathology there are two types of fatty liver: the macrovesicular type in which there are large fat deposits, and the microvesicular type. Imaging is unable to distinguish between the two types. Focal fatty liver on histology typically shows macrovesicular fat deposits. Generally, these lesions do not cause any symptoms and may be solitary or multiple. A general disposition to steatosis (see Table 2) or a localized hypoxia may be the cause, although focal fatty infiltration of the liver may also occur in patients after chemotherapy.

There is a distinct disease entity called non-alcohol induced steatohepatitis (NASH) which demonstrates the transition from steatosis to hepatitis and cirrhosis. This was first described in adipose patients after gastrointestinal bypass (see Table 3) [7].

Table 2. Causes of steatosis hepatis

Diabetes mellitus	Fatty liver in pregnancy
Obesity	Reye's syndrome
Kwashiorkor	Heat-stroke
Alcohol- or drug-induced liver injury	SIDS
Chronic inflammatory bowel disease	Insect bites
Hepatitis C	Chron. hepatitis B and C in transplanted livers
Malaria	Wolman's disease
Immotile cilia syndrome	Chemotherapy

Table 3. Causes of non-alcohol induced steatohepatitis (NASH)

Morbid obesity	Parenteral nutrition
Gastroplasty, gastro-intestinal bypass	Weber-Christian disease
Diabetes mellitus type II	Abetalipoproteinemie
Drug-induced liver injury	

3.8.4 Wilson's Disease

Wilson's disease is an inherited autosomal-recessive disease typically associated with an increased intestinal uptake of copper and subsequent deposition in the liver, basal ganglia and other organs. There may be an acute or even fulminant hepatitis, chronic inflammation or cirrhosis. In contrast to hemochromatosis, patients do not demonstrate an increased risk of developing HCC.

Wilson's disease should be considered when a low level of coeruloplasmin (less than 1.3 mmol/l) and an increased quantity of copper is present in the liver (greater than 250 mg/g dry weight) [159].

Clinical symptoms in patients suffering from Wilson's disease seem to be directly related to the accumulation of copper in the brain, cornea, liver and kidneys.

Liver cirrhosis induced by Wilson's disease is normally macronodular. However, a mixed type or a micronodular type can also be observed. Histology reveals nodules of variable size separated by fibrous septa with minimal cholangiolar proliferation and varying signs of inflammation [109].

However, the distribution of copper deposition does not correlate with the pattern of nodules [162].

The current treatment of choice is D-Penicillamin in order to chelate unbound copper for urinary excretion [146].

However, on occasion the ultimate therapeutic option of liver transplantation should also be taken into account [129].

3.8.5 Primary Sclerosing Cholangitis

An unspecific inflammatory fibrosis of the intermediate and large bile ducts leads to irregular stenosis and ectasia of the intra- and extrahepatic bile ducts. This often remains completely asymptomatic and is only diagnosed because of increased levels of alkaline phosphatase (AP), although chronic fatigue, stomach pain and intermittent jaundice may also result [104, 179, 189].

Typically, primary sclerosing cholangitis predominates among male patients in the fifth decade of life [188].

The clinical course can be variable, with many patients dying due to progressive hepatic insufficiency. The only curative treatment is liver transplantation. About ten percent of all patients with primary sclerosing cholangitis subsequently develop cholangiocarcinoma or HCC [32].

An association with chronic inflammatory bowel disease (like Colitis ulcerosa) has also been reported. Primary sclerosing cholangitis has to be distinguished from secondary types of sclerosing cholangitis, such as those induced by surgical intervention, cholelithiasis and even cholangiocarcinoma [128].

3.8.6 Cirrhosis

Hepatic cirrhosis is the endpoint of different toxic, autoimmune, congenital or infectious diseases (see Table 4). Typically it is a diffuse process involving fibrosis and the forming of nodules [13].

Macropathologically there are micronodular (nodules < 3 mm), macronodular (nodules > 3 mm) and mixed types of cirrhosis. In micronodular cirrhosis the liver normally displays no irregularity of shape and there is an increased fibrotic reaction compared to the macronodular type (Fig. 34). Although hepatomegaly is frequently seen in the early stages, the size of the liver later decreases. The macronodular type typically displays an irregular surface (Fig.35) and large fibrotic bands. A transition from the micro- to the macronodular type of cirrhosis sometimes occurs in patients under treatment or after alcoholic abstinence [14].
Although many definitions of cirrhosis can be found in the literature, the most appropriate and concise of these states that cirrhosis is *"a diffuse process characterized by fibrosis and a conversion of normal architecture into structurally abnormal nodules"*. Essential for the diagnosis of cirrhosis is the presence of both fibrosis and

Table 4. Different pathologies leading to hepatic cirrhosis

- Toxic	
Alcohol	Methotrexate
Isoniazid	Methyldopa
Amiodarone	
- Infections	
Hepatitis B and C	Schistosomiasis
- Autoimmune	
Chronic active hepatitis	Primary biliary cirrhosis
- Metabolic	
Wilson's disease	Hemochromatosis
α-1-antitrypsin-deficiency	Galactosemia
Glycogen storage disease	Tyrosinemia
Diseases of urea cycle	Abetalipoproteinemia
- Biliary obstruction	
Atresia	Cystic fibrosis
Cholelithiasis	Strictures
Sclerosing cholangitis	
- Vascular	
Budd-Chiari syndrome	Veno-occlusive disease
Chronic cardiac insufficiency	Hereditary hemorrhagic teleangiectasia with AV-shunts liver
- Others	
Neonatal hepatitis-syndrome	Indian childhood cirrhosis
Intestinal bypass	Sarcoidosis

nodules throughout the entire liver. However, regeneration should not be present and this must be taken into account when evaluating histopathologic specimens from needle biopsies. For this reason, liver cirrhosis is a diagnosis that should only be assigned by the pathologist; cross sectional imaging should indicate only the diffuse nature of the process.

Fibrosis is an integral part of cirrhosis and differentiates it from nodular regenerative hyperplasia. Structurally abnormal nodules may often occur but sometimes they can only be identified by means of subtle architectural changes, such as a disordered or compressed cell plate pattern. Although abnormalities in vasculature and blood flow are very important, they are not included in the definition since these changes are a consequence of the other pathologic features rather than primary abnormalities. Equally, true regenerative nodules can be a late occurrence in cirrhosis and therefore regeneration is also excluded from the definition. Although regeneration is not essential for the diagnosis of cirrhosis, it is important to point out that regeneration is a critical factor influencing the evolution of cirrhosis [13, 131, 147].

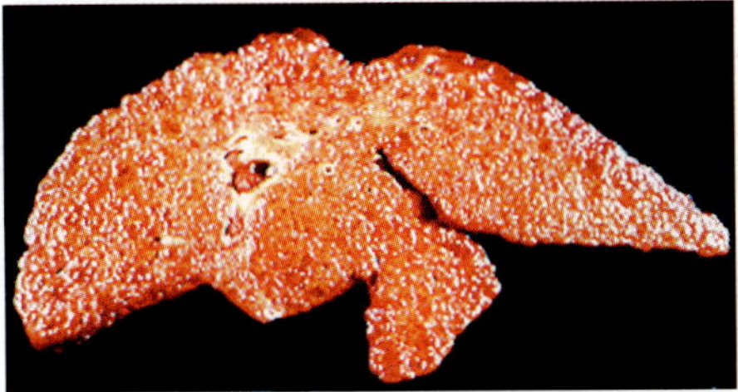

Fig. 34. Cut section of liver affected by macronodular cirrhosis with a marked variation in size and shape. This is accentuated by the intervening fibrous stroma which varies from broad scars to thin delicate bands of fibrosis tissue

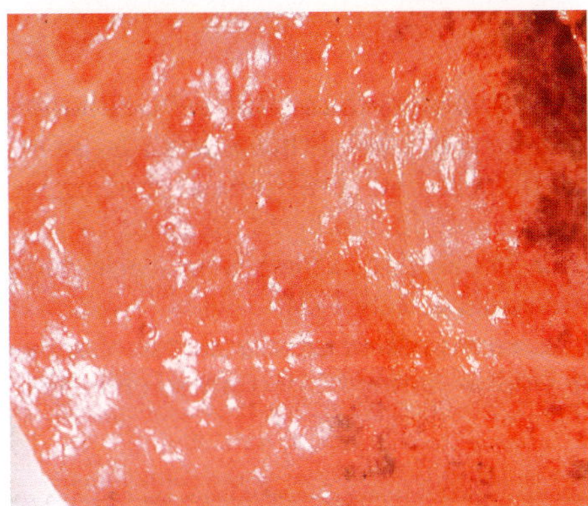

Fig. 35. Large nodules in a macronodular cirrhosis on the capsular surface of the liver

3.8.7 Primary Biliary Cirrhosis

This disease, whose etiology remains obscure, typically affects small hepatic ducts which become surrounded by chronic inflammatory infiltrations and are eventually destroyed. Microscopic examination frequently reveals portal tracts without bile ducts. Women in the fourth and fifth decades are affected to the greatest extent and there seems to be an association with autoimmune disorders such as Sjögren's syndrome, Sicca complex, CREST* syndrome and vasculitis. Typical symptoms include cholestasis, progredient fibrosis and cirrhosis [39, 86, 133].

3.8.8 Secondary Biliary Cirrhosis

This type of cirrhosis is induced by the obstruction of the extrahepatic bile ducts. Choledocholithiasis as well as benign strictures or malignant neoplasms may be the cause. Since regenerative nodules are typically absent, the condition is more a diffuse regenerative process than a true cirrhosis. Portal hypertension without typical morphological signs of liver cirrhosis is frequently observed [137, 151, 185].

---

*Calcinosis cutis, Raynauld's symptoms, esophageal motility disorder, sclerodactylia, teleangiectasia.

3.8.9 Reye's Syndrome

Reye's syndrome is an acute fatty degeneration of the liver occurring together with encephalopathy. It typically affects children with viral infections (influenza B or varicella) who have been treated with acetylic salicylic acid. There is only a limited hepatomegaly and the steatosis seems to be intermittent. Hence, the only decisive finding for prognosis is the extent of the neurological symptoms [31, 132].

3.8.10 Caroli's Syndrome

This cystic ectasia of small intrahepatic ducts is typically found diffusely, although cases of segmental occurrence may also be observed. Cholelithiasis leads to an intermittent obstructive jaundice with pain and fever and concomitant cholangitis. Possible complications are similar to those of choledochal cysts. In cases of segmental occurrence a partial hepatic resection is curative. There is an association with congenital hepatic fibrosis and Potter's sequence [28, 113].

Patients with Caroli's syndrome have an increased risk of intrahepatic cholangiocellular carcinoma, and thus regular imaging studies should be performed (Fig. 36).

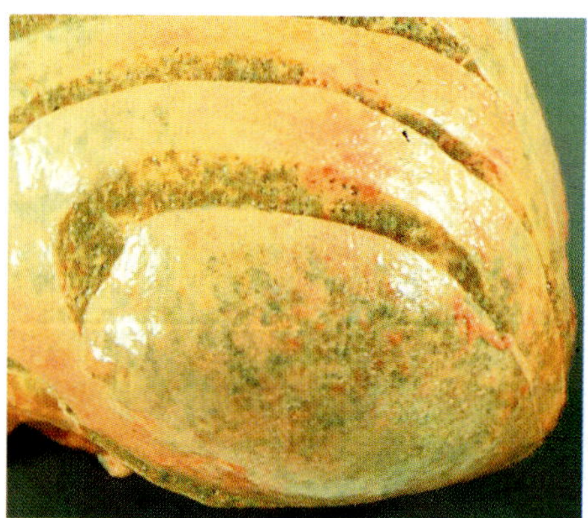

Fig. 36. Macroscopic aspect of a liver affected by Caroli's disease. The parenchyma shows yellowish changes due to cystically dilated bile ducts and congestion of bile

3.8.11 Liver Disease in Patients with Cystic Kidneys

3.8.11.1 Cystic Liver Disease in Combination with Cystic Kidney Disease

Liver cysts are associated with the autosomal dominant as well as the recessive type of renal cysts. In the dominant type there are hepatic cysts at birth of up to 10 cm in size, which usually become symptomatic in the fifth decade. Hepatomegaly, pain, and fever in cases of infection are the leading symptoms. Women seem to be affected more frequently than men, and there is a correlation with the number of pregnancies. Diverticles of the colon, a vitium cordis, ovarian cysts, inguinal herniation or intracranial aneurysms may occur concomitantly. Von Meyenburg complexes, which involve irregularly dilated bile ducts, seem to be associated with the development of liver cysts in autosomal dominant cystic kidney disease [112, 130].

In the autosomal recessive type of disease the degree of hepatic involvement may vary. Infants with the perinatal type typically do not live long because of pulmonary complications.

In the neonatal and infantile type there is a tendency to portal fibrosis and cystic dilation of bile ducts in combination with renal insufficiency. The juvenile type presents with portal hypertension. Microscopically, there is an increased number of bile ducts in the portal tracts, which are irregularly formed and linked together [21].

3.8.11.2 Congenital Hepatic Fibrosis and Cystic Kidneys

Congenital hepatic fibrosis together with cystic kidneys is a distinct entity. Symptoms of cholangitis and portal hypertension are relevant findings. Patients typically present late with esophageal variceal bleeding. Macroscopically, the liver seems to be enlarged and tough, and cysts are not visible. Concomitant congenital malformations may be found [64, 96] (see Table 5).

Table 5. Pathologies and syndromes with concomitant hepatic cirrhosis

Congenital hepatic fibrosis
Familial congenital heart disease
Pulmonary arterivenous fistula
Gastric ulcers
Protein-losing enteropathies syndr.
Laurence-Moon-Biedl-syndrome
Similar changes
Meckel's syndrome
Ivemark's syndrome
Ellis-van-Crefeld syndrome
Nephronophthisis – congenital hepatic fibrosis
Jeune syndrome
Vaginal atresia syndrome
Tuberous sclerosis
Medullary cystic disease

3.8.12 Langerhans Cell Histiocytosis

Liver involvement in histiocytosis is found in 29–71% of all cases. The leading symptoms are sclerosing cholangitis with cholestasis, progressive decrease of intrahepatic bile ducts and fibrosis with portal hypertension. Systemic chemotherapy may lead to an improvement, but in severe pediatric cases transplantation may be the only curative treatment [69, 120].

3.8.13 Storage Diseases

3.8.13.1 Glycogen Storage Disease

The different forms of glycogen storage disease are all inherited autosomal recessive. Glycogen storage disease should always be considered in children with hepatomegaly, hypoglycemia, growth retardation, an unproportional distribution of body fat and increased transaminases [117, 140] (see Table 6).

Table 6. Overview of glycogen storage diseases

Type	Hepatic manifestation	Other manifestations
Ia (von Gierke)	hepatomegaly, HCC, hepatic adenoma	growth retardation, seizures, hypoglycemia osteoporosis, gout, glomerulonephritis, amyloidosis
Ib	hepatomegaly, HCC, hepatic adenoma	growth retardation, seizures, hypoglycemia, osteoporosis, gout, glomerulonephritis, amyloidosis, neutropenia and frequent infections
II (Pompe)	microscopic changes, hepatomegaly	hypotonia, respiratory and cardiac insufficiency (infantile type)
III (Forbes)	hepatomegaly, cirrhosis, hepatic adenoma	hypoglycemia, muscle weakness, growth retardation
IV (Anderson)	hepatomegaly, cirrhosis, focal fatty areas	growth retardation, cardiac insufficiency
VI & IX	hepatomegaly	growth retardation, mild hypoglycemia, hyperlipidemia

3.8.13.2 Galactosemia

Galactosemia is an inherited autosomal-recessive condition that manifests primarily through the first exposure to galactose via lactose in fed milk. The cause and effect of this disease are mostly due to a defect in the enzyme galactose-1-phosphate uridyl transferase [82].

Children with this disease typically present shortly after birth with growth retardation, nausea, vomiting, diarrhea and jaundice. If untreated a cirrhosis may develop by the age of 6 months [156].

3.8.13.3 Hereditary Intolerance of Fructose

This inherited disorder of fructose metabolism is either caused by a deficiency of fructose-1-phosphate aldolase or is due to a dysfunction of the enzyme fructose-1,6-biphosphatase [15, 62].

Primary symptoms include poor feeding, vomiting and failure to thrive. Additionally, hepato-splenomegaly, hemorrhages, jaundice, fever and ascites can be found. Sometimes cases with acute liver failure may occur, and there is frequently a steatosis and subsequent cirrhosis [123].

3.8.13.4 Mucopolysaccharidosis

Mucopolysaccharidosis is due to the deficient activity of enzymes responsible for the catabolism of glucosaminoglycans. It involves the accumulation of excessive amounts of mucopolysaccharides in the somatic and visceral tissue and the excretion of partial metabolites in the urine. Additionally, accumulations of gangliosides can be found. Mucopolysaccharidosis may be subdivided into six different disorders with each one presenting different clinical features. Although the same catabolic pathway is affected, in each case the specific enzyme involved is different. The types to manifest in the liver are type I (Hurler), II (Hunter), III (Sanfilippo), VI (Maroteaux-Lamy) and VIIb. Macroscopically, the liver becomes enlarged and extensive fibrosis or cirrhosis may occur. When present, the fibrosis is generally diffuse with heavy deposits of collagen bundles and gradual microdissection of parenchyma into nodules. Cirrhosis in mucopolysaccharidosis can present as either a macronodular type or a micronodular type [180].

3.8.14   Viral Hepatitis

3.8.14.1 Acute Hepatitis

The various forms of viral hepatitis induced by different viruses have a similar morphology. Macroscopically, there is hepatomegaly with an edematous capsule, and distinct necrotic areas which lead to surface irregularities. In fulminant hepatitis, necrosis results in liver shrinkage and a relevant loss of parenchymal volume, however, there might be complete restitution. If necrosis occurs there may be scar formation, which is morphologically similar to that in cirrhosis. Cirrhosis typically develops in cases of chronic hepatitis [126, 169].

3.8.14.2 Chronic Hepatitis

An inflammatory process which lasts longer than six months without signs of regression is referred to as chronic hepatitis. Histologically, chronic hepatitis is a necro-inflammatory, primarily hepatocytic disease with or without cirrhosis, in which lymphocytes clearly dominate the inflammation. There is a gradation regarding the degree of inflammation, its localization and the subsequent fibrosis.

Macroscopically, an enlarged liver can be demonstrated in the acute phase caused by edematization. Ascites and splenomegaly are signs of a more fulminant course [45]. The main etiological categories for chronic hepatitis in addition to virus infection are listed in Table 7.

Table 7. Etiological categories of chronic hepatitis

– Viral (HBV, HDV, HCV)
– Autoimmune (classic lupoid-type and subtypes)
– Autoimmune overlap syndromes
– Drug induced (e.g. nitrofurantoin, alpha-methyldopa, isoniazid and others)
– Cryptogenic

3.8.15   Liver Disease in Congestive Heart Disease

A chronic failure of the right heart leads to an enlarged liver via congestion. Diffuse cell necrosis may develop due to the decreased blood flow, increased blood pressure and resulting hypoxemia (Fig. 37). Cell necrosis thereafter induces a fibrosis which resembles a micronodular cirrhosis. However, in contrast to other forms of cirrhosis the microscopic architecture remains intact [97].

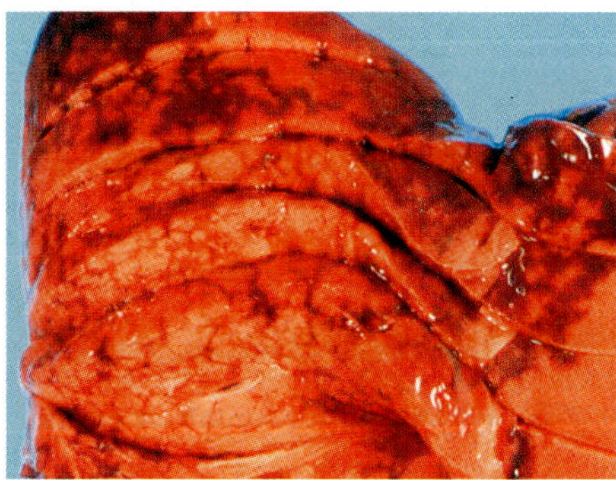

Fig. 37. Macroscopic aspect of cardiac liver cirrhosis based on congestive heart disease, leading to increased intrahepatic blood pressure and reduced flow with subsequent cirrhosis

3.9   Vascular Changes

3.9.1   Thrombosis of the Portal Vein

According to Virchow's trias there are three main mechanisms leading to a thrombosis: hypercoagulability, stasis and injury to the vascular endothelium (see Table 8). Obstruction of the portal vein may be intermittent, as can be shown in ultrasonographic and histologic studies. Recanalization is quite rare once the thrombus formation has reached the smaller portal branches [19, 168].

Table 8. Etiological factors leading to portal vein thrombosis

- Hypercoagulability	
Polycythaemia vera	Idiopathic thrombocytosis
Paroxysmal nocturnal hemoglobinuria	CML
Subclinical myeloproliferative disease	Oral contraceptive pills
Pregnancy	Protein C deficiency
Antithrombin III deficiency	
- Stasis	
Cirrhosis	HCC
Pancreatic carcinoma	Splenectomy
- Vascular injury	
Sepsis of the umbilical veins	Pylephlebitis
Trauma	Catheterization
Schistosomiasis	Chronic inflammatory bowel disease

3.9.2 Obstruction of Smaller Portal Branches

The type of portal hypertension caused by obliteration of the smaller portal branches sometimes occurs in systemic vasculitis or rheumatic disease and may be found prior to a manifest cirrhosis in primary sclerosing cholangitis (PSC), primary biliary cholangitis (PBC) or sarcoidosis. An infection with schistosoma – with eggs of the parasite causing a chronic inflammatory reaction – may lead to thrombosis and fibrosis. Acute thrombosis of a small portal vein causes a so-called pseudo-infarction (Zahn Infarction), while thrombosis of larger branches may induce a more diffuse atrophy with subsequent regenerative hyperplasia [6, 51, 134].

3.9.3 Budd-Chiari Syndrome

The combination of portal hypertension and hepatomegaly caused by an obstruction of the venous drainage was first described by Budd in 1845. This obstruction may be located intrahepatically in the small hepatic veins or extrahepatically in the larger veins or the inferior caval vein (Fig. 38). The type of obliterative endophlebitis of small hepatic veins described by Chiari is called "veno-occlusive disease". A principal clinical symptom is slowly increasing portal hypertension. Only a few patients develop a fulminant disease with acute liver failure, hepatic encephalopathy and coagulopathy, and this arises from the sudden obstruction of all larger hepatic veins. This may be caused by any coagulation disorder which predisposes subjects to a thrombosis, or by a growing neoplasm, a hypertrophied caudate lobe or membrane formation in the inferior caval vein. Treatment options include anticoagulation, resection of a mechanical obstruction or porto-systemic shunting. The last approach may involve liver transplantation. In acute obstruction the liver seems to be enlarged because of a dilation of the sinusoids. If there is only a partial obstruction there might be hypertrophy of the areas with diminished drainage [92, 114, 175] (see Table 9).

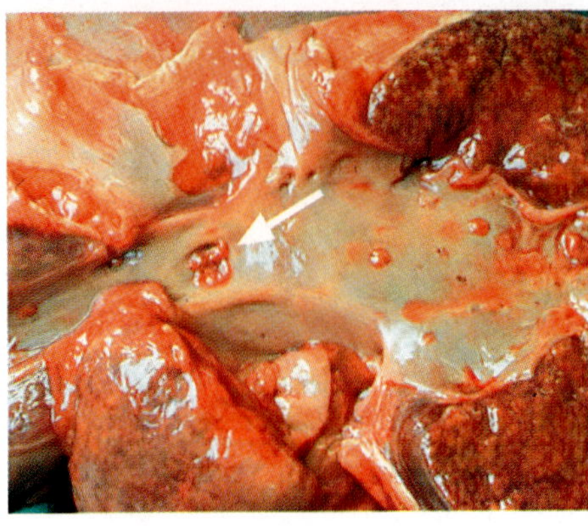

Fig. 38. Cut section of a liver from a patient with Budd-Chiari syndrome demonstrating thrombus formation in a large hepatic vein (*arrow*)

Table 9. Etiological factors leading to thrombosis of the hepatic veins

- Hypercoagulability

Polycythemia vera	Subclinical myeloid dysplasia
Paroxysmal nocturnal hemoglobinuria	Promyelocytic leukemia
Chronic myeloid leukemia	Oral contraceptive pills
Preganancy	Anticardiolipin antibodies
Idiopathic thrombozytopenic purpura	Protein C deficiency
Antithrombin III deficiency	

- Stasis

Membranous obstruction of the inferior caval vein	Congenital anomalies
Cirrhosis	Cardiac insufficiency
Constrictive pericarditis	Obstruction of the sup. caval vein
Atrial myxoma	Sickle cell anemia
HCC	Hypernephroma
Adrenal carcinoma	Hodgkin's disease
Wilms' tumor	Leiomyoma and leiomyosarcoma
Metastasizing neoplasms	Hydatid cysts
Abscess formation	Hematoma

- Vascular injury

Trauma	Catheterization
Amyloidosis	Vasculitis
Tuberculosis	Behçet's disease
Sarcoidosis	Filariasis

- Others

Chronic inflammatory bowel disease	Protein-losing enteropathy
Multiple myeloma	

3.9.4 Veno-Occlusive Disease (VOD)

A fibrotic obstruction of the small (< 1 mm) liver veins leads to hepatomegaly with congestion of the sinusoids. If longstanding, this results in liver fibrosis. Causative agents include pyrrolizidine alkaloids, which are found in exotic teas and as contamination in cereals. Azathioprin and cysteamin are also known to induce VOD, while whole body irradiation, together with intensive chemotherapy, is thought to lead to injury of the endothelium of small hepatic veins. Acute symptoms include sudden onset of pain with hepatomegaly and ascites. More than 50% of all bone marrow-transplanted patients show signs of VOD. Typical symptoms in these cases are weight gain, jaundice, thrombocytopenia and early stage liver failure. A similar disease is seen in patients under Dacarbazine, but histologically there is no fibrotic obstruction but a thrombosis, probably induced by an allergic reaction [23, 40, 57, 186].

3.9.5 Lobular or Segmental Atrophy

Thrombosis of the portal or hepatic veins may lead to focal atrophy with subsequent compensatory hypertrophy of the neighboring segments. This is especially common in patients with cirrhotic livers. Syphilis and metastatic carcinoma are known to cause a so-called hepar lobatum. Segmental atrophy may also be due to a congenital anomaly [71, 127].

3.9.6 Infarction / Ischemia

Usually, an obstruction of the hepatic artery does not induce hepatic ischemia, as the blood flow via the portal vein is sufficient to guarantee parenchymal supply. Large infarcts are only possible if both vessels have a diminished flow, as in shock, chronic portal vein thrombosis or cirrhotic livers. Here, the increased portal tension induces a reduction of blood flow in the portal vessels. Intravasal coagulation may also cause liver infarctions [33, 141].

3.10 HIV-associated Liver Diseases

The liver in HIV is mainly affected by opportunistic infections. About half of all patients with seroconversion into mononucleose-like disease have hepatomegaly. In almost 100% of HIV patients there are non-specific hepatic findings such as granulomatous inflammation, peliosis hepatis or amyloidosis [37, 41].

Kaposi Sarcoma
About 20% of all HIV-infected patients develop a Kaposi's sarcoma of the liver, typically growing from the portal tracts along the bile ducts. Parenchymal lesions are typically small (5–10 mm), and are located subcapsularly [74].

Primary Lymphoma of the Liver
Primary liver lymphomas are found more frequently in HIV-infected patients than in non-infected individuals. There may be focal lesions with necrotic centers or a more diffuse infiltration of the liver parenchyma as well as lymphoma of bile ducts, which may resemble a sclerosing cholangitis [27, 85].

Cholangitis
Cryptosporidiae and microsporidiae may induce a cholangitis especially if CD4+ counts are below $4/mm^3$. Sclerosis leads to pain, fever and cholestasis. Furthermore, there is an increased incidence of bacterial cholangitis, induced by gram-negative agents [17, 110].

Fungal Infections
Generally, fungal infections are a major problem in HIV-positive patients or in patients with manifest AIDS. In these cases fungal infections may occur as focal as well as disseminated infections in which the liver may be affected. The most important pathogenic germs are *Candida albicans*, *Cryptococcus neoformans*, *Histoplasma capsulatum*, *Pneumocystis carinii* and *Aspergillus*. For an accurate diagnosis a liver biopsy should be performed. However, the most sensitive techniques to classify the fungi responsible for the infection are blood culture and blood antigenemia tests [73, 190].

Protozoal infections
Protozoal infections which may affect the liver in HIV-positive patients include *Toxoplasma gondii*, *Leishmania species* and *Cryptosporidium parvum*.

HIV-associated Toxoplasmosis usually presents with focal lesions in the brain. Disseminated toxoplasmosis outside this location is uncommon in AIDS patients and is only occasionally found by chance or in autopsy material [22].

As the infection with *Leishmania* depends on the geographical distribution of this pathogenic germ, HIV-associated Leishmaniosis only occurs in endemic regions such as southern Europe, South America and Africa. Inocculated parasites may persist latently in the body for several years manifesting only in a more progressed state of immunodeficiency [4].

Bacterial infections
Bacterial infections which show an increased incidence in HIV-positive patients and which may manifest in the liver include tuberculosis, infections with atypical Mycobacteria, bacillery angiomatosis, cat-scratch disease and Q fever.

Hepatic foci of tuberculosis may appear as single or multiple mass lesions as well as miliary tuberculosis. Recent studies have revealed that active tuberculosis is present in 50% of adults dying of AIDS and that the liver is involved in 85% of these cases. Thus, tuberculosis represents the most important and most frequent hepatotropic HIV-associated disease [103].

HIV-associated infection with atypical Mycobacteria, such as *M. avium* and *M. intracellulare*, depends on the geographic distribution and correlates with the CD4+ lymphocyte count. Infections within the liver manifest with increased serum alkaline phosphatase indicating either an obstruction of the bile ducts by enlarged lymph nodes in the liver hilum, or obstruction of the terminal ductules by intrahepatic *M. avium* granulomas. Thus, infections with atypical Mycobacteria should also be considered in cases of intrahepatic abscess formation in HIV-positive patients [106, 174].

3.11 Hepatic Traumatization

The spleen and liver are the most frequently involved organs in traumatization by car accident or penetration. Up to 60% of all patients with hepatic trauma are hemodynamically unstable and up to 45% have concomitant splenic involvement. The right liver lobe is the most frequently traumatized area. Subcapsular hematoma often results in a more restricted blood loss. These are typically lens-shaped and cause compression of the neighboring parenchyma. Rib fractures are a frequent finding. Parenchymal contusions and hematoma are less sharply demarcated. Parenchymal tears of the area nuda typically run parallel to hepatic veins and may remain undiscovered in peritoneal lavage. There may be some intra-parenchymal or subcapsular air formation one to two days after traumatization in necrotic areas. Traumatization of the bile ducts may cause bile leakage which, on occasion, leads to formation of a demarcated bilioma. Hemorrhage in bile ducts may be suspected in cases of increased bile density. Generally, acute trauma most often presents with areas of high bile density, which in the course of time may lead to the development of more cystic lesions [29, 30, 44].

3.12 Metastases

Liver metastases are the most frequent malignant liver lesions. Between 24% and 36% of all patients who die of a malignancy are known to have hepatic metastases which frequently are below 1 cm in size [148].

In order of decreasing frequency the principal organs which harbor the primary tumors of origin are the colon, stomach, pancreas, breast and lung. Hematogeneous spread via the portal vein is usually found in malignancies of the gastrointestinal tract, whereas lymphogeneous spread occurs in bile duct and pancreatic carcinoma. Primary tumors such as lung cancer seem to metastasize via the arterial blood supply of the liver. Hematologic disease such as lymphoma or leukemia may also infiltrate the hepatic parenchyma.

Metastases vary in size, consistency, uniformity of growth, stromal response and vascularity and can be either infiltrative or expansive. The appearance of metastases depends on the primary source and mode of propagation. Metastatic adenocarcinomas from the gallbladder and colon often contain calcifications and have a slimy cut surface because of mucin production. Tumors that are expanding and massive, such as colon cancer metastases, often have central liquefactive necrosis (Fig. 39). Metastases that have significant necrosis and/or fibrosis can umbilicate the surface of the liver capsule, which is helpful for differentiation from HCCs which rarely cause umbilication. Poorly differentiated tumors such as seminomas, oat-cell carcinomas, non-Hodgkin's lymphomas and undifferentiated sarcomas tend to have a uniformly soft, "fish flesh-like" consistency. Squamous cell carcinomas have a granular and caseous central portion that lacks the shiny appearance of

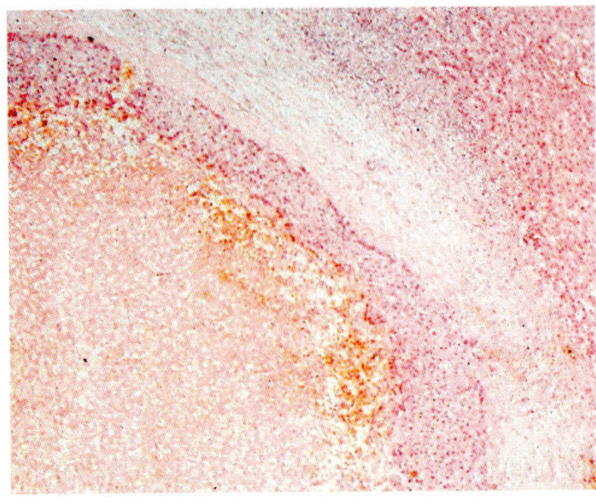

Fig. 39. Histology of a liver metastasis of a colorectal adenocarcinoma. Note the central necrosis surrounded by a rim of viable tumor tissue

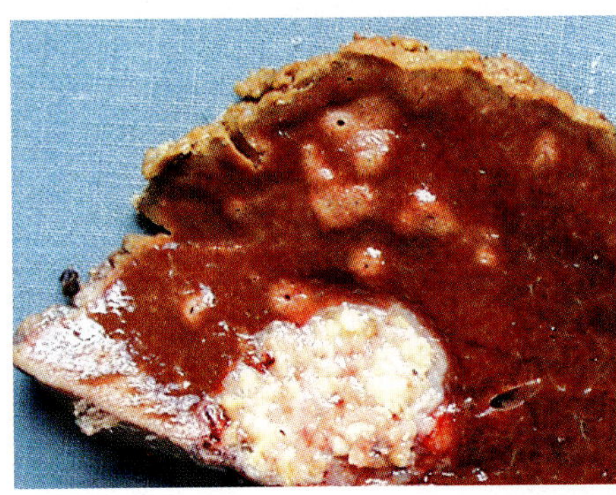

Fig. 40. Cut section of the liver in metastatic liver disease in a patient with primary colon carcinoma, demonstrating subcapsular as well as diffuse intrahepatic metastases

most adenocarcinomas. Individual metastases in the same liver can vary greatly in appearance because of differences in blood supply, hemorrhage, cellular differentiation, fibrosis and necrosis.

Most metastases maintain the microscopic features of the primary tumor, including the degree of stromal growth. Approximately 7–15% of patients with metastatic liver disease have tumor thrombi that occlude the portal and/or hepatic veins. Metastases that penetrate the large portal veins disseminate through peripheral portal branches. The vascular supply of liver metastases is virtually all arterial and this is the basis of imaging strategies and therapeutic modalities. Although hepatic metastases from the splanchnic bed originally derive their blood supply from the portal vein, the blood supply becomes progressively arterial.

Metastases of Colorectal Adenocarcinoma

Colorectal carcinoma is the second most common carcinoma in men and women. 15% of all patients initially present with hepatic metastases due to vascular drainage via the portal vein (Fig. 40). Thereafter, local recurrence or distant metastases can occur during the first two years after the intended curative resection of the primary tumor. Their prevalence depends on TNM* stage and is about 14% [191, 197].

---

* TNM= T, extent of tumor compared to surrounding tissue; N, number of lymph nodules affected by tumor cells; M, metastases present or not.

A second surgical intervention is the only treatment that seems to be beneficial to patients with hepatic metastases despite a relatively low 5-year survival rate of 25% [145]. It seems that survival increases with the latency of the recurrent tumor growth [158].

Alternative palliative treatment modalities which may be relevant include chemotherapy with 5-Fluorouracil and Levamisol [115], embolization of arterial tumor vessels [35], and cryotherapeutic intervention [138].

Liver Metastases of Breast Carcinoma
Breast cancer is one of the most frequent malignancies in female patients in the western world. Patients with known hepatic metastases die rapidly if no therapy is initiated [75]. However, regional chemotherapy alone or in combination with partial hepatic resection does not seem to be of benefit [102]. Systemic chemotherapy only induces a partial remission in 30–40% of all patients.

Carcinoid Metastases
Almost two thirds of all carcinoids are found in the appendix, while up to one third are located in some other part of the small intestine. The course of disease and hence both life expectancy and quality is mainly dependent upon the extent of metastatic growth. Typical flush symptoms can often be relieved by a reduction of the hepatic tumor burden. The 5-year survival of patients with hepatic metastases is about 21% if no therapy is initiated [116]. Hemihepatectomy or segmental resection in patients with metastatic growth in one liver lobe and intermittent embolization of hepatic arteries in disseminated disease may improve the survival to up to 70% [1]. As carcinoid tumors usually display relatively slow tumor growth, liver transplantation in patients with diffuse metastases may be another treatment modality. Chemotherapy with 5-Fluorouracil, Streptozotocine, Doxorubicine or Dacarbacine as a monotherapy is of no benefit alone [116], although there may be some tumor regression when conducted in combination with embolization (Fig. 41).

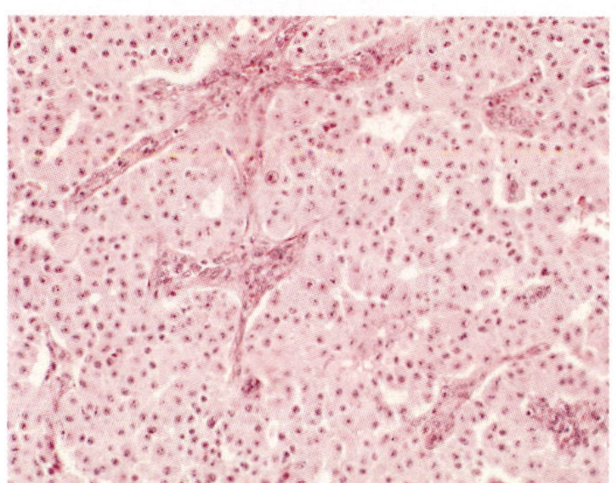

Fig. 41. Histology of hepatic metastasis of a neuroendocrine pancreatic tumor with glandular differentiation and no signs of tumor necrosis

3.13 Infiltration of the Liver in Hematologic Diseases

3.13.1 Non-Hodgkin's Lymphoma (NHL)

The primary hepatic manifestation in NHL must be distinguished from secondary involvement. Patients with primary lymphoma seem to have a favorable prognosis when initial resection is followed by chemotherapy. Typically, well demarcated lesions with surrounding necrosis are found, and diffuse infiltration is rare [150].

However, a secondary liver infiltration, seems to occur quite frequently. Well-differentiated B-cell lymphomas tend to form multiple small nodules, whereas more undifferentiated types show a more diffuse manifestation which is hard to identify on imaging studies. Unlike other solid metastatic diseases to the liver, an involvement of both liver and spleen is typically found in lymphoma [90].

3.13.2 Hepatic Hodgkin's Lymphoma

Secondary infiltration of the hepatic parenchyma also seems to occur in patients with Hodgkin's lymphoma. Fever and hepatomegaly with jaundice may be the consequence. The morphology varies from diffuse infiltration to large well-demarcated areas or small nodules. In some patients there may be concomitant peliosis hepatis [83, 97].

SECTION 2

3.14 Radiological Classification on MRI

Liver lesions can be classified on the basis of both unenhanced and contrast-enhanced images (Table 10). On unenhanced imaging classification can be based upon the signal intensity and delineation of lesions on conventional T2w and T1w images as well as on opposed phase T1w images or T1w images acquired with fat suppression. Tables 11 and 12 show the characteristic appearances of many of the more common lesion types on unenhanced T2w and T1w images, respectively. Thus, on unenhanced imaging lesions with a high fluid content, lesions containing fat and lesions with internal hemorrhage can be detected and readily diagnosed. Unfortunately, unenhanced imaging alone cannot always differentiate reliably between benign and malignant lesions and, in many cases, additional information from contrast-enhanced imaging is necessary for accurate differential diagnosis.

The availability of contrast agents with markedly different properties means that lesions can be classified on the basis of different enhancement patterns on contrast-enhanced imaging (Table 10). Thus, lesions can be classified according to their behavior on dynamic imaging following the administration of extracellular contrast agents (in a similar manner to that which occurs on dual phase spiral CT imaging), and on their behavior on delayed imaging following the administration of contrast agents targeted either to the hepatocytes or the Kupffer cells.

In the dynamic phase of contrast enhancement after the administration of gadolinium-based contrast agents, lesions can be classified according to whether they demonstrate hypervascular or hypovascular enhancement patterns or delayed persistent enhancement on T1w acquisitions during the arterial, portal-venous and equilibrium phases, respectively (Table 13). Within these three major groups of lesions, lesions can be classified further according to the presence or absence of certain characteristic features. For example, a central scar within a hypervascular lesion in a non-cirrhotic liver that shows low signal intensity on T1w images and high signal intensity on T2w images may be indicative of focal nodular hyperplasia (Table 14). Similarly, a hypovascular lesion with a hypervascular rim that shows contrast agent washout at 10-15 min post-injection and a doughnut or halo sign on T2w images may be indicative of a metastasis of adenocarcinoma (Table 15). Finally, a lesion that shows nodular enhancement in the arterial phase followed by centripetal filling-in in the subsequent phases and high signal intensity on T2w images may be indicative of a hemangioma (Table 16).

Whereas the enhancement seen on dynamic T1w imaging gives information on the morphologic characteristics of lesions, that seen on delayed phase images after the injection of agents targeted either to the hepatocytes (e.g. Gd-BOPTA; Table 17 or Mn-DPDP; Table 18) or Kupffer cells (e.g. iron oxide agents; Table 19) gives information on the cellular content and cellular functionality of lesions. In the case of Gd-BOPTA, the information gained in the delayed phase is additional to that seen in the dynamic phase and may serve to distinguish lesions of hepatocellular origin that may be able to take up the agent such as FNH from lesions of hepatocellular origin that have lost this ability such as HCC and lesions of non-hepatocellular origin that are also unable to take up the agent (Table 17).

Similarly, lesions can be classified into different groups on the basis of their ability to take up Mn-DPDP (Table 18) and iron oxide particles (Table 19). However, the lack of a dynamic imaging capability combined with the sometimes overlapping levels of enhancement of different primary benign and malignant liver lesions often makes accurate differential diagnosis difficult with these agents.

The tables that follow demonstrate schematically an approach to the classification of liver lesions based on imaging features on unenhanced MR imaging and enhanced imaging after administration of both extracellular and liver-specific contrast agents.

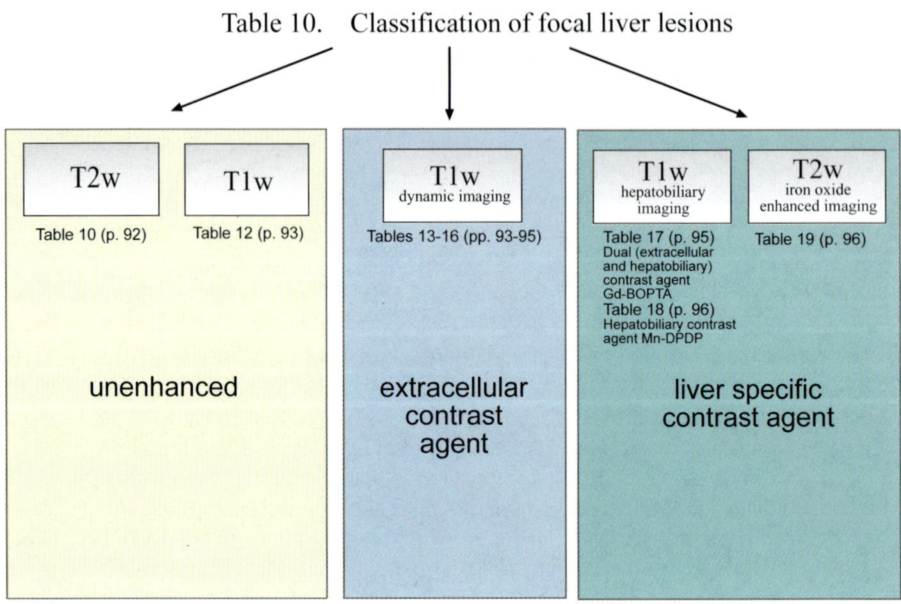
Table 10.   Classification of focal liver lesions
T2w
Table 10 (p. 92)
T1w
Table 12 (p. 93)
unenhanced
T1w
dynamic imaging
Tables 13-16 (pp. 93-95)
extracellular contrast agent
T1w
hepatobiliary imaging
Table 17 (p. 95)
Dual (extracellular and hepatobiliary) contrast agent Gd-BOPTA
Table 18 (p. 96)
Hepatobiliary contrast agent Mn-DPDP
T2w
iron oxide enhanced imaging
Table 19 (p. 96)
liver specific contrast agent

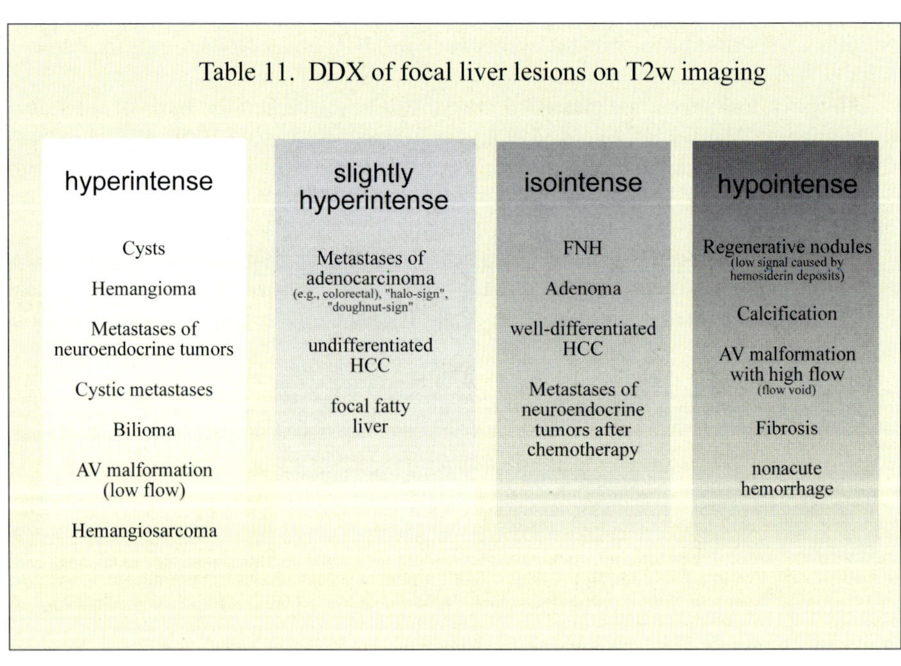
Table 11. DDX of focal liver lesions on T2w imaging
hyperintense
Cysts
Hemangioma
Metastases of neuroendocrine tumors
Cystic metastases
Bilioma
AV malformation (low flow)
Hemangiosarcoma
slightly hyperintense
Metastases of adenocarcinoma (e.g., colorectal), "halo-sign", "doughnut-sign"
undifferentiated HCC
focal fatty liver
isointense
FNH
Adenoma
well-differentiated HCC
Metastases of neuroendocrine tumors after chemotherapy
hypointense
Regenerative nodules (low signal caused by hemosiderin deposits)
Calcification
AV malformation with high flow (flow void)
Fibrosis
nonacute hemorrhage

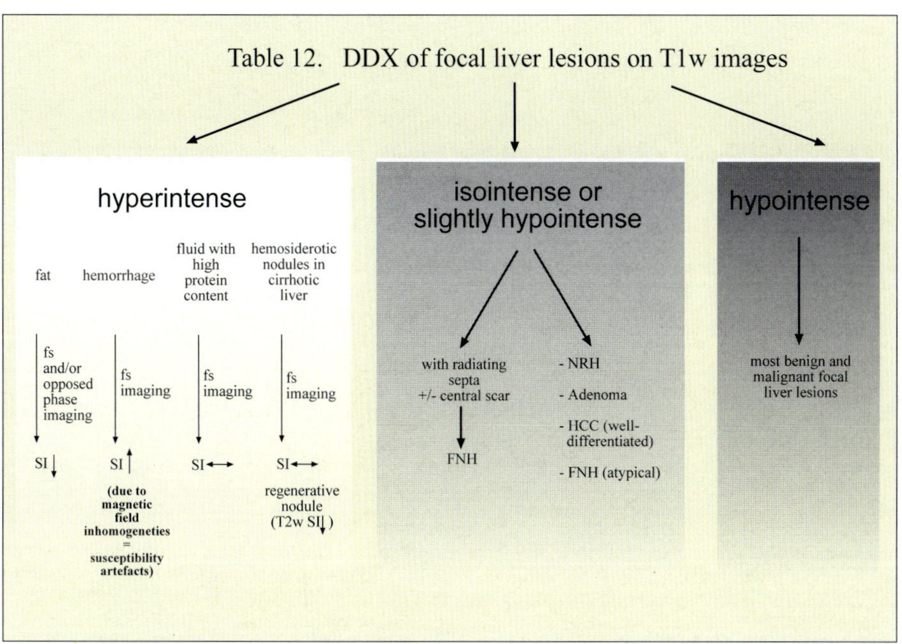

Table 12.   DDX of focal liver lesions on T1w images
hyperintense
isointense or slightly hypointense
hypointense
fat
hemorrhage
fluid with high protein content
hemosiderotic nodules in cirrhotic liver
fs and/or opposed phase imaging
fs imaging
fs imaging
fs imaging
SI ↓
SI ↑
SI ↔
SI ↔
(due to magnetic field inhomogeneties = susceptibility artefacts)
regenerative nodule (T2w SI↓)
with radiating septa +/- central scar
- NRH
- Adenoma
- HCC (well-differentiated)
- FNH (atypical)
FNH
most benign and malignant focal liver lesions

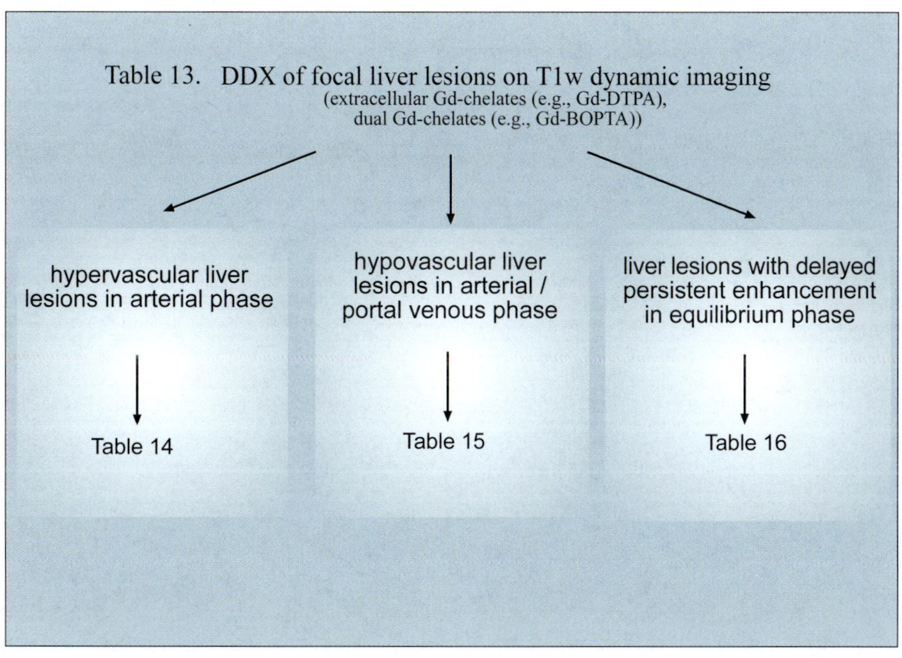

Table 13.   DDX of focal liver lesions on T1w dynamic imaging
(extracellular Gd-chelates (e.g., Gd-DTPA),
dual Gd-chelates (e.g., Gd-BOPTA))
hypervascular liver lesions in arterial phase
hypovascular liver lesions in arterial / portal venous phase
liver lesions with delayed persistent enhancement in equilibrium phase
Table 14
Table 15
Table 16

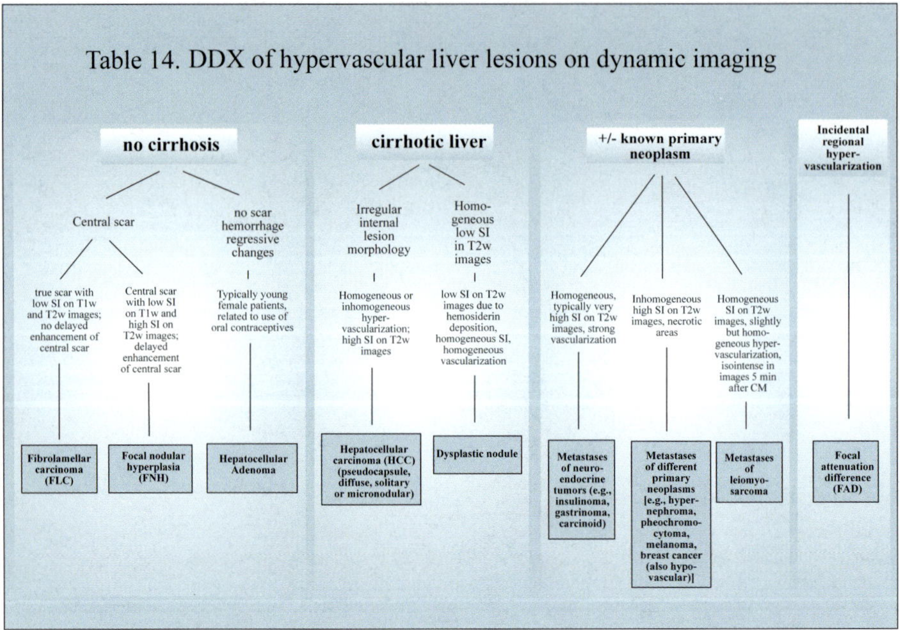
Table 14. DDX of hypervascular liver lesions on dynamic imaging

no cirrhosis
cirrhotic liver
+/- known primary neoplasm
Incidental regional hyper-vascularization

Central scar
no scar hemorrhage regressive changes
Irregular internal lesion morphology
Homo-geneous low SI in T2w images

true scar with low SI on T1w and T2w images; no delayed enhancement of central scar
Central scar with low SI on T1w and high SI on T2w images; delayed enhancement of central scar
Typically young female patients, related to use of oral contraceptives
Homogeneous or inhomogeneous hyper-vascularization; high SI on T2w images
low SI on T2w images due to hemosiderin deposition, homogeneous SI, homogeneous vascularization
Homogeneous, typically very high SI on T2w images, strong vascularization
Inhomogeneous high SI on T2w images, necrotic areas
Homogeneous SI on T2w images, slightly but homo-geneous hyper-vascularization, isointense in images 5 min after CM

Fibrolamellar carcinoma (FLC)
Focal nodular hyperplasia (FNH)
Hepatocellular Adenoma
Hepatocellular carcinoma (HCC) (pseudocapsule, diffuse, solitary or micronodular)
Dysplastic nodule
Metastases of neuro-endocrine tumors (e.g., insulinoma, gastrinoma, carcinoid)
Metastases of different primary neoplasms [e.g., hyper-nephroma, pheochromo-cytoma, melanoma, breast cancer (also hypo-vascular)]
Metastases of leiomyo-sarcoma
Focal attenuation difference (FAD)

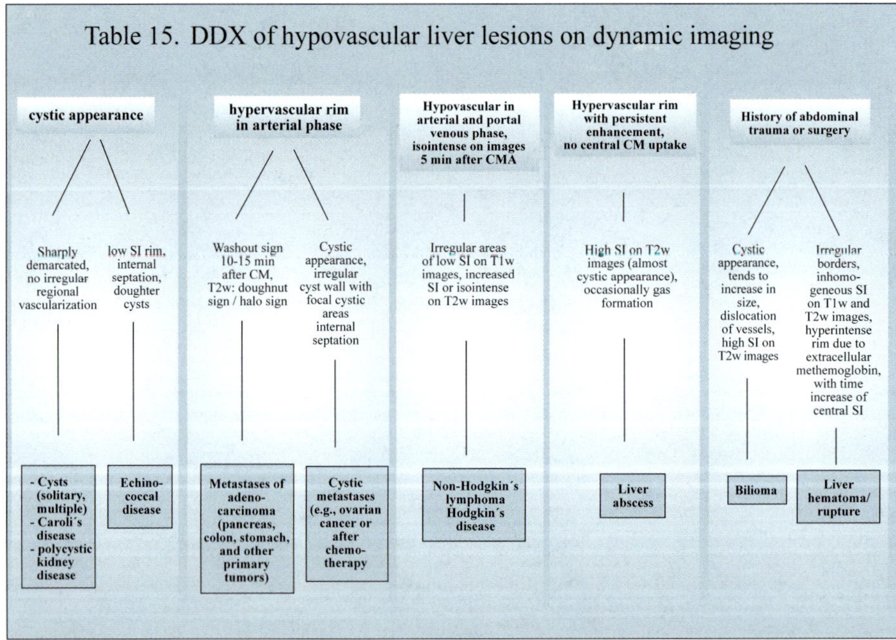
Table 15. DDX of hypovascular liver lesions on dynamic imaging

cystic appearance
hypervascular rim in arterial phase
Hypovascular in arterial and portal venous phase, isointense on images 5 min after CMA
Hypervascular rim with persistent enhancement, no central CM uptake
History of abdominal trauma or surgery

Sharply demarcated, no irregular regional vascularization
low SI rim, internal septation, doughter cysts
Washout sign 10-15 min after CM, T2w: doughnut sign / halo sign
Cystic appearance, irregular cyst wall with focal cystic areas internal septation
Irregular areas of low SI on T1w images, increased SI or isointense on T2w images
High SI on T2w images (almost cystic appearance), occasionally gas formation
Cystic appearance, tends to increase in size, dislocation of vessels, high SI on T2w images
Irregular borders, inhomo-geneous SI on T1w and T2w images, hyperintense rim due to extracellular methemoglobin, with time increase of central SI

- Cysts (solitary, multiple)
- Caroli´s disease
- polycystic kidney disease
Echino-coccal disease
Metastases of adeno-carcinoma (pancreas, colon, stomach, and other primary tumors)
Cystic metastases (e.g., ovarian cancer or after chemo-therapy)
Non-Hodgkin´s lymphoma Hodgkin´s disease
Liver abscess
Bilioma
Liver hematoma/ rupture

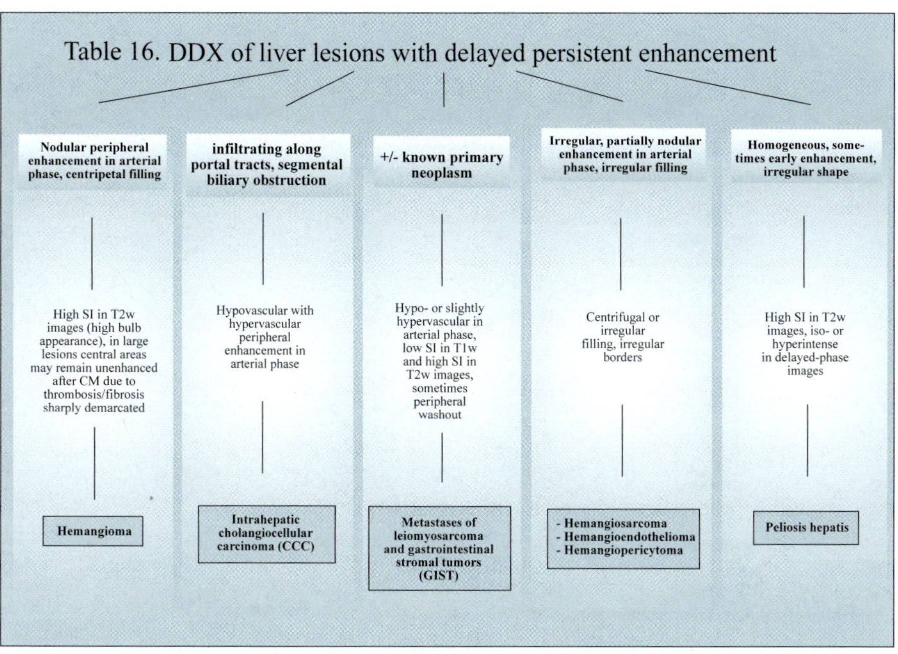

Table 16. DDX of liver lesions with delayed persistent enhancement

Nodular peripheral enhancement in arterial phase, centripetal filling

infiltrating along portal tracts, segmental biliary obstruction

+/- known primary neoplasm

Irregular, partially nodular enhancement in arterial phase, irregular filling

Homogeneous, sometimes early enhancement, irregular shape

High SI in T2w images (high bulb appearance), in large lesions central areas may remain unenhanced after CM due to thrombosis/fibrosis sharply demarcated

Hypovascular with hypervascular peripheral enhancement in arterial phase

Hypo- or slightly hypervascular in arterial phase, low SI in T1w and high SI in T2w images, sometimes peripheral washout

Centrifugal or irregular filling, irregular borders

High SI in T2w images, iso- or hyperintense in delayed-phase images

Hemangioma

Intrahepatic cholangiocellular carcinoma (CCC)

Metastases of leiomyosarcoma and gastrointestinal stromal tumors (GIST)

- Hemangiosarcoma
- Hemangioendothelioma
- Hemangiopericytoma

Peliosis hepatis

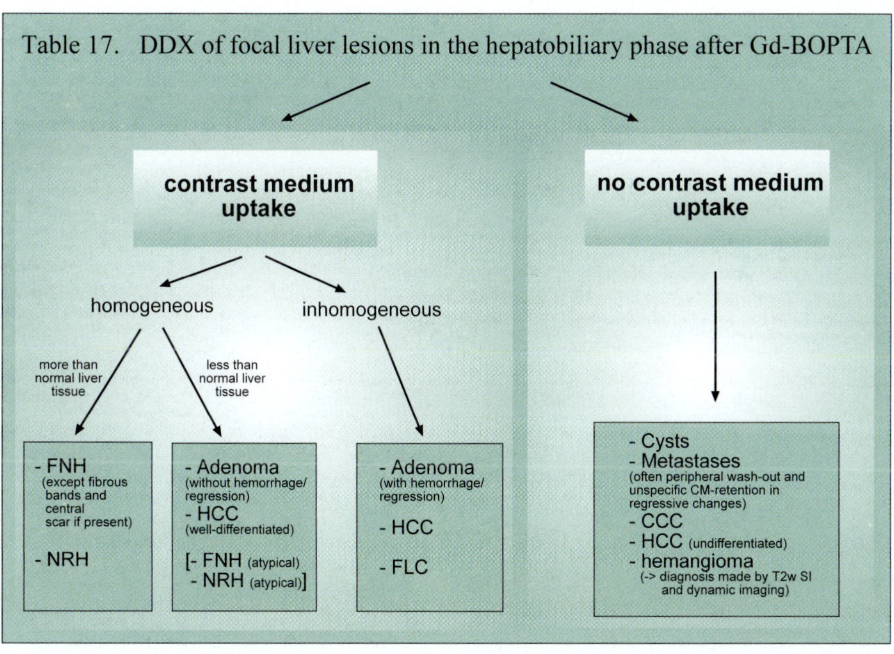

Table 17.   DDX of focal liver lesions in the hepatobiliary phase after Gd-BOPTA

contrast medium uptake

no contrast medium uptake

homogeneous

inhomogeneous

more than normal liver tissue

less than normal liver tissue

- FNH
(except fibrous bands and central scar if present)

- NRH

- Adenoma
(without hemorrhage/ regression)
- HCC
(well-differentiated)

[- FNH (atypical)
- NRH (atypical)]

- Adenoma
(with hemorrhage/ regression)

- HCC

- FLC

- Cysts
- Metastases
(often peripheral wash-out and unspecific CM-retention in regressive changes)
- CCC
- HCC (undifferentiated)
- hemangioma
(-> diagnosis made by T2w SI and dynamic imaging)

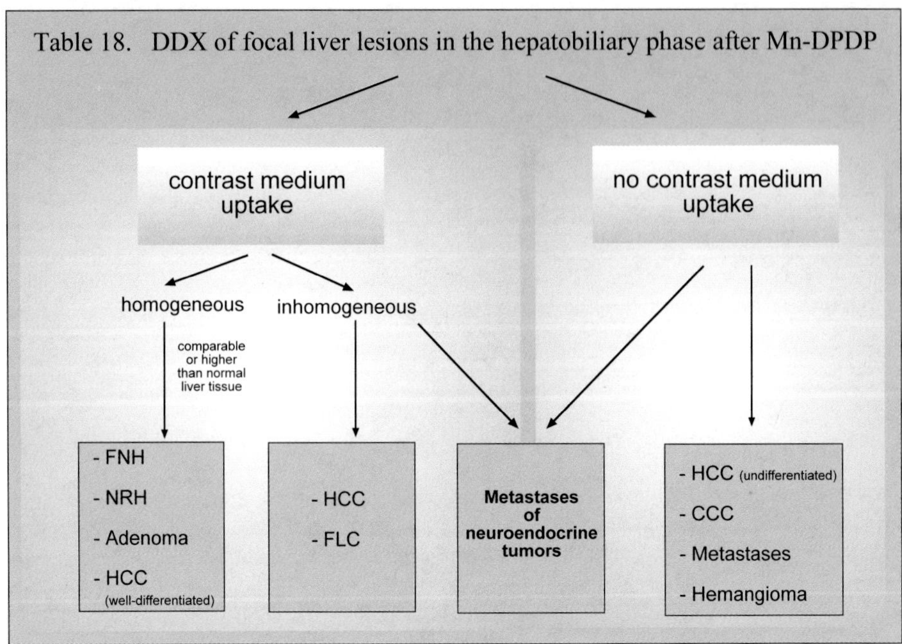

Table 18.   DDX of focal liver lesions in the hepatobiliary phase after Mn-DPDP
contrast medium uptake
no contrast medium uptake
homogeneous
inhomogeneous
comparable or higher than normal liver tissue
- FNH
- NRH
- Adenoma
- HCC (well-differentiated)
- HCC
- FLC
Metastases of neuroendocrine tumors
- HCC (undifferentiated)
- CCC
- Metastases
- Hemangioma

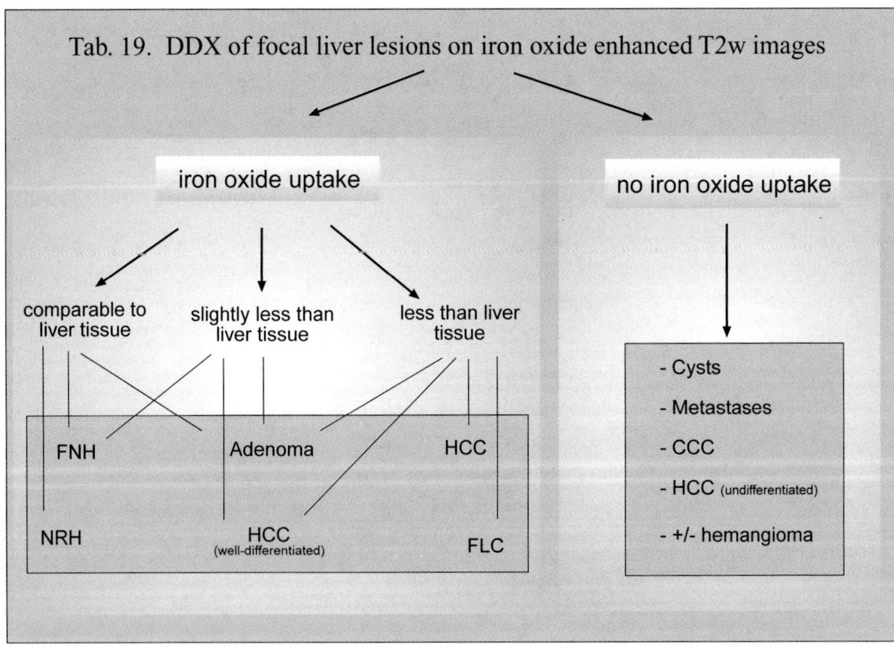

Tab. 19.   DDX of focal liver lesions on iron oxide enhanced T2w images
iron oxide uptake
no iron oxide uptake
comparable to liver tissue
slightly less than liver tissue
less than liver tissue
FNH
Adenoma
HCC
NRH
HCC (well-differentiated)
FLC
- Cysts
- Metastases
- CCC
- HCC (undifferentiated)
- +/- hemangioma

References

1. Ahlman H, Westberg G, Wangberg B, Nilsson O, Tylen U, Schersten T, Tisell LE. Treatment of liver metastases of carcinoid tumors. World J Surg 1996 Feb;20(2):196-202
2. Akinoglu A, Demiryurek H, Guzel C. Alveolar hydatid disease of the liver: a report on thirty-nine surgical cases in eastern Anatolia, Turkey. Am J Trop Med Hyg 1991 Aug;45(2):182-9
3. Allaire GS, Rabin L, Ishak KG, Sesterhenn IA. Bile duct adenoma. A study of 152 cases. Am J Surg Pathol 1988 Sep;12(9):708-15
4. Alvar J, Gutierrez-Solar B, Molina R, Lopez-Velez R, Garcia-Camacho A, Martinez P, Laguna F, Cercenado E, Galmes A. Prevalence of Leishmania infection among AIDS patients. Lancet 1992 Jun 6;339(8806):1427
5. Anderson JB, Cooper MJ, Williamson RC. Adenocarcinoma of the extrahepatic biliary tree. Ann R Coll Surg Engl 1985 May;67(3):139-43
6. Andrade ZA, Peixoto E, Guerret S, Grimaud JA. Hepatic connective tissue changes in hepatosplenic schistosomiasis. Hum Pathol 1992 May;23(5):566-73
7. Angulo P. Nonalcoholic fatty liver disease. N Engl J Med 2002 Apr 18;346(16):1221-31
8. Anonymious. Hepatocellular cancer: differences between high and low incidence regions. Lancet 1987 Nov 21;2(8569):1183-4
9. Anthony PP. Primary carcinoma of the liver: a study of 282 cases in Ugandan Africans. J Pathol 1973 May;110(1):37-48
10. Anthony PP. A guide to the histological identification of fungi in tissues. J Clin Pathol 1973 Nov;26(11):828-31
11. Anthony PP. Inflammatory pseudotumour (plasma cell granuloma) of lung, liver and other organs. Histopathology 1993 Nov;23(5):501-3
12. Anthony PP, Vogel CL, Barker LF. Liver cell dysplasia: a premalignant condition. J Clin Pathol 1973 Mar;26(3):217-23
13. Anthony PP, Ishak KG, Nayak NC, Poulsen HE, Scheuer PJ, Sobin LH. The morphology of cirrhosis: definition, nomenclature, and classification. Bull World Health Organ 1977;55(4):521-40
14. Anthony PP, Ishak KG, Nayak NC, Poulsen HE, Scheuer PJ, Sobin LH. The morphology of cirrhosis. Recommendations on definition, nomenclature, and classification by a working group sponsored by the World Health Organization. J Clin Pathol 1978 May;31(5):395-414
15. Baker L, Winegrad AI. Fasting hypoglycaemia and metabolic acidosis associated with deficiency of hepatic fructose-1,6-diphosphatase activity. Lancet 1970 Jul 4;2(7662):13-6
16. Baum JK, Bookstein JJ, Holtz F, Klein EW. Possible association between benign hepatomas and oral contraceptives. Lancet 1973 Oct 27;2(7835):926-9
17. Beaugerie L, Teilhac MF, Deluol AM, Fritsch J, Girard PM, Rozenbaum W, Le Quintrec Y, Chatelet FP. Cholangiopathy associated with Microsporidia infection of the common bile duct mucosa in a patient with HIV infection. Ann Intern Med 1992 Sep 1;117(5):401-2
18. Belamaric J. Intrahepatic bile duct carcinoma and C. sinensis infection in Hong Kong. Cancer 1973 Feb;31(2):468-73
19. Belli L, Romani F, Sansalone CV, Aseni P, Rondinara G. Portal thrombosis in cirrhotics. A retrospective analysis. Ann Surg 1986 Mar;203(3):286-91
20. Bloustein PA, Silverberg SG. Squamous cell carcinoma originating in an hepatic cyst. Case report with a review of the hepatic cyst-carcinoma association. Cancer 1976 Nov;38(5):2002-5
21. Blyth H, Ockenden BG. Polycystic disease of kidney and liver presenting in childhood. J Med Genet 1971 Sep;8(3):257-84
22. Bonacini M, Kanel G, Alamy M. Duodenal and hepatic toxoplasmosis in a patient with HIV infection: review of the literature. Am J Gastroenterol 1996 Sep;91(9):1838-40
23. Brooks SE, Miller CG, McKenzie K, Audretsch JJ, Bras G. Acute veno-occlusive disease of the liver. Fine structure in Jamaican children. Arch Pathol 1970 Jun;89(6):507-20
24. Bruneton JN, Kerboul P, Drouillard J, Menu Y, Normand F, Santini N. Hepatic lipomas: ultrasound and computed tomographic findings. Gastrointest Radiol 1987;12(4):299-303
25. Bryan RT, Schantz PM. Echinococcosis (hydatid disease). J Am Vet Med Assoc 1989 Nov 1;195(9):1214-7
26. Buhler H, Pirovino M, Akobiantz A, Altorfer J, Weitzel M, Maranta E, Schmid M. Regression of liver cell adenoma. A follow-up study of three consecutive patients after discontinuation of oral contraceptive use. Gastroenterology 1982 Apr;82(4):775-82
27. Caccamo D, Pervez NK, Marchevsky A. Primary lymphoma of the liver in the acquired immunodeficiency syndrome. Arch Pathol Lab Med 1986 Jun;110(6):553-5
28. Caroli J. Diseases of the intrahepatic biliary tree. Clin Gastroenterol 1973 Jan;2(1):147-61
29. Carrillo EH, Richardson JD. The current management of hepatic trauma. Adv Surg 2001;35:39-59
30. Carrillo EH, Wohltmann C, Richardson JD, Polk HC Jr. Evolution in the treatment of complex blunt liver injuries. Curr Probl Surg 2001 Jan;38(1):1-60

31. Casteels-Van Daele M, Van Geet C, Wouters C, Eggermont E. Reye's syndrome. Lancet 2001 Jul 28;358(9278):334

32. Chapman RW. Aetiology and natural history of primary sclerosing cholangitis—a decade of progress? Gut 1991 Dec;32(12):1433-5

33. Chen V, Hamilton J, Qizilbash A. Hepatic infarction. A clinicopathologic study of seven cases. Arch Pathol Lab Med 1976 Jan;100(1):32-6

34. Cheuk W, Woo PCY, Yuen KY, Yu PH, Chan JKC, Intestinal inflammatory pseudotumour with regional lymph node involvement: identification of a new bacterium as the aetiological agent. J Pathol 2000; 192: 289-292.

35. Chuang VP, Wallace S. Hepatic artery embolization in the treatment of hepatic neoplasms. Radiology 1981 Jul;140(1):51-8

36. Coffin CM, Humphrey PA, Dehner LP. Extrapulmonary inflammatory myofibroblastic tumor: a clinical and pathological survey. Semin Diagn Pathol. 1998; 15: 85-101

37. Cozzi PJ, Abu-Jawdeh GM, Green RM, Green D. Amyloidosis in association with human immunodeficiency virus infection. Clin Infect Dis 1992 Jan;14(1):189-91

38. Craig JR, Peters RL, Edmondson HA, Omata M. Fibrolamellar carcinoma of the liver: a tumor of adolescents and young adults with distinctive clinico-pathologic features. Cancer 1980 Jul 15;46(2):372-9

39. Culp KS, Fleming CR, Duffy J, Baldus WP, Dickson ER. Autoimmune associations in primary biliary cirrhosis. Mayo Clin Proc 1982 Jun;57(6):365-70

40. Culvenor CC, Edgar JA, Smith LW, Kumana CR, Lin HJ. Heliotropium lasiocarpum Fisch and Mey identified as cause of veno-occlusive disease due to a herbal tea. Lancet 1986 Apr 26;1(8487):978

41. Czapar CA, Weldon-Linne CM, Moore DM, Rhone DP. Peliosis hepatis in the acquired immunodeficiency syndrome. Arch Pathol Lab Med 1986 Jul;110(7):611-3

42. Da Silva LC, Carrilho FJ. Hepatosplenic schistosomiasis. Pathophysiology and treatment. Gastroenterol Clin North Am 1992 Mar;21(1):163-77

43. Daldrup HE, Reimer P, Rummeny EJ, Fischer H, Bocker W, Peters PE. The regression of a hepatocellular adenoma after the withdrawal of hormonal contraception. Rofo Fortschr Geb Rontgenstr Neuen Bildgeb Verfahr 1995 Nov;163(5):449-51

44. David Richardson J, Franklin GA, Lukan JK, Carrillo EH, Spain DA, Miller FB, Wilson MA, Polk HC Jr, Flint LM. Evolution in the management of hepatic trauma: a 25-year perspective. Ann Surg 2000 Sep;232(3):324-30

45. De Groote J. Classification of Chronic Hepatitis. Ann Clin Res 1976 Jun;8(3):130-8

46. Dehner LP, Ishak KG. Vascular tumors of the liver in infants and children. A study of 30 cases an review of the literature. Arch Pathol 1971 Aug;92(2):101-11

47. Dehner LP. The enigmatic inflammatory pseudotumour: the current state of our understanding or misunderstanding. J Pathol. 2000. Nov, 192(3): 277-9

48. Delas N, Faurel JP, Wechsler B, Adotti F, Leroy O, Lemerez M. Association of peliosis and necrotizing vasculitis. Nouv Presse Med 1982 Sep 25;11(37):2787

49. DeMaioribus CA, Lally KP, Sim K, Isaacs H, Mahour GH. Mesenchymal hamartoma of the liver. A 35-year review. Arch Surg 1990 May;125(5):598-600

50. Desmet VJ. Cholangiopathies: past, present, and future. Semin Liver Dis 1987 May;7(2):67-76

51. Devaney K, Goodman ZD, Epstein MS, Zimmerman HJ, Ishak KG. Hepatic sarcoidosis. Clinicopathologic features in 100 patients. Am J Surg Pathol 1993 Dec;17(12):1272-80

52. Deziel DJ, Rossi RL, Munson JL, Braasch JW, Silverman ML. Management of bile duct cysts in adults. Arch Surg 1986 Apr;121(4):410-5

53. Di Bisceglie AM. Hepatitis C and hepatocellular carcinoma. Semin Liver Dis 1995 Feb;15(1):64-9

54. Dietze O, Davies SE, Williams R, Portmann B. Malignant epithelioid haemangioendothelioma of the liver: a clinicopathological and histochemical study of 12 cases. Histopathology 1989 Sep;15(3):225-37

55. Ducreux M, Lartigau E, Eschwege F, Etienne JP. Radiotherapy of malignant tumors of the liver. Gastroenterol Clin Biol 1995 Apr;19(4):350-60

56. Edwards CQ, Dadone MM, Skolnick MH, Kushner JP. Hereditary haemochromatosis. Clin Haematol 1982 Jun;11(2):411-35

57. Fajardo LF, Colby TV. Pathogenesis of veno-occlusive liver disease after radiation. Arch Pathol Lab Med 1980 Nov;104(11):584-8

58. Farber E. Hepatocyte proliferation in stepwise development of experimental liver cell cancer. Dig Dis Sci 1991 Jul;36(7):973-8

59. Ferrell L, Wright T, Lake J, Roberts J, Ascher N. Incidence and diagnostic features of macroregenerative nodules vs. small hepatocellular carcinoma in cirrhotic livers. Hepatology 1992 Dec;16(6):1372-8

60. Foster JH, Berman MM. The malignant transformation of liver cell adenomas. Arch Surg 1994 Jul;129(7):712-7

61. Foster JH, Donohue TA, Berman MM. Familial liver-cell adenomas and diabetes mellitus. N Engl J Med 1978 Aug 3;299(5):239-41

62. Froesch ER, Wolf HP, Baitsch H. Hereditary fructose intolerance. An inborn defect of hepatic fructose-1-phosphatase splitting aldolase. Am J Med 1963;34:151-167

63. Furuta T, Yoshida Y, Saku M, Honda H, Muranaka T, Oshiumi Y, Kanematsu T, Sugimachi K. Treatment of symptomatic non-parasitic liver cysts—surgical treatment versus alcohol injection therapy. HPB Surg 1990 Oct;2(4):269-77; discussion 277-9

64. Gang DL, Herrin JT. Infantile polycystic disease of the liver and kidneys. Clin Nephrol 1986 Jan;25(1):28-36

65. Gonzalez A, Canga F, Cardenas F, Castellano G, Garcia H, Cuenca B, Sanchez F, Solis-Herruzo JA. An unusual case of hepatic adenoma in a male. J Clin Gastroenterol 1994 Sep;19(2):179-81

66. Goodman ZD, Ishak KG. Angiomyolipomas of the liver. Am J Surg Pathol 1984 Oct;8(10):745-50

67. Grasso S, Manusia M, Sciacca F. Unusual liver lesion in tuberous sclerosis. Arch Pathol Lab Med 1982 Jan;106(1):49

68. Greenstein AJ, Lowenthal D, Hammer GS, Schaffner F, Aufses AH Jr. Continuing changing patterns of disease in pyogenic liver abscess: a study of 38 patients. Am J Gastroenterol 1984 Mar;79(3):217-26

69. Grundy P, Ellis R. Histiocytosis X: a review of the etiology, pathology, staging, and therapy. Med Pediatr Oncol 1986;14(1):45-50

70. Guo KJ, Yamaguchi K, Enjoji M. Undifferentiated carcinoma of the gallbladder. A clinicopathologic, histochemical, and immunohistochemical study of 21 patients with a poor prognosis. Cancer 1988 May 1;61(9):1872-9

71. Hadjis NS, Blumgart LH. Clinical aspects of liver atrophy. J Clin Gastroenterol 1989 Feb;11(1):3-7

72. Haratake J, Koide O, Takeshita H. Hepatic lymphangiomatosis: report of two cases, with an immunohistochemical study. Am J Gastroenterol 1992 Jul;87(7):906-9

73. Harding CV. Blastomycosis and opportunistic infections in patients with acquired immunodeficiency syndrome. An autopsy study. Arch Pathol Lab Med 1991 Nov; 115(11): 1133-6

74. Hasan FA, Jeffers LJ, Welsh SW, Reddy KR, Schiff ER. Hepatic involvement as the primary manifestation of Kaposi's sarcoma in the acquired immune deficiency syndrome. Am J Gastroenterol 1989 Nov;84(11):1449-51

75. Hoe AL, Royle GT, Taylor I. Breast liver metastases—incidence, diagnosis and outcome. J R Soc Med 1991 Dec;84(12):714-6

76. Horowitz ME, Etcubanas E, Webber BL, Kun LE, Rao BN, Vogel RJ, Pratt CB. Hepatic undifferentiated (embryonal) sarcoma and rhabdomyosarcoma in children. Results of therapy. Cancer 1987 Feb 1;59(3):396-402

77. Ishak KG, Glunz PR. Hepatoblastoma and hepatocarcinoma in infancy and childhood. Report of 47 cases. Cancer 1967 Mar;20(3):396-422

78. Ishak KG, Rabin L. Benign tumors of the liver. Med Clin North Am 1975 Jul;59(4):995-1013

79. Ishak KG, Willis GW, Cummins SD, Bullock AA. Biliary cystadenoma and cystadenocarcinoma: report of 14 cases and review the literature. Cancer 1977 Jan;39(1):322-38

80. Ishak KG, Sesterhenn IA, Goodman ZD, Rabin L, Stromeyer FW. Epithelioid hemangioendothelioma of the liver: a clinicopathologic and follow-up study of 32 cases. Hum Pathol 1984 Sep;15(9):839-52

81. Ishak KG, Anthony PP, Sobin LH. Histological typing of tumours of the liver. World Health Organization International Histological Classification of Tumours, 2nd edn. Berlin: Springer-Verlag, 1994.

82. Isselbacher KJ, Anderson ER, Kurakoski K, Kalckar HM. Congenital galactosemia, a single enzymatic block in galactose metabolism. Science 1956; 123: 635

83. Jaffe ES. Malignant lymphomas: pathology of hepatic involvement. Semin Liver Dis 1987 Aug;7(3):257-68

84. Jones RS. Carcinoma of the gallbladder. Surg Clin North Am 1990 Dec;70(6):1419-28

85. Kaplan LD, Kahn J, Jacobson M, Bottles K, Cello J. Primary bile duct lymphoma in the acquired immunodeficiency syndrome (AIDS). Ann Intern Med 1989 Jan 15;110(2):161-2

86. Kaplan MM. Primary biliary cirrhosis. N Engl J Med 1987 Feb 26;316(9):521-8

87. Karasawa T, Itoh K, Komukai M, Ozawa U, Sakurai I, Shikata T. Squamous cell carcinoma of gallbladder—report of two cases and review of literature. Acta Pathol Jpn 1981 Mar;31(2):299-308

88. Kerlin P, Davis GL, McGill DB, Weiland LH, Adson MA, Sheedy PF 2nd. Hepatic adenoma and focal nodular hyperplasia: clinical, pathologic, and radiologic features.Gastroenterology 1983 May;84(5 Pt 1):994-1002

89. Khuroo MS, Zargar SA, Mahajan R. Hepatobiliary and pancreatic ascariasis in India. Lancet 1990 Jun 23;335(8704):1503-6

90. Kim H, Dorfman RF. Morphological studies of 84 untreated patients subjected to laparotomy for the staging of non-Hodgkin's lymphomas. Cancer 1974 Mar;33(3):657-74

91. Klatskin G. Adenocarcinoma of the hepatic duct at its bifurcation within the porta hepatis. Am J Med 1965; 38: 241-256.

92. Klein AS, Sitzmann JV, Coleman J, Herlong FH, Cameron JL. Current management of the Budd-Chiari syndrome. Ann Surg 1990 Aug;212(2):144-9

93. Koga A, Ichimiya H, Yamaguchi K, Miyazaki K, Nakayama F. Hepatolithiasis associated with cholangiocarcinoma. Possible etiologic significance. Cancer 1985 Jun 15;55(12):2826-9

94. Kurathong S, Lerdverasirikul P, Wongpaitoon V, Pramoolsinsap C, Kanjanapitak A, Varavithya W,

Phuapradit P, Bunyaratvej S, Upatham ES, Brockelman WY. Opisthorchis viverrini infection and cholangiocarcinoma. A prospective, case-controlled study. Gastroenterology 1985 Jul;89(1):151-6

95. Lack EE, Neave C, Vawter GF. Hepatoblastoma. A clinical and pathologic study of 54 cases. Am J Surg Pathol 1982 Dec;6(8):693-705

96. Landing BH, Wells TR, Claireaux AE. Morphometric analysis of liver lesions in cystic diseases of childhood. Hum Pathol 1980 Sep;11(5 Suppl):549-60

97. Lefkowitch JH, Falkow S, Whitlock RT. Hepatic Hodgkin's disease simulating cholestatic hepatitis with liver failure. Arch Pathol Lab Med. 1985 May;109(5):424-6.

98. Lewis WD, Jenkins RL, Rossi RL, Munson L, ReMine SG, Cady B, Braasch JW, McDermott WV. Surgical treatment of biliary cystadenoma. A report of 15 cases. Arch Surg 1988 May;123(5):563-8

99. Ley TJ, Griffith P, Nienhuis AW. Transfusion haemosiderosis and chelation therapy. Clin Haematol 1982 Jun;11(2):437-64

100. Libbrecht L, Craninx M, Nevens F, Desmet V, Roskams T. Predictive value of liver cell dysplasia for development of hepatocellular carcinoma in patients with non-cirrhotic and cirrhotic chronic viral hepatitis. Histopathology 2001 Jul;39(1):66-73

101. Logani S, Lucas DR, Cheng JD, Ioachim HL, Adsay NV. Spindle cell tumours associated with mycobacteria in lymph nodes of HIV-positive patients: 'Kaposi sarcoma with mycobacteria' and 'mycobacterial pseudotumour'. Am J Surg Pathol; 23: 656-661.

102. Lorenz M, Wiesner J, Staib-Sebler E, Encke A. Regional therapy breast cancer liver metastases. Zentralbl Chir 1995;120(10):786-90

103. Lucas SB, Hounnou A, Peacock C, Beaumel A, Djomand G, N'Gbichi JM, Yeboue K, Honde M, Diomande M, Giordano C, et al. The mortality and pathology of HIV infection in a west African city. AIDS 1993 Dec;7(12):1569-79

104. Ludwig J, MacCarty RL, LaRusso NF, Krom RA, Wiesner RH. Intrahepatic cholangiectases and large-duct obliteration in primary sclerosing cholangitis. Hepatology 1986 Jul-Aug;6(4):560-8

105. Mackay IR, Gershwin ME. Primary biliary cirrhosis: current knowledge, perspectives, and future directions. Semin Liver Dis 1989 May;9(2):149-57

106. Massenkeil G, Opravil M, Salfinger M, von Graevenitz A, Luthy R. Disseminated coinfection with Mycobacterium avium complex and Mycobacterium kansasii in a patient with AIDS and liver abscess. Clin Infect Dis 1992 Feb;14(2):618-9

107. Mathieu D, Zafrani ES, Anglade MC, Dhumeaux D. Association of focal nodular hyperplasia and hepatic hemangioma. Gastroenterology 1989 Jul;97(1):154-7

108. Matsumoto J, Kondo S, Okushiba S, Morikawa T, Sugiura H, Omi A, Hirano S, Ambo Y, Katoh H, Fujita M, Shimizu M. Biliary cystadenocarcinoma with superficial spread to the extrahepatic bile duct. Hepatogastroenterology 2001 May-Jun;48(39):647-9

109. McCullough AJ, Fleming CR, Thistle JL, Baldus WP, Ludwig J, McCall JT, Dickson ER. Diagnosis of Wilson's disease presenting as fulminant hepatic failure. Gastroenterology 1983 Jan;84(1):161-7

110. McGowan I, Hawkins AS, Weller IV. The natural history of cryptosporidial diarrhoea in HIV-infected patients.AIDS 1993 Mar;7(3):349-54

111. McLean CA, Pedersen JS. Endocrine cell carcinoma of the gallbladder. Histopathology 1991 Aug;19(2):173-6

112. Melnick PJ. Polycystic liver. Arch Pathol 1955; 59: 162-172

113. Mercadier M, Chigot JP, Clot JP, Langlois P, Lansiaux P. Caroli's disease. World J Surg 1984 Feb;8(1):22-9

114. Mitchell MC, Boitnott JK, Kaufman S, Cameron JL, Maddrey WC. Budd-Chiari syndrome: etiology, diagnosis and management. Medicine (Baltimore) 1982 Jul;61(4):199-218

115. Moertel CG, Fleming TR, Macdonald JS, Haller DG, Laurie JA, Goodman PJ, Ungerleider JS, Emerson WA, Tormey DC, Glick JH, et al. Levamisole and fluorouracil for adjuvant therapy of resected colon carcinoma. N Engl J Med 1990 Feb 8;322(6):352-8

116. Moertel CG, Johnson CM, McKusick MA, Martin JK Jr, Nagorney DM, Kvols LK, Rubin J, Kunselman S. The management of patients with advanced carcinoid tumors and islet cell carcinomas. Ann Intern Med 1994 Feb 15;120(4):302-9

117. Moses SW. Pathophysiology and dietary treatment of the glycogen storage diseases. J Pediatr Gastroenterol Nutr 1990 Aug;11(2):155-74

118. Nakanuma Y. Nodular regenerative hyperplasia of the liver: retrospective survey in autopsy series. J Clin Gastroenterol 1990 Aug;12(4):460-5

119. Nakhleh RE, Glock M, Snover DC. Hepatic pathology of chronic granulomatous disease of childhood. Arch Pathol Lab Med 1992 Jan;116(1):71-5

120. Nezelof C, Frileux-Herbet F, Cronier-Sachot J. Disseminated histiocytosis X: analysis of prognostic factors based on a retrospective study of 50 cases. Cancer 1979 Nov;44(5):1824-38

121. Nichols FC 3rd, van Heerden JA, Weiland LH. Benign liver tumors. Surg Clin North Am1989 Apr;69(2):297-314

122. Nishizaki T, Kanematsu T, Matsumata T, Yasunaga C, Kakizoe S, Sugimachi K. Myelolipoma of the liver. A case report. Cancer 1989 Mar 1;63(5):930-4

123. Odievre M, Gentil C, Gautier M, Alagille D. Hereditary fructose intolerance in childhood. Diagnosis, management, and course in 55 patients. Am J Dis Child 1978 Jun;132(6):605-8

124. Okulski EG, Dolin BJ, Kandawalla NM. Intrahepatic biliary papillomatosis. Arch Pathol Lab Med 1979 Nov;103(12):647-9

125. Popper H, Thomas LB, Telles NC, Falk H, Selikoff IJ. Development of hepatic angiosarcoma in man induced by vinyl chloride, thorotrast, and arsenic. Comparison with cases of unknown etiology. Am J Pathol 1978 Aug;92(2):349-69

126. Proujansky R, Vinton N. Acute Hepatitis. Adolesc Med 1995 Oct;6(3):437-446

127. Qizilbash A, Kontozoglou T, Sianos J, Scully K. Hepar lobatum associated with chemotherapy and metastatic breast cancer. Arch Pathol Lab Med 1987 Jan;111(1):58-61

128. Rabinovitz M, Gavaler JS, Schade RR, Dindzans VJ, Chien MC, Van Thiel DH. Does primary sclerosing cholangitis occurring in association with inflammatory bowel disease differ from that occurring in the absence of inflammatory bowel disease? A study of sixty-six subjects. Hepatology 1990 Jan;11(1):7-11

129. Rakela J, Kurtz SB, McCarthy JT, Ludwig J, Ascher NL, Bloomer JR, Claus PL. Fulminant Wilson's disease treated with postdilution hemofiltration and orthotopic liver transplantation. Gastroenterology 1986 Jun;90(6):2004-7

130. Ramos A, Torres VE, Holley KE, Offord KP, Rakela J, Ludwig J. The liver in autosomal dominant polycystic kidney disease. Implications for pathogenesis. Arch Pathol Lab Med 1990 Feb;114(2):180-4

131. Rappaport AM, MacPhee PJ, Fisher MM, Phillips MJ. The scarring of the liver acini (Cirrhosis). Tridimensional and microcirculatory considerations. Virchows Arch A Pathol Anat Histopathol 1983;402(2):107-37

132. Reye RDK, Morgan G, Baral J. Encephalopathy and fatty degeneration of the viscera, a disease entity in chikdhood. Lancet 1963;2:749-752

133. Reynolds TB, Denison EK, Frankl HD, Lieberman FL, Peters RL. Primary biliary cirrhosis with scleroderma, Raynaud's phenomenon and telangiectasia. New syndrome. Am J Med 1971 Mar;50(3):302-12

134. Reynolds WJ, Wanless IR. Nodular regenerative hyperplasia of the liver in a patient with rheumatoid vasculitis: a morphometric study suggesting a role for hepatic arteritis in the pathogenesis. J Rheumatol 1984 Dec;11(6):838-42

135. Riegler JL. Preneoplastic conditions of the liver. Semin Gastrointest Dis 1996 Apr;7(2):74-87

136. Rossi RL, Silverman ML, Braasch JW, Munson JL, ReMine SG. Carcinomas arising in cystic conditions of the bile ducts. A clinical and pathologic study. Ann Surg 1987 Apr;205(4):377-84

137. Rubin E, Popper H. The evolution of human cirrhosis deduced from observations in experimental animals. Medicine (Baltimore) 1967 Mar;46(2):163-83

138. Ruers T, Bleichrodt RP. Treatment of liver metastases, an update on the possibilities and results. Eur J Cancer 2002 May;38(7):1023-33

139. Ryan J, Straus DJ, Lange C, Filippa DA, Botet JF, Sanders LM, Shiu MH, Fortner JG. Primary lymphoma of the liver. Cancer 1988 Jan 15;61(2):370-5

140. Ryman BE. The glycogen storage diseases. J Clin Pathol Suppl (R Coll Pathol) 1974;8:106-21

141. Saegusa M, Takano Y, Okudaira M. Human hepatic infarction: histopathological and postmortem angiological studies. Liver 1993 Oct;13(5):239-45

142. Sakamoto M, Hirohashi S, Shimosato Y. Early stages of multistep hepatocarcinogenesis: adenomatous hyperplasia and early hepatocellular carcinoma. Hum Pathol 1991 Feb;22(2):172-8

143. Sanfelippo PM, Beahrs OH, Weiland LH. Cystic disease of the liver. Ann Surg 1974 Jun;179(6):922-5

144. Schafer AI, Cheron RG, Dluhy R, Cooper B, Gleason RE, Soeldner JS, Bunn HF. Clinical consequences of acquired transfusional iron overload in adults. N Engl J Med 1981 Feb 5;304(6):319-24

145. Scheele J, Stang R, Altendorf-Hofmann A, Paul M. Resection of colorectal liver metastases. World J Surg 1995 Jan-Feb;19(1):59-71

146. Scheinberg IH, Sternlieb I, Schilsky M, Stockert RJ. Penicillamine may detoxify copper in Wilson's disease. Lancet 1987 Jul 11;2(8550):95

147. Scheuer PJ. Liver biopsy in the diagnosis of cirrhosis. Gut 1970 Mar;11(3):275-8

148. Schulz W, Borchard F. The size of the liver metastases in a low metastatic count. A quantitative study of postmortem livers. Rofo Fortschr Geb Rontgenstr Neuen Bildgeb Verfahr 1992. Apr;156(4):320-4

149. Scoazec JY, Marche C, Girard PM, Houtmann J, Durand-Schneider AM, Saimot AG, Benhamou JP, Feldmann G. Peliosis hepatis and sinusoidal dilation during infection by the human immunodeficiency virus (HIV). An ultrastructural study. Am J Pathol 1988 Apr;131(1):38-47

150. Scoazec JY, Degott C, Brousse N, Barge J, Molas G, Potet F, Benhamou JP. Non-Hodgkin's lymphoma presenting as a primary tumor of the liver: presentation, diagnosis and outcome in eight patients. Hepatology 1991 May;13(5):870-5

151. Scobie BA, Summerskill WHJ. Hepatic cirrhosis secondary to obstruction of the biliary system. Am J Dig Dis 1965;10:135-146

152. Selinger M, Koff RS. Thorotrast and the liver: a reminder. Gastroenterology 1975 Apr;68(4 Pt 1):799-803

153. Senninger N, Langer R, Klar E, Otto G, Kraus T, Baas J, Herfarth C. Liver transplantation for hepatocellular carcinoma. Transplant Proc 1996 Jun;28(3):1706-7

154. Shortell CK, Schwartz SI. Hepatic adenoma and focal nodular hyperplasia. Surg Gynecol Obstet 1991 Nov;173(5):426-31

155. Simon DM, Krause R, Galambos JT. Peliosis hepatis in a patient with marasmus. Gastroenterology 1988 Sep;95(3):805-9

156. Smetana HF, Olen Olen E. Hereditary galactose disease. Am J Clin Pathol 1962;38:3-25

157. Stanley P, Geer GD, Miller JH, Gilsanz V, Landing BH, Boechat IM. Infantile hepatic hemangiomas. Clinical features, radiologic investigations and treatment of 20 patients. Cancer 1989 Aug 15;64(4):936-49

158. Steele G Jr, Ravikumar TS, Benotti PN. New surgical treatments for recurrent colorectal cancer. Cancer 1990 Feb 1;65(3 Suppl):723-30

159. Sternlieb I. Evolution of the hepatic lesion in Wilson's disease (hepatolenticular degeneration). Prog Liver Dis 1972;4:511-25

160. Stocker JT, Ishak KG. Undifferentiated (embryonal) sarcoma of the liver: report of 31 cases. Cancer 1978 Jul;42(1):336-48

161. Stocker JT, Ishak KG. Mesenchymal hamartoma of the liver: report of 30 cases and review of the literature. Pediatr Pathol 1983 Jul-Sep;1(3):245-67

162. Stromeyer FW, Ishak KG. Histology of the liver in Wilson's disease: a study of 34 cases. Am J Clin Pathol 1980 Jan;73(1):12-24

163. Tamburro CH. Relationship of vinyl monomers and liver cancers: angiosarcoma and hepatocellular carcinoma. Semin Liver Dis 1984 May;4(2):158-69

164. Tavill AS, Wood EJ, Kreel L, Jones EA, Gregory M, Sherlock S. The Budd-Chiari syndrome: correlation between hepatic scintigraphy and the clinical, radiological, and pathological findings in nineteen cases of hepatic venous outflow obstruction. Gastroenterology 1975 Mar;68(3):509-18

165. Terada T, Terasaki S, Nakanuma Y. A clinicopathologic study of adenomatous hyperplasia of the liver in 209 consecutive cirrhotic livers examined by autopsy. Cancer 1993 Sep 1;72(5):1551-6

166. Trampert L, Benz P, Ruth T, Oberhausen E. Nuclear medicine diagnosis of focal liver lesions. Nuklearmedizin 1993 Aug;32(4):174-7

167. Ueyama T, Ding J, Hashimoto H, Tsuneyoshi M, Enjoji M. Carcinoid tumor arising in the wall of a congenital bile duct cyst. Arch Pathol Lab Med 1992 Mar;116(3):291-3

168. Valla D, Casadevall N, Huisse MG, Tulliez M, Grange JD, Muller O, Binda T, Varet B, Rueff B, Benhamou JP. Etiology of portal vein thrombosis in adults. A prospective evaluation of primary myeloproliferative disorders.Gastroenterology 1988 Apr;94(4):1063-9

169. Valla D, Flejou JF, Lebrec D, Bernuau J, Rueff B, Salzmann JL, Benhamou JP. Portal hypertension and ascites in acute hepatitis: clinical, hemodynamic and histological correlations. Hepatology 1989 Oct;10(4):482-7

170. Van Steenbergen W, Joosten E, Marchal G, Baert A, Vanstapel MJ, Desmet V, Wijnants P, De Groote J. Hepatic lymphangiomatosis. Report of a case and review of the literature. Gastroenterology 1985 Jun;88(6):1968-72

171. Van Wijk HB, Elias EA. Heptatic and rectal pathology in Schistosoma intercalatum infection. Trop Geogr Med 1975 Sep;27(3):237-48

172. Wada K, Kondo F, Kondo Y. Large regenerative nodules and dysplastic nodules in cirrhotic livers: a histopathologic study. Hepatology 1988 Nov-Dec;8(6):1684-8

173. Walker NI, Horn MJ, Strong RW, Lynch SV, Cohen J, Ong TH, Harris OD. Undifferentiated (embryonal) sarcoma of the liver. Pathologic findings and long-term survival after complete surgical resection. Cancer 1992 Jan 1;69(1):52-9

174. Wallace JM, Hannah JB. Mycobacterium avium complex infection in patients with the acquired immunodeficiency syndrome. A clinicopathologic study.Chest 1988 May;93(5):926-32

175. Wang ZG. Recognition and management of Budd-Chiari syndrome. Experience with 143 patients. Chin Med J (Engl) 1989 May;102(5):338-46

176. Wanless IR. Micronodular transformation (nodular regenerative hyperplasia) of the liver: a report of 64 cases among 2,500 autopsies and a new classification of benign hepatocellular nodules. Hepatology 1990 May;11(5):787-97

177. Wanless IR. Portal vein thrombosis is associated with large regenerative nodules and diffuse nodular hyperplasia in cirrhotic livers. Hepatology 1994;20:412A

178. Wanless IR, Albrecht S, Bilbao J, Frei JV, Heathcote EJ, Roberts EA, Chiasson D. Multiple focal nodular hyperplasia of the liver associated with vascular malformations of various organs and neoplasia of the brain: a new syndrome. Mod Pathol 1989 Sep;2(5):456-62

179. Warren KW, Athanassiades S, Monge JI. Primary sclerosing cholangitis. A study of forty-two cases. Am J Surg 1966 Jan;111(1):23-38

180. Warzok R, Seidlitz G. Mucopolysaccharidoses. Genetics, clinical pathology, therapeutic regimes Zentralbl Pathol 1992 Jun;138(3):226-34

181. Watanabe S, Okita K, Harada T, Kodama T, Numa Y, Takemoto T, Takahashi T. Morphologic stud-

ies of the liver cell dysplasia. Cancer 1983 Jun 15;51(12):2197-205
182. Wedig MP, Altmann C. Hormonal contraception and focal nodular hyperplasia. Zentralbl Gynakol 1991;113(24):1399-402
183. Weinberg AG, Finegold MJ. Primary hepatic tumors of childhood. Hum Pathol 1983 Jun;14(6):512-37
184. Weinbren K, Mutum SS. Pathological aspects of diffuse nodular hyperplasia of the liver. J Pathol 1984 Jun;143(2):81-92
185. Weinbren K, Hadjis NS, Blumgart LH. Structural aspects of the liver in patients with biliary disease and portal hypertension. J Clin Pathol 1985 Sep;38(9):1013-20
186. Weitz H, Gokel JM, Loeschke K, Possinger K, Eder M. Veno-occlusive disease of the liver in patients receiving immunosuppressive therapy. Virchows Arch A Pathol Anat Histol 1982;395(3):245-56
187. White JE, Chase CW, Kelley JE, Brock WB, Clark MO, Inflammatory pseudotumour of the liver associated with extrahepatic infection. South Med J 1997; 90: 23-29.
188. Wiesner RH, LaRusso NF. Clinicopathologic features of the syndrome of primary sclerosing cholangitis. Gastroenterology 1980 Aug;79(2):200-6
189. Wiesner RH, LaRusso NF, Ludwig J, Dickson ER. Comparison of the clinicopathologic features of primary sclerosing cholangitis and primary biliary cirrhosis. Gastroenterology 1985 Jan;88(1 Pt 1):108-14
190. Wilkins MJ, Lindley R, Dourakis SP, Goldin RD. Surgical pathology of the liver in HIV infection. Histopathology 1991 May;18(5):459-64
191. Willett CG, Tepper JE, Cohen AM, Orlow E, Welch CE. Failure patterns following curative resection of colonic carcinoma. Ann Surg 1984 Dec;200(6):685-90
192. Yamagata M, Kanematsu T, Matsumata T, Utsunomiya T, Ikeda Y, Sugimachi K. Management of haemangioma of the liver: comparison of results between surgery and observation. Br J Surg 1991 Oct;78(10):1223-5
193. Yasuma T, Yanaka M. Primary sarcoma of the gallbladder—report of three cases. Acta Pathol Jpn 1971 May;21(2):285-304
194. Zafrani ES. Update on vascular tumours of the liver. J Hepatol 1989 Jan;8(1):125-30
195. Zafrani ES, Degos F, Guigui B, Durand-Schneider AM, Martin N, Flandrin G, Benhamou JP, Feldmann G. The hepatic sinusoid in hairy cell leukemia: an ultrastructural study of 12 cases. Hum Pathol 1987 Aug;18(8):801-7
196. Zak FG. Peliosis hepatis. Am J Pathol 1950; 26: 1-15
198. Zavadsky KE, Lee YT. Liver metastases from colorectal carcinoma: incidence, resectability, and survival results. Am Surg 1994 Dec;60(12):929-33
197. Zhang ZD, Myles J, Pai RP, Howard JM. Malignant melanoma of the biliary tract: a case report. Surgery 1991 Mar;109(3 Pt 1):323-8
199. Zieren J, Zieren HU, Muller JM. Liver resections for primary liver malignancies. Personal results and analysis of the literature. Langenbecks Arch Chir 1994;379(3):159-67

4   Imaging of Benign Focal Liver Lesions

Contents

4.1 Primary Benign Liver Lesions

Benign tumors can arise from each of the cellular components of the liver: hepatocytes, biliary epithelium and mesenchymal tissue. The following classification summarizes the cellular origin of the principal lesions:

Hepatocellular origin
    Hepatocellular adenoma
    Hepatocellular hyperplasia
        Focal nodular hyperplasia (FNH)
        Nodular regenerative hyperplasia
Cholangiocellular origin
    Hepatic cyst
        Simple hepatic cyst
        Congenital hepatic fibrosis or polycystic liver disease
    Biliary cystadenoma

Mesenchymal origin
  Mesenchymal hamartoma
  Hemangioma
  Peliosis Hepatis
  Infantile hemangioendothelioma
  Lipoma, Angiomyolipoma, Myelolipoma
  Leiomyoma

Most benign tumors are discovered incidentally during abdominal ultrasonography, and the most common entities are simple cysts, cavernous hemangiomas, FNH and adenomas.

4.1.1 Hemangioma

Hepatic hemangioma is the most common primary liver tumor, the incidence of which in the general population varies in published reports from 0.4–20%. Hemangiomas may be multiple in up to 50% of cases or arise in conjunction with other neoplasms. An association with focal nodular hyperplasia is observed in 15–20% of cases [13, 28, 56].

There are two forms of hemangioma, those that occur in childhood and those that occur in adults. Infantile hepatic hemangioma frequently resolves spontaneously. However, it may also become life-threatening if associated with arteriovenous shunting and cardiac failure. In such cases, the lesion requires aggressive surgical intervention. Hemangioma in adults occurs most frequently in the fourth and fifth decades of life and there is a higher incidence in women (about 80%). Estrogen replacement therapy may play a role in the pathogenesis of this type of tumor [22]. Hemorrhage is the most common reason for prophylactic resection although this occurs relatively infrequently.

Hemengioma, whether solitary or multiple, is a well-defined lesion which ranges in size from a few mm to more than 20 cm. Hemangiomas larger than 10 cm are considered "giant" hemangiomas. Microscopically it is a tumor composed of multiple vascular channels lined by a single layer of endothelial cells supported by a thin, fibrous stroma. Large lesions almost always have a heterogeneous composition with areas of fibrosis, necrosis, cystic changes and intratumoral coarse calcifications. In some cases, abundant fibrous tissue completely replaces the lesion [2, 123].

A large proportion of hemangiomas are asymptomatic, and liver function tests are normal. Rarely, however, patients present with abdominal pain, and in exceptional cases, with fever, leukocytosis, thrombocytopenia, consumptive coagulopathy (Kasabach-Merritt Syndrome) or cholestasis. Occasionally, very large hemangiomas may cause symptoms by compressing adjacent organs [90].

On ultrasound (US), hemangiomas are typically homogeneously hyperechoic with well-defined margins, and may exibit faint acoustic enhancement. The echogenicity may vary because these tumors contain cystic and fibrotic regions, especially when large (Fig. 1). Color Doppler US demonstrates filling vessels in the periphery of the tumor but no significant color Doppler flow deep within the hemangioma itself (Fig. 2). Power Doppler, however, may detect flow within heman-

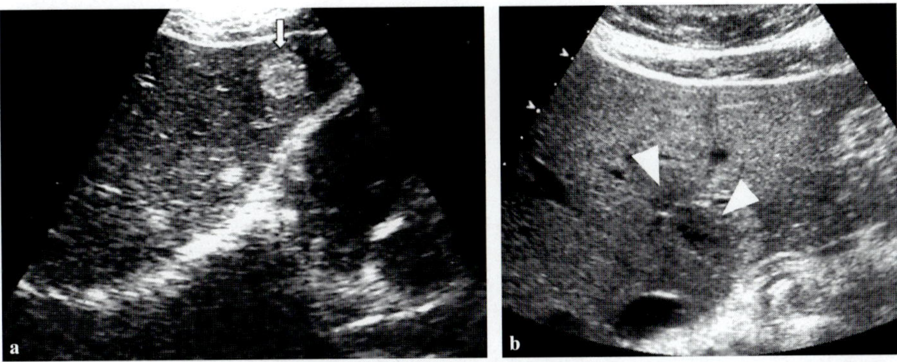

Fig. 1a,b. Hemangioma. Ultrasound reveals either a well-defined homogeneously hyperechoic lesion (*arrow in* **a**), or a tumor with heterogeneous echogenicity (*arrowheads in* **b**)

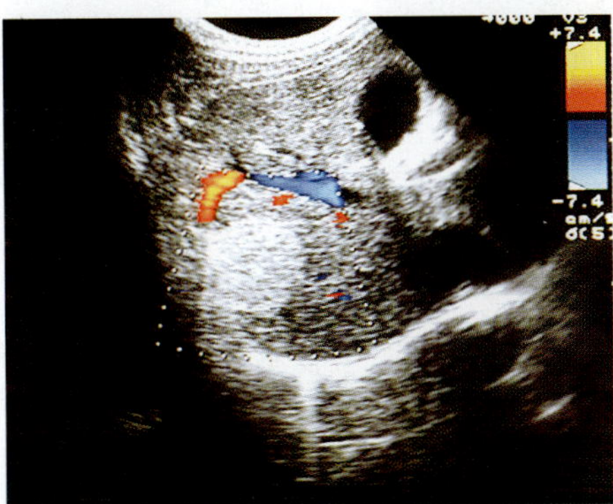

Fig. 2. Hemangioma. On color Doppler ultrasound the lesion demonstrates an homogeneous structure without flow within the nodule

giomas but the pattern is non-specific and can be seen in other primary hepatic liver lesions such as hepatocellular carcinoma (HCC) and FNH [21].

Hemangiomas appear as low density masses with well-defined lobulated margins on unenhanced computed tomography (CT) scans. During the arterial phase on spiral CT, hemangiomas demonstrate initial peripheral enhancement that progresses centrally. On delayed scans the lesion becomes hyperintense or isointense to the liver (Fig. 3). Early globular peripheral enhancement corresponding to large peripheral feeding vessels can also be observed. The presence of globular enhancement, which is isodense with the aorta, has been found to be about 70% sensitive and 100% specific for differentiating hemangioma from hepatic metastases [63]. Although small lesions often fill in completely (Fig. 4), large tumors may have central unenhanced zones corresponding to scar tissue or cystic cavities (Fig. 3) [136]. Hemangiomas cause a focal defect on both hepatobiliary and sulfur colloid scans. The underlying liver has normal isotope uptake. Tagged red blood cell scans can be virtually diagnostic of this lesion; there is a defect in the early phases that shows prolonged and persistent "filling in" on delayed scans [43].

On unenhanced T1-weighted magnetic resonance (MR) images, hemangiomas are most commonly visualized as well-defined homogeneous slightly hypointense masses, with lobulated borders. On T2-weighted images, they characteristically

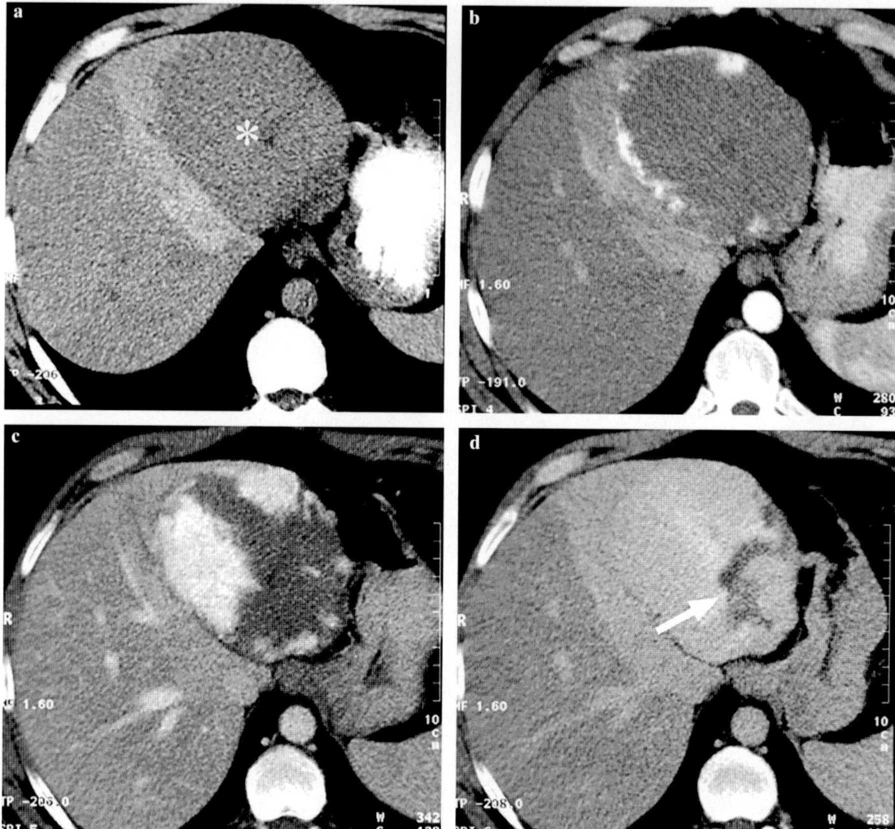

Fig. 3a-d. Cavernous hemangioma. On the unenhanced CT scan (**a**) the lesion (*asterisk*) is homogeneously hypodense with well-defined margins. During the arterial phase (**b**) hyperdense peripheral nodular enhancement is seen, which progresses centrally during the portal-venous phase (**c**). Stromal components within the lesion are demonstrated during the equilibrium phase (**d**) as areas of incomplete filling-in (*arrow*)

show marked homogeneous hyperintensity with occasional areas of low intensity that correspond to regions of fibrosis (Fig. 5) [68, 104]. After contrast agent administration, three types of enhancement pattern may be seen, depending on the size of the lesion. The majority of lesions under 1.5 cm in diameter show uniform enhancement during the arterial phase at 25–30 sec post-contrast (Fig. 6). Medium-sized lesions between 1.5 and 5 cm in diameter show either uniform early enhancement or peripheral nodular enhancement progressing centripetally to uniform enhancement by the equilibrium phase at 5–6 min post-contrast. Large hemangiomas (>5 cm), on the other hand, demonstrate peripheral nodular enhancement with persistent central hypointensity that correlates with regions of fibrosis and/or cystic areas (Fig. 7). The peripheral nodular enhancement, detected during the arterial phase of the dynamic series, is very useful for differentiating hemangioma from metastases. On occasions, it may be difficult to differentiate hemangiomas that enhance uniformly from vascular metastases that frequently demonstrate a similar enhancement pattern. For these lesions the combination of T2-weighted and serial

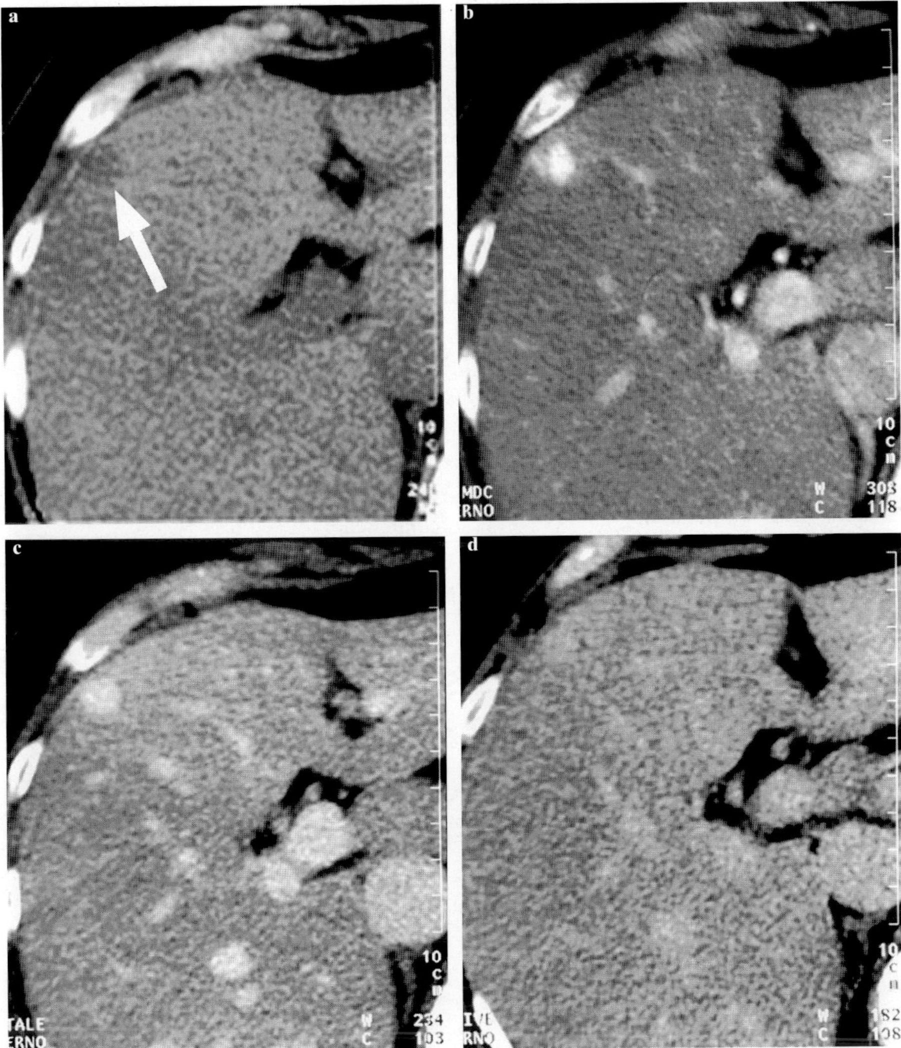

Fig. 4a-d. Hypervascular hemangioma. On the unenhanced CT scan (**a**) the hemangioma (*arrow*) appears slightly hypodense. Rapid filling-in is seen in the arterial phase (**b**) which persists into the portal-venous phase (**c**). During the delayed phase (**d**) the hemangioma is isodense as compared with the surrounding liver tissue

dynamic post-contrast T1-weighted images facilitates a confident diagnosis of hemangioma [105]. Alternatively, contrast agents with liver-specific properties, such as Gd-BOPTA, are highly specific for hemangioma. In this case, a pattern of "nodular" enhancement is frequently seen on images after Gd-BOPTA, rather than the rim enhancement typical of metastases. During the delayed liver-specific phase, hemangiomas tend to be isointense or slightly hypointense compared with the surrounding liver parenchyma (Fig. 7e), and to contain low intensity areas, indicative of fibrotic or cystic components.

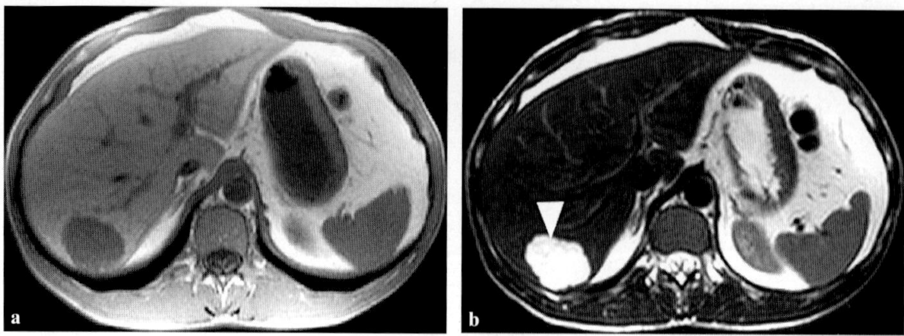

Fig. 5a,b. Hemangioma. On the unenhanced GE T1-weighted MR image (**a**), the hemangioma is seen as a well-defined hypointense mass. Conversely, on the T2-weighted image (**b**), the lesion (*arrowhead*) is markedly hyperintense

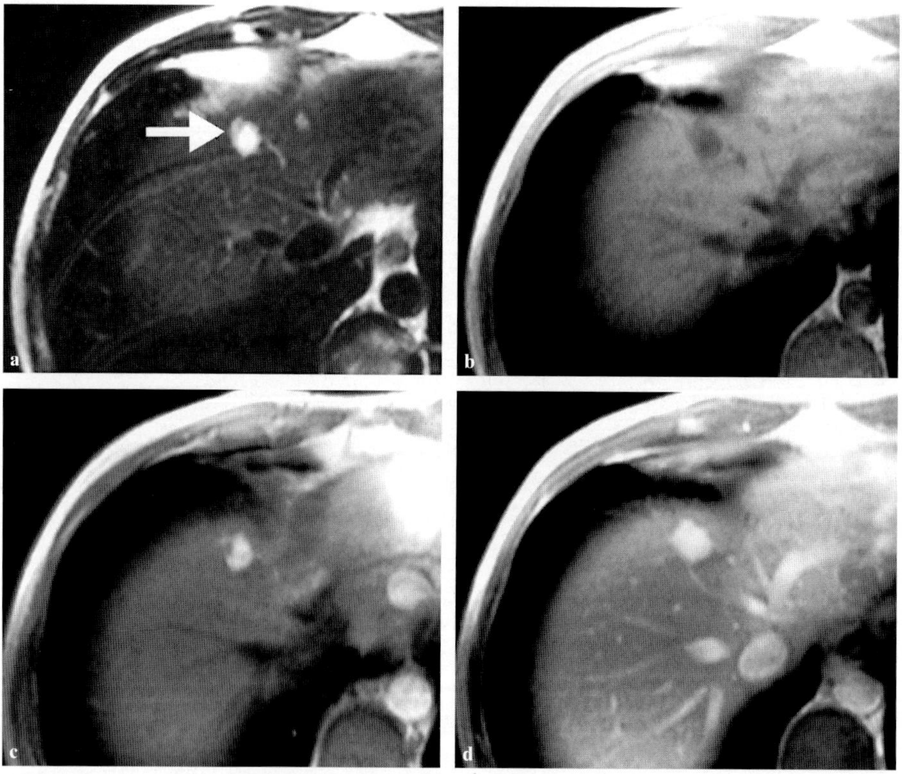

Fig. 6a-d. Hypervascular hemangioma after Gd-BOPTA. The lesion (*arrow*) is markedly hyperintense on the unenhanced Turbo SE T2-weighted image (**a**), and hypointense on the unenhanced GE T1-weighted image (**b**). Rapid enhancement on images acquired during the arterial phase (**c**) after the bolus injection of Gd-BOPTA becomes homogeneous during the portal venous phase (**d**)

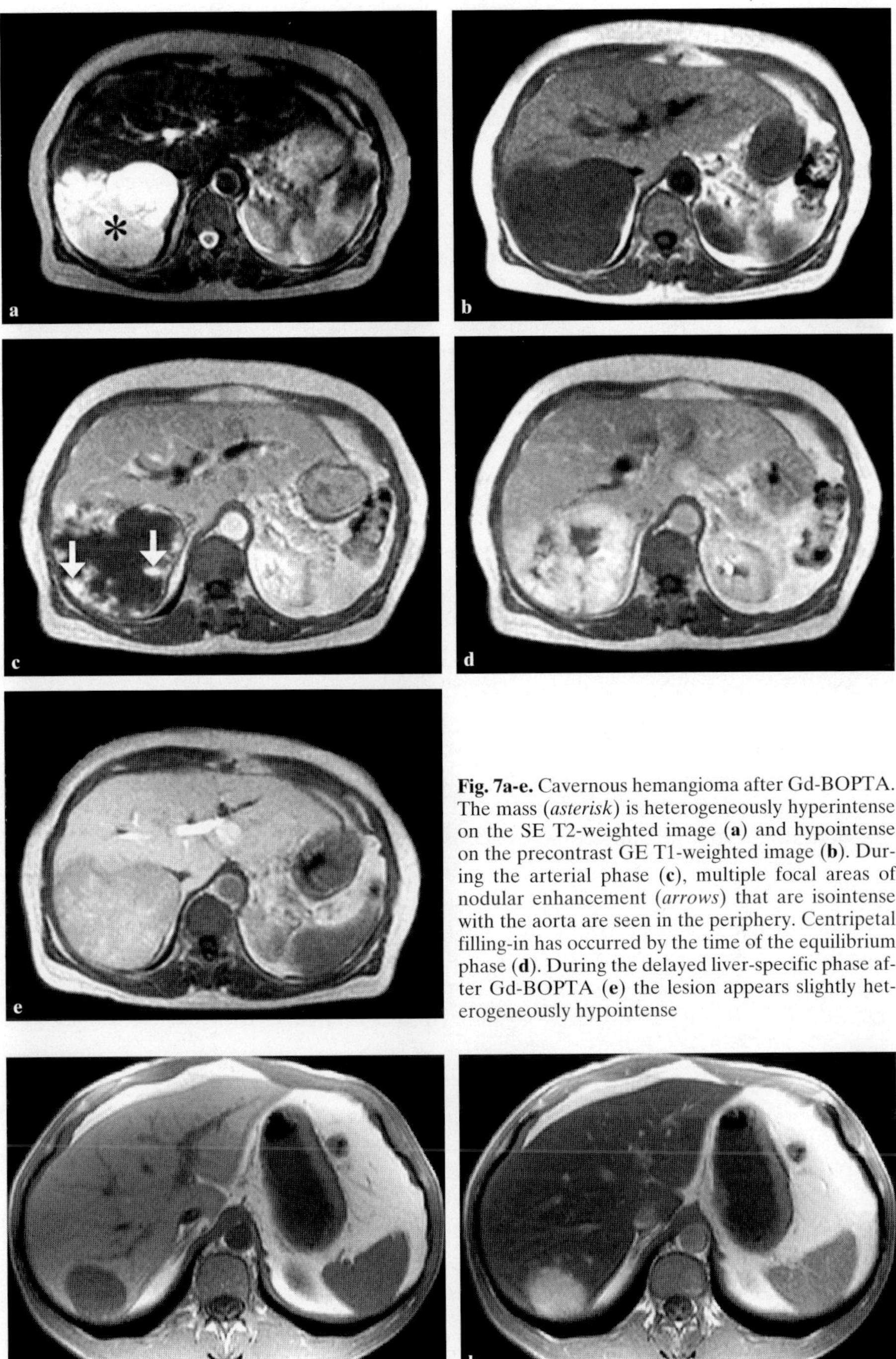

Fig. 7a-e. Cavernous hemangioma after Gd-BOPTA. The mass (*asterisk*) is heterogeneously hyperintense on the SE T2-weighted image (**a**) and hypointense on the precontrast GE T1-weighted image (**b**). During the arterial phase (**c**), multiple focal areas of nodular enhancement (*arrows*) that are isointense with the aorta are seen in the periphery. Centripetal filling-in has occurred by the time of the equilibrium phase (**d**). During the delayed liver-specific phase after Gd-BOPTA (**e**) the lesion appears slightly heterogeneously hypointense

Fig. 8a,b. Hemangioma after SPIO. On the unenhanced GE T1-weighted image the hemangioma appears hypointense (**a**). On the post-contrast T1-weighted image after SPIO administration (**b**) the lesion shows increased signal intensity compared to the surrounding liver tissue (T1 effect)

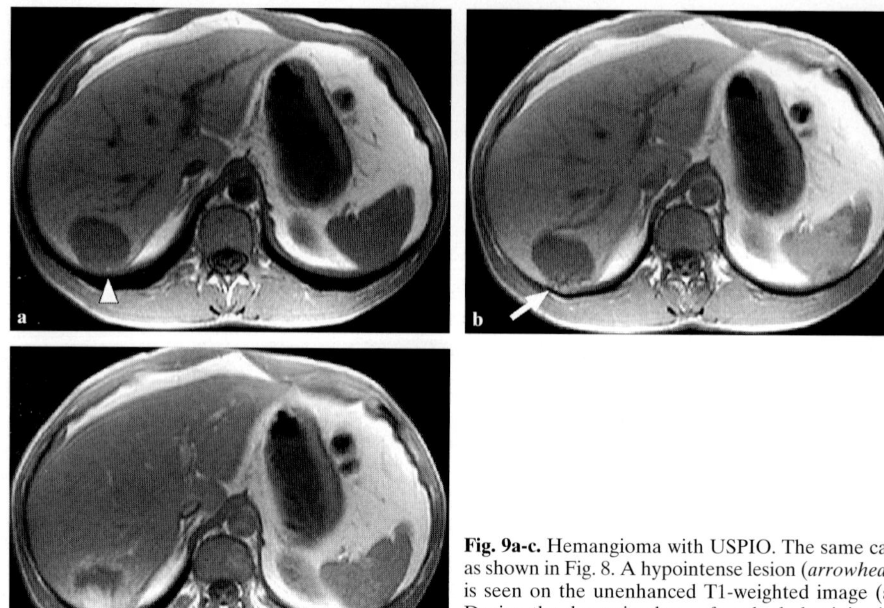

Fig. 9a-c. Hemangioma with USPIO. The same case as shown in Fig. 8. A hypointense lesion (*arrowhead*) is seen on the unenhanced T1-weighted image (**a**). During the dynamic phase after the bolus injection of SHU 555 A, the hemangioma (*arrows*) demonstrates weak nodular peripheral enhancement (**b, c**)

After administration of superparamagnetic iron oxide (SPIO) contrast agents, hemangiomas show an increased signal intensity on post-contrast T1-weighted images and appear hyperintense compared to the surrounding liver (Fig. 8) [39]. On T1-weighted dynamic phase images acquired after the administration of ultrasmall superparamagnetic iron oxide (USPIO) contrast agents, hemangiomas are enhanced becoming hyperintense relative to the normal liver (Fig. 9). On T2-weighted images, the lesions demonstrate decreased signal intensity, and may become isointense to the liver, particularly at higher doses of USPIO [102]. Since these lesions do not usually contain significant numbers of Kupffer cells or normal hepatocytes, they do not usually show uptake of SPIO particles or Mn-DPDP.

4.1.2 Peliosis Hepatis

Peliosis hepatis is a rare entity characterized by widespread blood-filled cystic cavities in the liver. Peliosis frequently develops in association with malignancies and chronic wasting diseases, such as tubercolosis. However, it has also been described in association with renal transplantation, hematological at disorders and infection with human immunodeficiency virus (*Rochalimaea hensela*), as well as in patients on long-term treatment with anabolic steroids, oral contraceptives, hormones, estrogen or Azathiaprine. Regression is generally observed after such agents have been stopped or after appropriate antibiotic therapy [122, 137].

Macroscopically, peliosis is characterized by cystic dilated sinusoids filled with red blood cells and bound by cords of liver cells. Two varieties have been described: the phlebectatic type, in which the blood-filled spaces are lined with endothelium and are based on aneurysmal dilatation of the central veins, and the parenchymal type, in which the blood spaces are not lined with endothelium and are usually associated with hemorrhagic parenchymal necrosis. Peliosis can be differentiated from hemangioma by the presence of portal tracts within the fibrous stroma of the blood-filled spaces. Numerous theories have been proposed for the cause of peliosis hepatis, including outflow obstruction and hepatocellular necrosis leading to cystic blood-filled formations. Peliosis hepatis is usually found incidentally at autopsy but, rarely, it can cause hepatic failure or liver rupture with hemoperitoneum or shock. Patients sometimes have non-specific signs such as hepatomegaly and portal hypertension [122].

Ultrasound findings are not specific for the diagnosis of peliosis hepatis; the hepatic echopattern is usually non-homogeneous with both hyperechoic and hypoechoic areas [66].

On CT images after the bolus administration of iodinated contrast material, these lesions usually appear hypodense initially, becoming isodense with time (88).

On unhenhanced T2-weighted MR images peliosis hepatis frequently demonstrates high signal intensity similar to that seen with hemangioma. Conversely, low signal intensity is usually seen on unenhanced T1-weighted images. After gadolinium administration, the lesions may show homogeneous hypervascularization depending on flow, and may appear iso- or hyperintense on equilibrium phase images after Gd-BOPTA (Fig. 10). In the hepatobiliary phase after Gd-BOPTA or Mn-DPDP, the lesion again appears hypointense.

4.1.3 Focal Nodular Hyperplasia

Focal nodular hyperplasia (FNH) is a benign tumor-like lesion of the liver considered to be the result of a hyperplastic response to the presence of a pre-existing vascular malformation. It is thought that increased arterial flow hyperperfuses the local parenchyma leading to secondary hepatocellular hyperplasia [131]. FNH is the second most common benign hepatic tumor after hemangioma and has been shown to constitute about 8% of primary hepatic tumors at autopsy [18]. It usually occurs in women of childbearing and middle age, but cases have been reported in men and children. Most investigators agree that oral contraceptives are not the causal agents of FNH [8]. However, estrogens could have a trophic effect on FNH by increasing the size of the nodule and contributing to the vascular changes [131].

Clinically, this tumor is usually an incidental finding discovered at autopsy, during elective surgery, or on diagnostic imaging performed for other reasons. Clinical symptoms include right upper quadrant or epigastric pain. However, most patients are asymptomatic at discovery: fewer than one third of cases are discovered because of clinical symptoms. When present, the clinical symptoms are usually caused by larger lesions which expand the Glisson capsule or have a focal mass effect on surrounding organs. The natural history of FNH is characterized by the absence of complications. Therefore, typical asymptomatic FNH should be managed conservatively in association with the discontinuation of oral contraceptives. Surgical resection is only rarely indicated, when the symptoms are particularly severe.

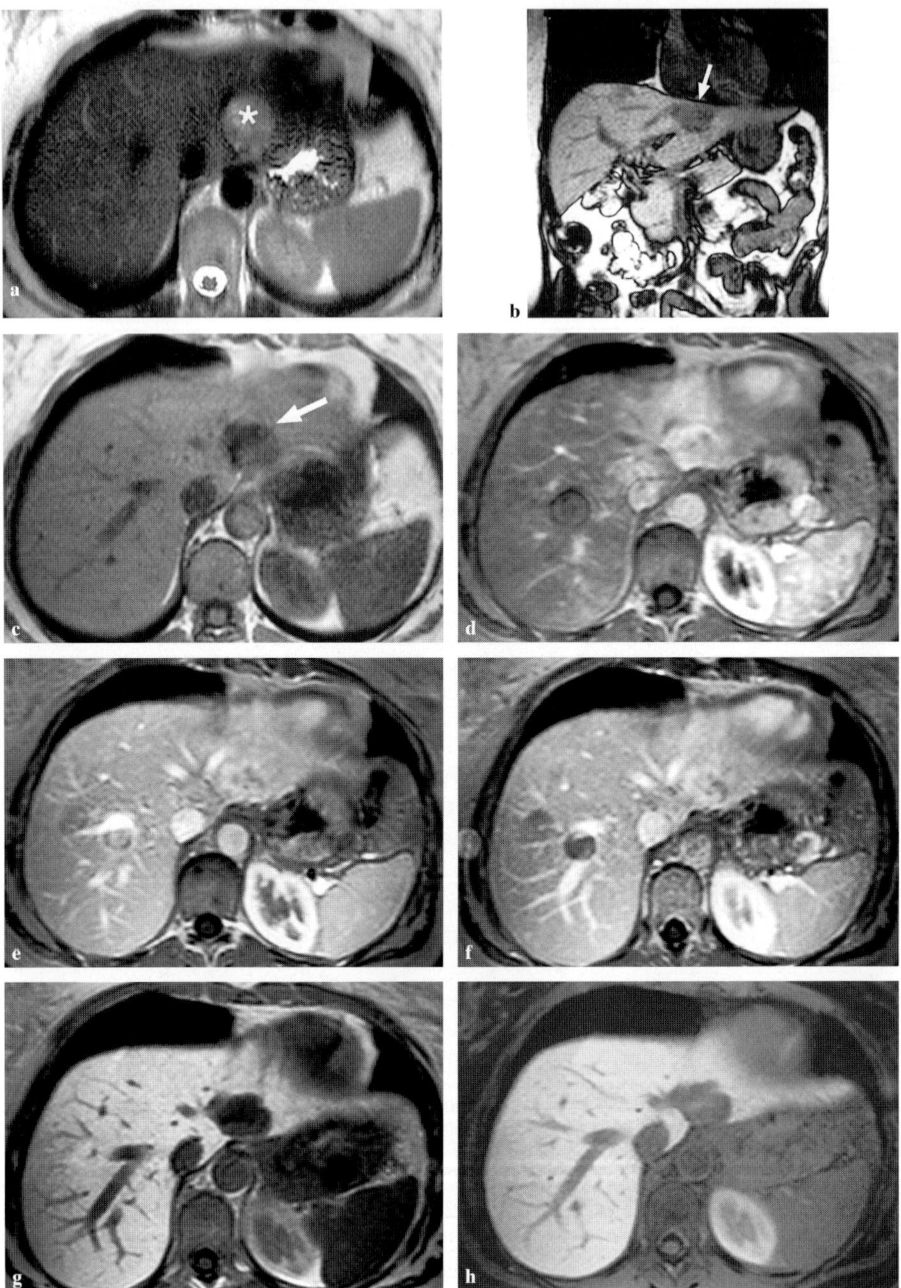

Fig. 10a-h. Peliosis hepatis. The lesion (*asterisk*) shows heterogeneous high signal intensity on the T2-weighted HASTE image (**a**) and appears hypointense (*arrows*) on unenhanced coronal and axial GE T1 weighted images (**b** and **c**, respectively). Early heterogeneous enhancement at the periphery of the lesion is seen on T1-weighted images acquired during the arterial phase after the bolus administration of Gd-BOPTA (**d**). Thereafter, heterogeneous hyperintensity is seen during the portal-venous and equilibrium phases (**e** and **f**, respectively). On delayed phase images the peliosis hepatis shows low signal intensity (**g**). The lesion appears hypointense on late phase GE T1-weighted Fat. Sat. images after mangafodipir administration (**h**)

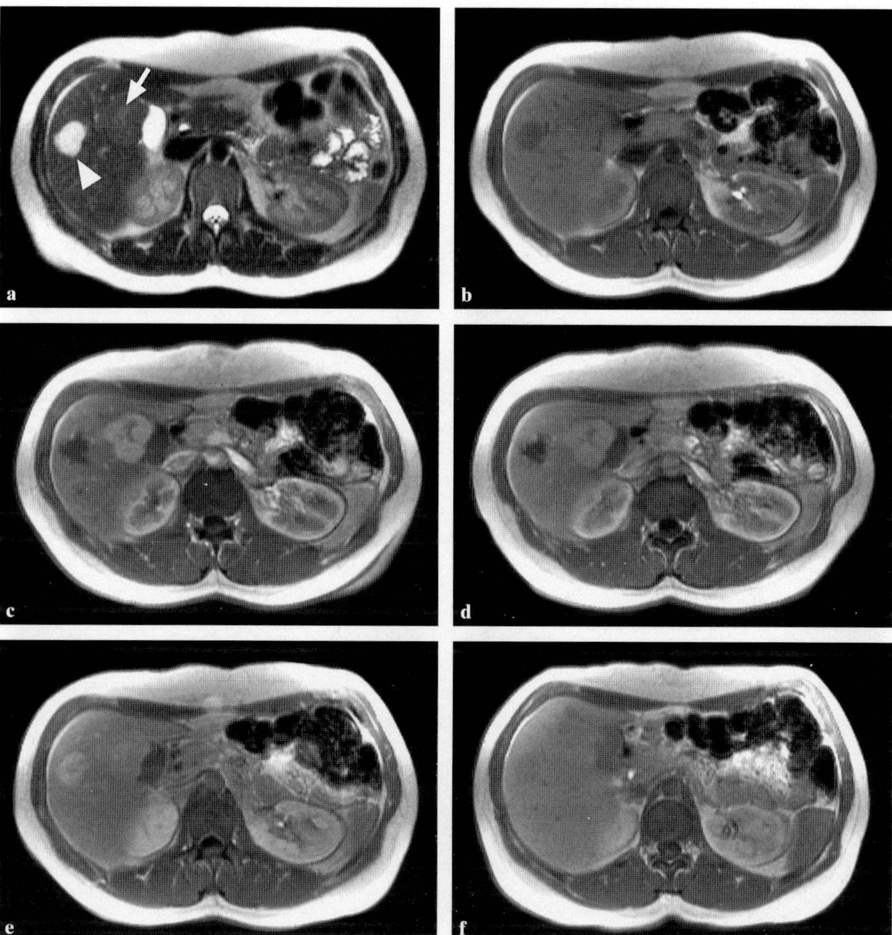

Fig. 11a-f. FNH/Hemangioma. Unenhanced T2w images (**a**) show a slightly hyperintense lesion with a small hyperintense central scar (*arrow*) compressing the gallbladder. An additional subcapsular lesion (*arrowhead*) with homogeneous high signal intensity (light-bulb phenomenon indicative of hemangioma) can be seen. On the unenhanced T1w gradient echo image (**b**), the suspected hemangioma appears homogeneously hypointense with distinct borders while the lesion compressing the gallbladder shows isointense signal intensity and lobulation. On arterial phase images after the bolus administration of Gd-BOPTA (**c**), the lesion located near the gallbladder shows strong hyperintensity with a central hypointense scar. On portal-venous phase images (**d**), this lesion is still hyperintense and clearly delineated and the central scar is still hypointense. The second lesion demonstrates nodular peripheral enhancement typical of hemangioma. Imaging during the equilibrium phase at 5 min after Gd-BOPTA administration (**e**) reveals enhancement of the central scar, a typical enhancement pattern of pseudoscar formation in FNH. The second lesion shows homogeneous contrast agent uptake. In the hepatobiliary phase (**f**), the lesion close to the gallbladder appears isointense to the surrounding parenchyma, indicating a lesion consisting of functioning hepatocytes able to take up Gd-BOPTA. The imaging pattern is consistent with that of an FNH. The second lesion is again hypointense and the imaging pattern is consistent with that of a hemangioma

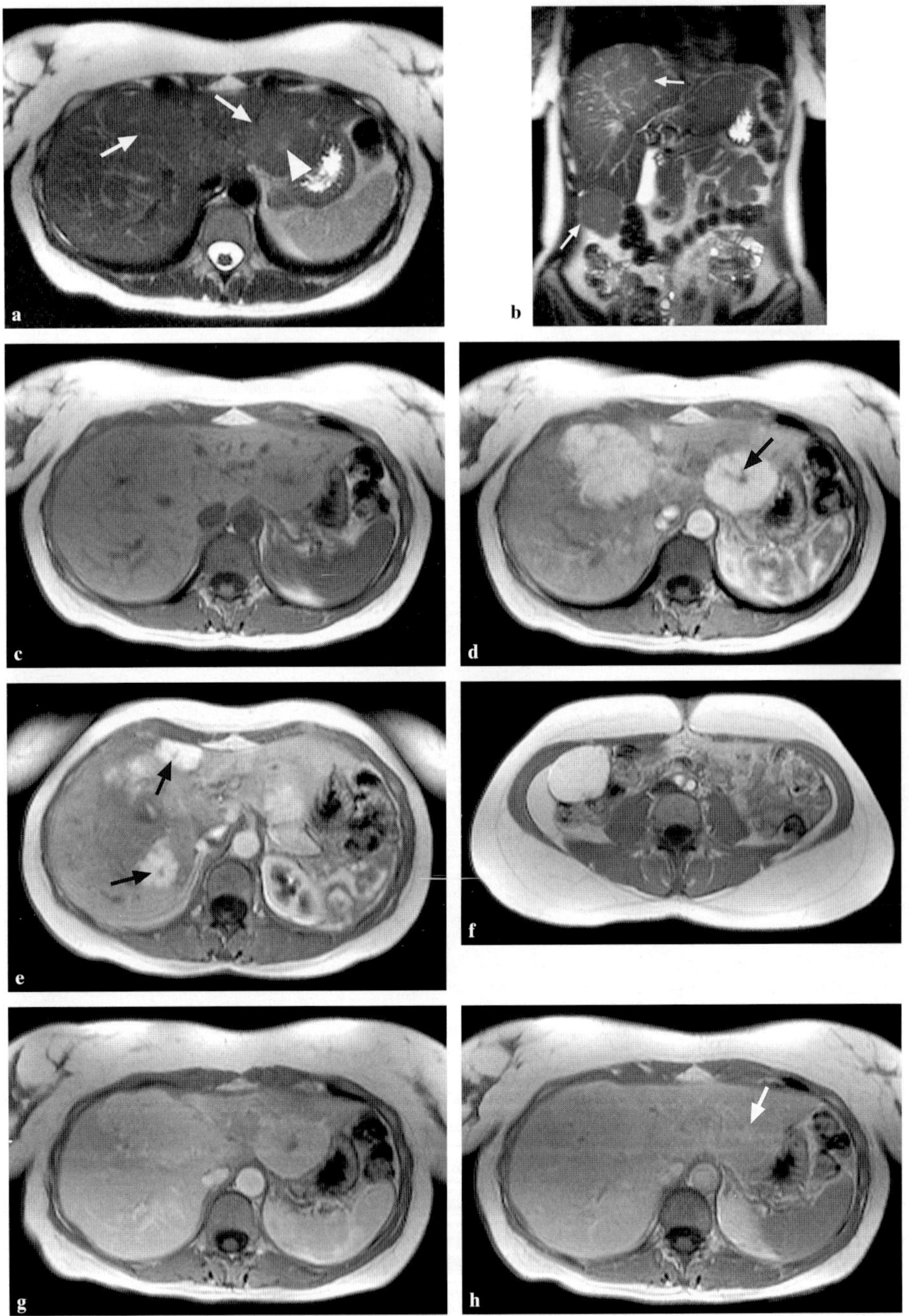

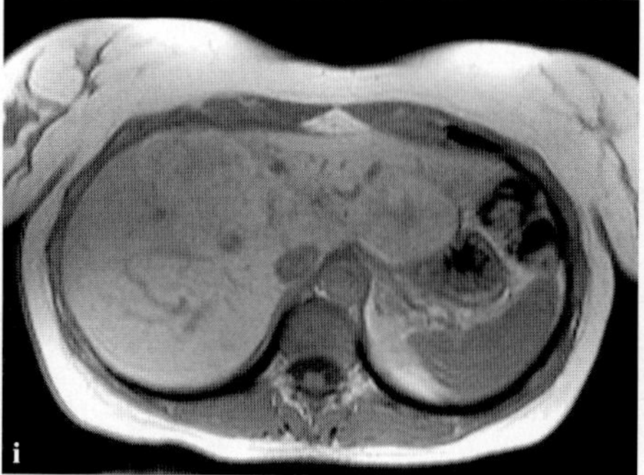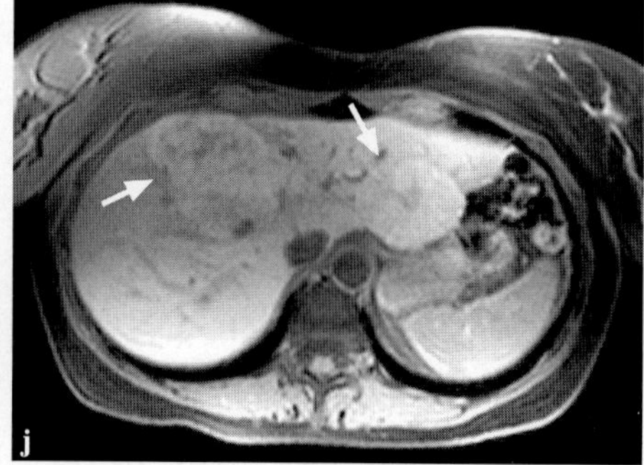

Fig. 12a-j. Multiple focal nodular hyperplasia (FNH). Unenhanced axial and coronal T2w images (**a**, **b**) reveal several slightly hyperintense liver lesions (*arrows*) with one lesion in the left liver lobe demonstrating a central scar (*arrowhead*). On unenhanced T1w images the lesions are slightly hypointense (**c**). Arterial phase images acquired after the bolus injection of Gd-BOPTA reveal strong hypervascularization of all the lesions (**d-f**), and a central scar in three of the lesions (*arrows*). In the portal-venous phase the lesions are slightly hyperintense (**g**). In the equilibrium phase (**h**), the central scar of the lesion in the left liver lobe shows late enhancement (*arrow*). This is typical for FNH in which the central scar is more an arterio-venous malformation than a true scar. T1w images acquired during the hepatobiliary phase (**i**), show enhancement of the liver lesions. This is more obvious on T1w fs images (*arrows*) acquired at the same time point (**j**) and is indicative of the lesions containing functioning hepatocytes that are able to take up Gd-BOPTA. The fact that the lesions enhance to a higher degree than the surrounding liver tissue is indicative of the benign nature of the lesions and of the fact that the biliary system of FNH is malformed leading to a slowing of biliary excretion

FNH is usually a solitary, homogeneous, subcapsular nodular mass which only infrequently undergoes hemorrhage and necrosis. On cut sections, the majority of these tumors have a central fibrous scar and sharp margins with no capsule [18]. Often they have a mean diameter of around 5 cm at the time of diagnosis, although sometimes it is possible to find lesions that replace an entire lobe of the liver.

The classical form of FNH with a central stellate scar is seen in < 50% of cases. Variant, often small lesions, with atypical features such as the absence of a central scar, the presence of a portal vein, or telangiectatic changes, are being detected with increasing frequency. FNH lesions are composed of nearly normal hepatocytes arranged in plates that are one or two cells thick. FNH almost always demonstrate ductular differentiation and malformed vessels in a nodular architecture. Thus, accurate diagnosis can frequently be made even in the absence of a scar [8].

Evidence to support the theory that FNH is the result of a hyperplastic response to the presence of a pre-existing vascular malformation comes from the frequent finding of FNH in association with cavernous hemangiomas (Fig. 11). Moreover, when multiple (Fig. 12), FNH lesions are often associated with other lesions, such as meningioma, astrocytoma and teleangiectasia of the brain, and systemic arterial dysplasia [8, 18, 131]. FNH has also been described in association with hepatocellular adenoma and liver adenomatosis [31]. In these conditions, it appears that FNH lesions may be secondary to systemic and local abnormalities of vascular growth induced by oral contraceptives, tumor-induced growth factors, thrombosis and local arterio-venous shunting [8].

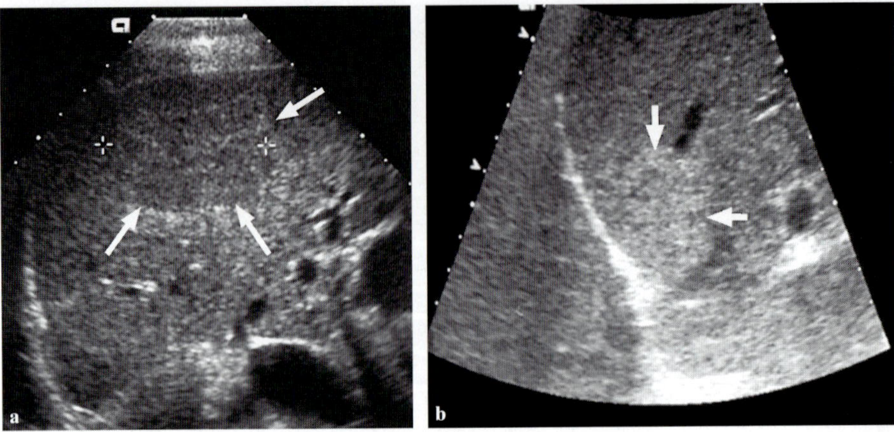

Fig.13a,b. Focal nodular hyperplasia. The ultrasound examination reveals a homogeneous lesion (*arrows*) that is either hypoechoic (**a**) or hyperechoic (**b**) compared to the surrounding normal liver

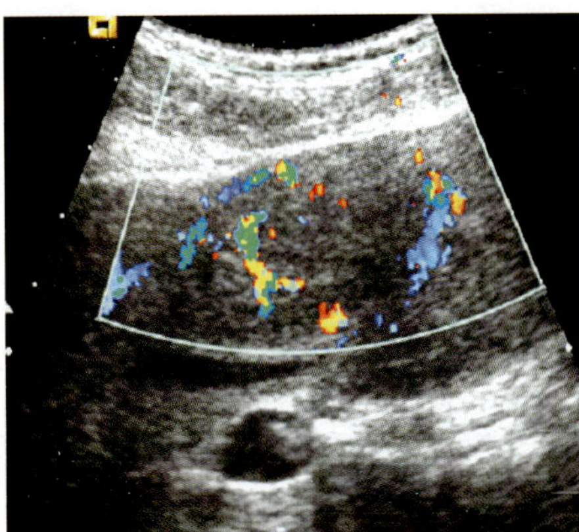

Fig. 14. Focal nodular hyperplasia. The arterial hypervascularity of the lesion and large feeding arteries from the periphery to the center are demonstrated on color Doppler ultrasound examination

On ultrasound (US) images, FNH appears well-demarcated and either isoechoic or slightly hypo- or hyperechoic relative to the normal liver (Fig. 13). Displacement of contiguous hepatic vessels may be the only detectable abnormality. The central scar and septa are often difficult to visualize on US; however, when apparent, they are usually hyperechoic areas that may demonstrate hypervascularity on color Doppler US. In some cases, color Doppler US reveals a central hypervascular nidus, corresponding to the scar. Large draining vessels may sometimes be identified in the periphery at the tumor margins (Fig. 14) [107, 116].

FNH is usually isoattenuating or slightly hypoattenuating on unenhanced CT (Fig. 15a). The lesions generally only appear hyperattenuating to unenhanced liver when there is hepatic steatosis or when the liver is otherwise abnormally decreased in attenuation. However, FNH may still be isoattenuating or hypoattenuating on unenhanced CT in patients with hepatic steatosis when there is fatty infiltration of the FNH itself [74]. A low density central area, corresponding to the

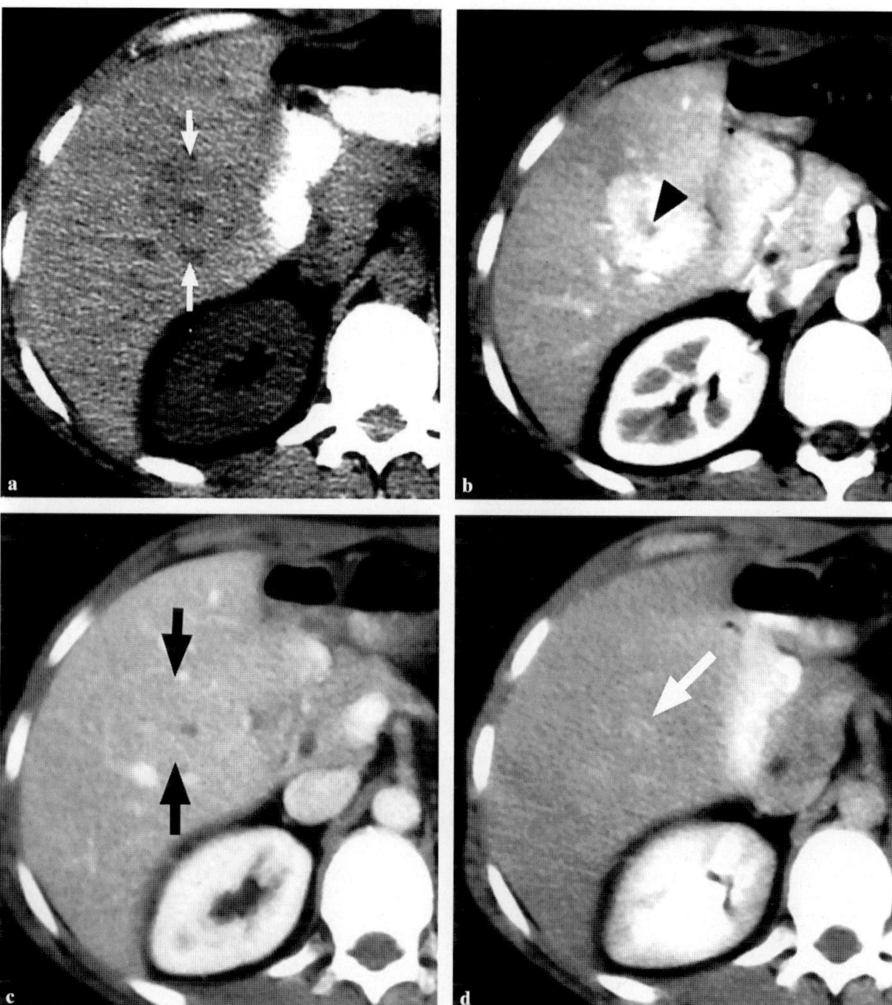

Fig. 15a-d. Focal nodular hyperplasia. On unenhanced CT (**a**), the FNH (*arrows*) is isoattenuating to the liver. During the arterial phase (**b**) after contrast medium administration, the nodule enhances rapidly and homogenously, while the central scar (*arrowhead*) remains hypodense. In the portal-venous and equilibrium phases (**c** and **d**, respectively) the FNH (*arrows*) appears isodense compared to normal liver parenchyma. In the later phase the central scar (*arrow*) is revealed as hyperattenuating

scar, may be seen in approximately one third of cases [107]. During the arterial phase of contrast-enhanced CT, FNH lesions enhance rapidly, becoming hyperdense relative to the normal liver (Fig. 15b). The low attenuation scar is then conspicuous against the hyperdense tissue. Foci of enhancement within the scar are indicative of arteries. In the portal-venous phase of enhancement, the difference in attenuation between FNH and normal liver decreases such that the lesions may become isodense with normal liver (Fig. 15c). The central scar is almost always seen as hypoattenuating to the remainder of the FNH on unenhanced and enhanced dynamic phase scans. On delayed scans, however, there is retention of contrast material within the fibrous scar giving it an isoattenuating or, more frequently, a hyperattenuating appearance (Fig. 15d). Detection of the central scar is related to the size of the FNH: whereas a central scar may be identified in as many as 65% of FNH greater than 3 cm in diameter, it may be seen in only about 25% of lesions smaller than 3 cm in diameter [12, 18].

On MR imaging, FNH are considered typical when they appear as homogeneously isointense or slightly hyperintense on T2-weighted images and isointense or slightly hypointense on T1-weighted images before contrast medium administration. Typical behavior during the dynamic phase of contrast enhancement is characterized by a marked and homogeneous signal intensity enhancement during the arterial phase, rapid and homogeneous signal intensity washout during the portal-venous phase, and signal isointensity (with the exception of the scar) during the equilibrium phase (Fig. 16). When present, the central stellate scar generally appears as hyperintense on T2-weighted images and hypointense on unenhanced T1-weighted images. During the dynamic phase of contrast enhancement, the scar appears as hypointense during the arterial and portal-venous phases and slightly hyperintense in the equilibrium phase (Fig. 16).

Atypical features of FNH can consist of lesion heterogeneity, hypointensity in the portal-venous or equilibrium phases, the absence of a central scar in lesions greater than 3 cm, scar hypointensity on T2-weighted images, and scar hypointensity in the equilibrium phase following injection of contrast agent. Other atypical features include the presence of hemorrhage, calcification or necrosis, or a pseudocapsule presenting as a complete hyperintense perilesional ring during the equilibrium phase (Fig. 17) [42].

The use of contrast-enhanced dynamic phase MR imaging with traditional extracellular gadolinium-based contrast agents provides the greatest diagnostic sensitivity among the techniques in current use, especially when combined with the information available on pre-contrast T1- and T2-weighted images. However, the high frequency of atypical features does not permit the accurate characterization of FNH in every case, and current diagnosis by MR imaging relies on the same morphologic and hemodynamic features as helical CT [42]. The availability of MR contrast agents with liver-specific properties increases the potential for accurate lesion characterization. FNH are depicted as either hyperintense or isointense during the delayed phase after administration of Gd-BOPTA, Gd-EOB-DTPA or Mn-DPDP reflecting the abnormal biliary drainage within the lesion (Fig. 18, 19). Gd-BOPTA and Gd-EOB-DTPA in particular offer both a dynamic and delayed phase imaging capability, thereby permitting both morphological and functional information to be acquired for the characterization of these lesions (Figs. 20, 21, 22, 23) [42, 67].

On T2-weighted images after SPIO administration, typical FNH demonstrate a signal loss due to the uptake of iron oxide particles by Kupffer cells within the lesion (Fig. 24) [38]. The degree of signal loss seen in FNH lesions using SPIO-enhanced T2-weighted sequences is significantly greater than that in other focal liver lesions, such as HCC and hepatic adenoma [83], however, overlap may occur due to the lack of function of Kupffer cells in FNH.

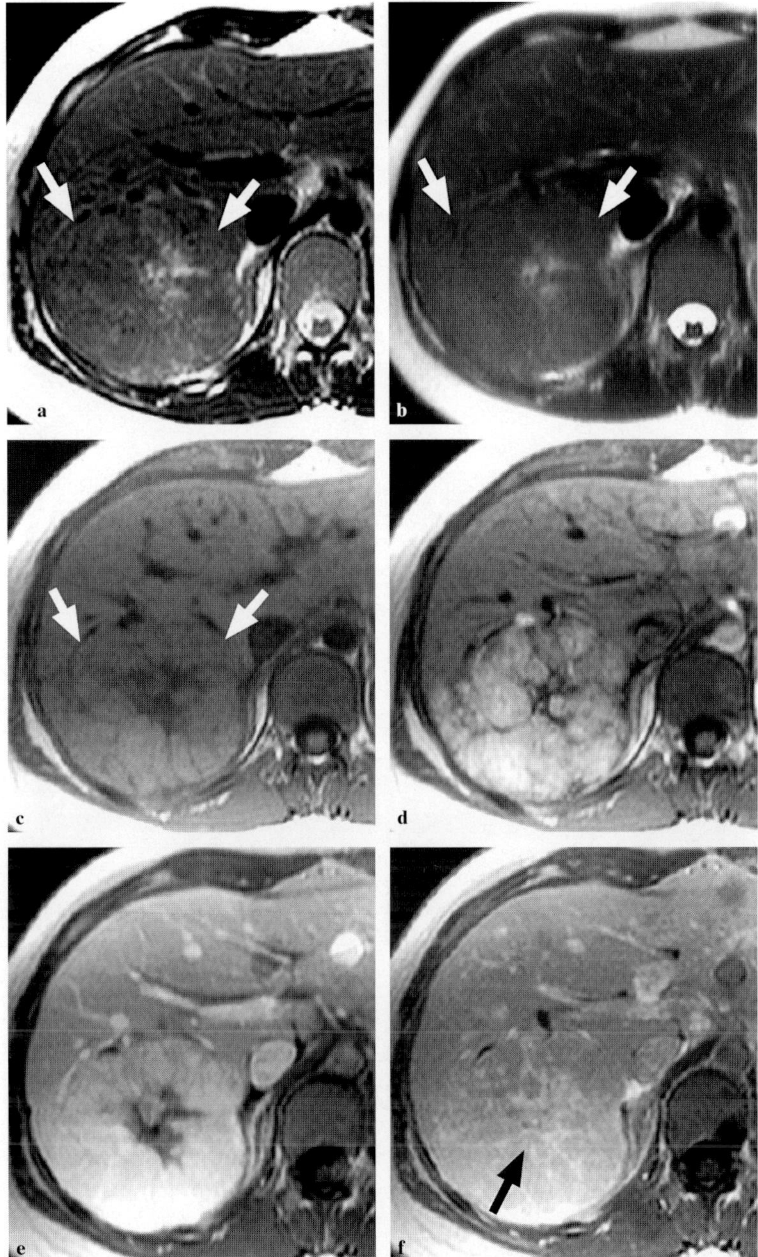

Fig. 16a-f. Focal nodular hyperplasia with Gd-DTPA. On the Turbo SE T2-weighted and HASTE T2-weighted images (**a** and **b**, respectively), the nodule (*arrows*) is isointense to the surrounding liver tissue and possesses a hyperintense "stellate" central scar. On the unenhanced T1-weighted image (**c**), the FNH (*arrows*) appears as an isointense lesion. This lesion shows intense and homogeneous enhancement during the arterial phase after contrast medium administration (**d**) and rapid washout in the portal-venous phase (**e**). In the equilibrium phase (**f**), the lesion is seen as isointense again. The central scar is typically hypointense on the unenhanced image as well as during the arterial and portal-venous phases. However, it appears hyperintense in the equilibrium phase (*arrow*) comparable to that seen in CT imaging

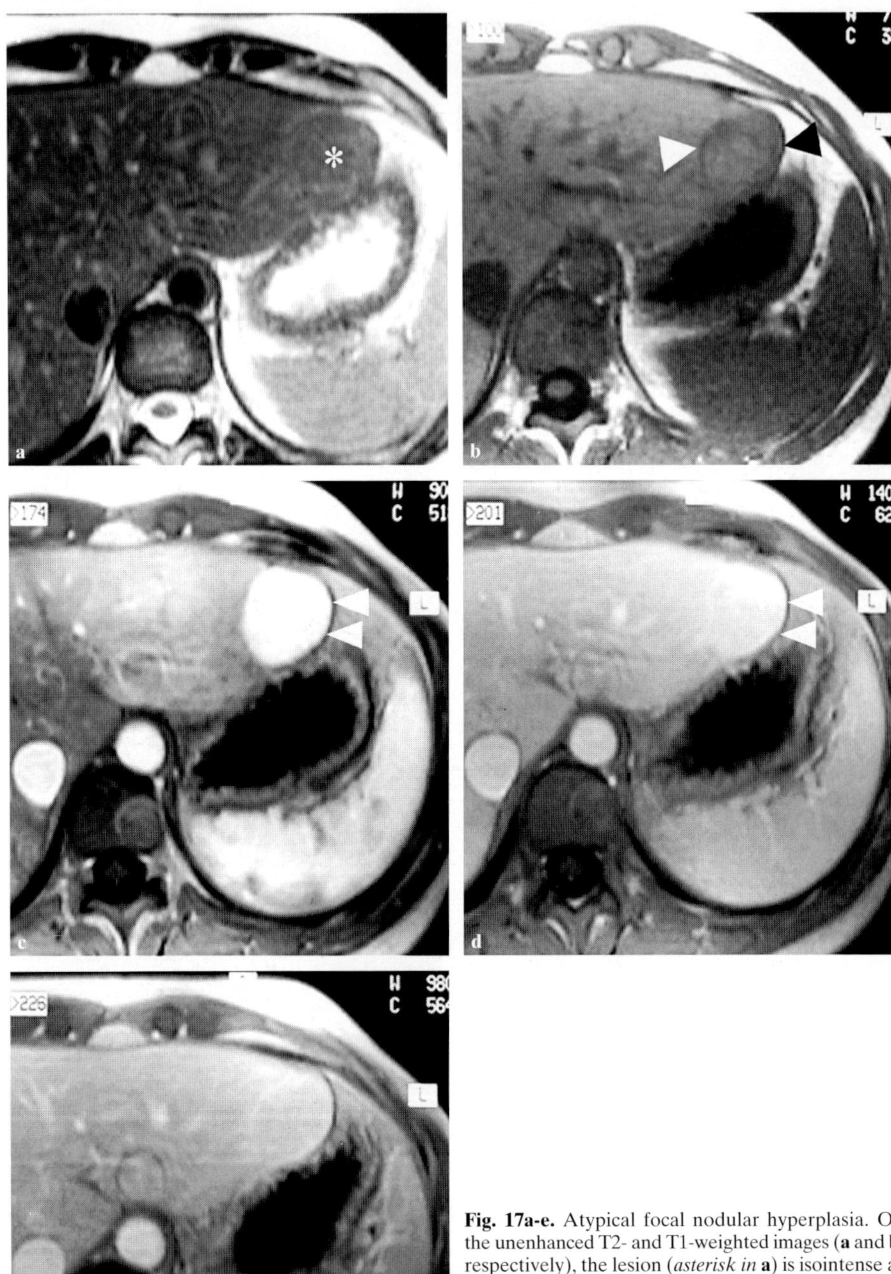

Fig. 17a-e. Atypical focal nodular hyperplasia. On the unenhanced T2- and T1-weighted images (**a** and **b**, respectively), the lesion (*asterisk in* **a**) is isointense as compared with the normal liver tissue and is delineated by a thin hypointense rim (*arrowheads in* **b**). During the early arterial (**c**) and portal-venous (**d**) phases after contrast medium administration, the lesion is seen as highly vascularized. The lesion remains slightly hyperintense in the equilibrium phase (**e**) when a hyperintense peripheral rim can also be seen

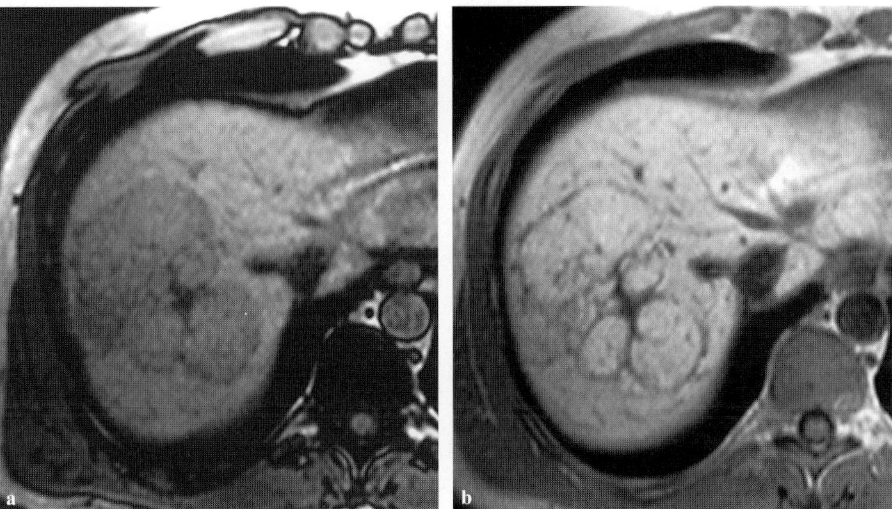

Fig. 18a,b. Focal nodular hyperplasia after Mn-DPDP. On the precontrast T1-weighted image (**a**), the FNH is seen as isointense with a stellate hypointense central scar. On the delayed image after mangafodipir administration (**b**), the lesion is again isointense as compared to the surrounding parenchyma

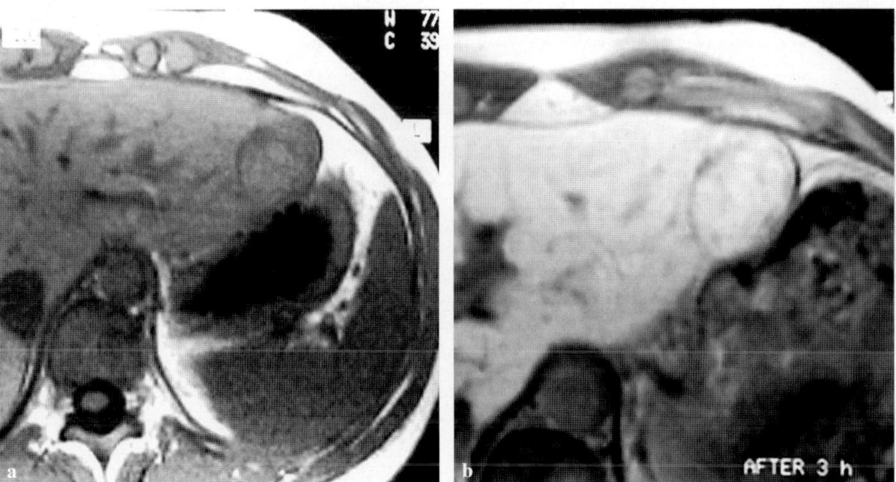

Fig. 19a,b. Atypical focal nodular hyperplasia after Gd-BOPTA. The same case as presented in Fig. 17. On the precontrast T1-weighted image (**a**) the FNH is isointense to partially slightly hypointense compared to the normal liver tissue. During the hepatobiliary phase at 3 h after the bolus administration of Gd-BOPTA (**b**), the lesion is again isointense to the surrounding liver parenchyma, indicating functioning hepatocytes. This enables the diagnosis of FNH

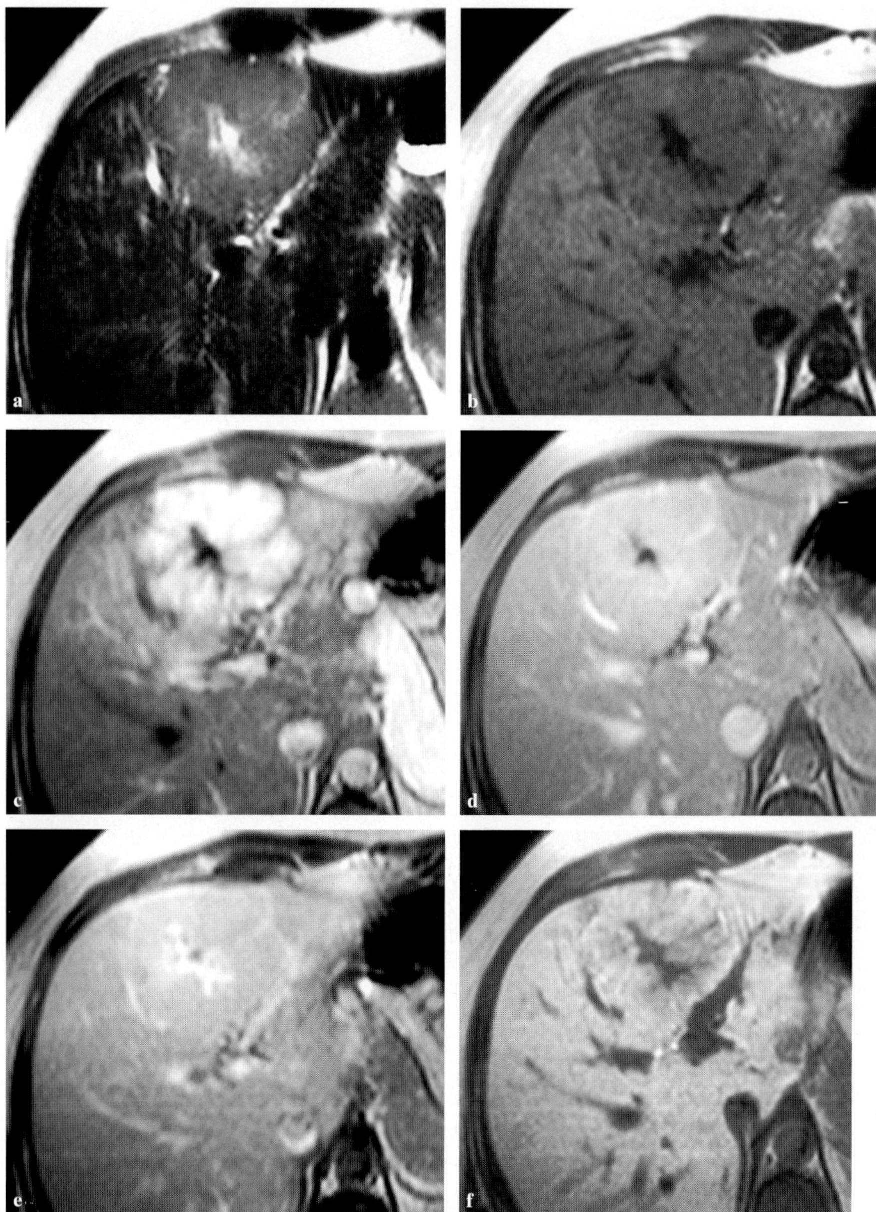

Fig. 20a-f. The unenhanced T2-weighted HASTE image (**a**) reveals a typically hyperintense lesion with a strongly hyperintense central area corresponding to scar. The unenhanced T1-weighted GE image (**b**) reveals a lesion that is slightly hypointense to the surrounding parenchyma. On this image, a more strongly hypointense scar is seen. T1-weighted imaging during the arterial (**c**), portal-venous (**d**), equilibrium (**e**) and delayed (**f**) phases after Gd-BOPTA administration reveals an enhancement pattern that is typical of FNH

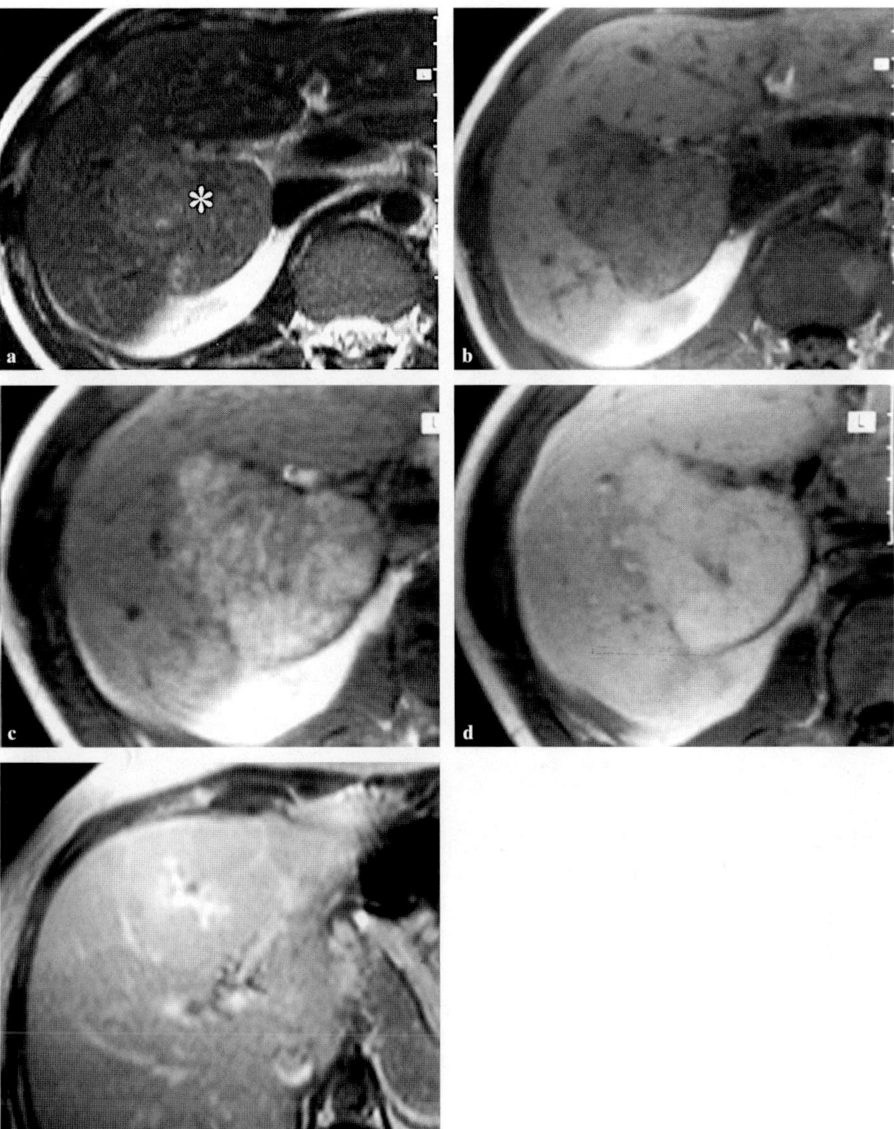

Fig. 21a-e. Atypical focal nodular hyperplasia after Gd-BOPTA. On the unenhanced SE T2-weighted image (**a**), the lesion (*asterisk*) shows lobulated margins, exophytic growth and heterogeneous hyperintensity. On the pre-contrast GE T1-weighted image (**b**), the lesion appears with heterogeneous hypointensity. During the arterial phase (**c**) after Gd-BOPTA administration, the nodule shows intense but heterogeneous enhancement. The lesion remains slightly hyperintense during the equilibrium phase (**d**). The signal intensity and enhancement pattern are not typical for FNH. On the hepatobiliary phase image (**e**), however, the lesion appears slightly hyperintense due to the uptake of Gd-BOPTA by normal hepatocytes and subsequent impaired biliary excretion. This finding is consistent with the characterization of FNH

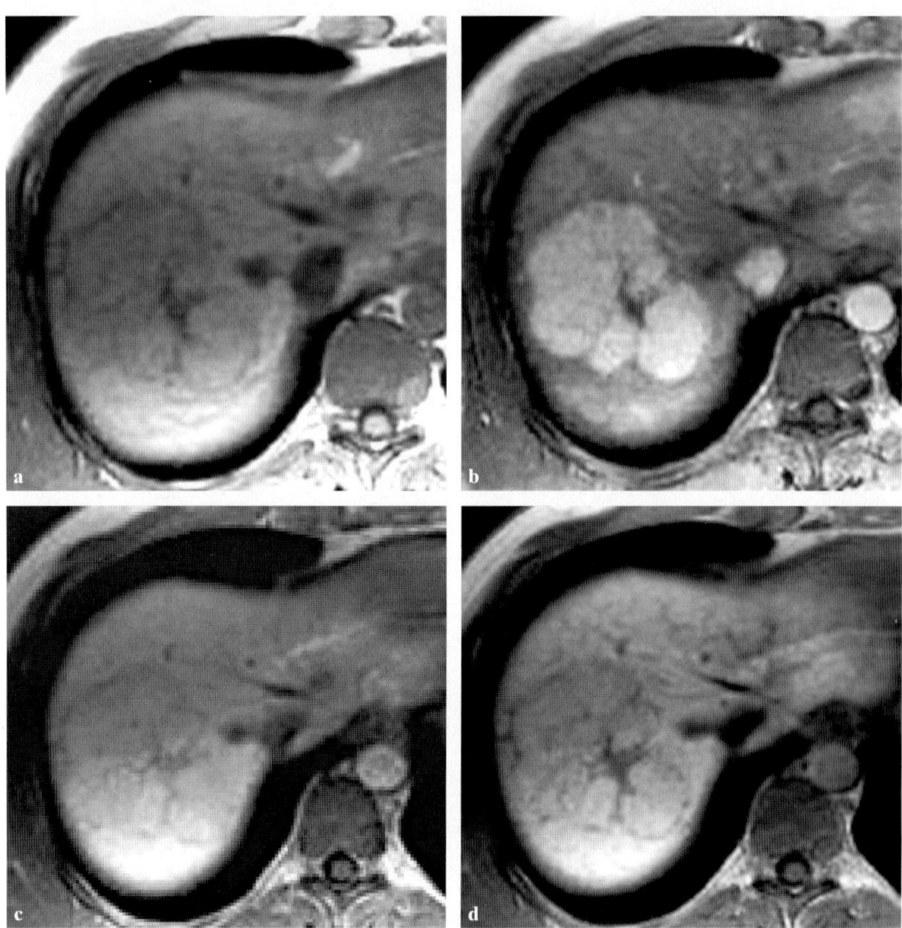

Fig. 22a-d. Focal nodular hyperplasia after Gd-BOPTA. On the pre-contrast T1-weighted image (**a**), the FNH is seen as isointense as compared with surrounding liver tissue. The intense and homogeneous enhancement seen during the arterial phases (**b**) as well as the isointensity demonstrated during the portal-venous (**c**) and hepatobiliary (**d**) phases is typical for FNH

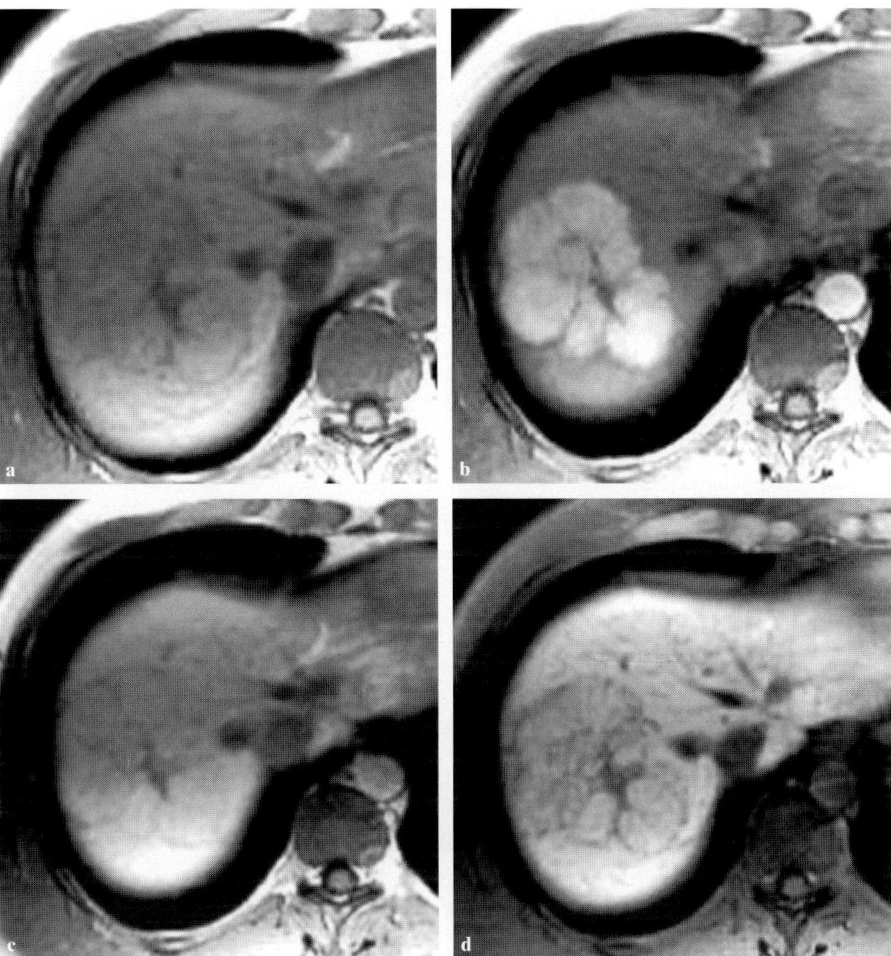

Fig. 23a-d. Focal nodular hyperplasia after Gd-EOB-DTPA. The same case as shown in Fig. 22. The enhancement pattern after Gd-EOB-DTPA is very similar to that observed after Gd-BOPTA; a slightly hypointense lesion on the unenhanced T1-weighted image (**a**) demonstrates strong hypointensity during the arterial phase (**b**) after the administration of Gd-EOB-DTPA. The subsequent portal-venous phase image (**c**) reveals the rapid washout typical of FNH. On the hepatobiliary phase image (**d**) the lesion demonstrates an iso/slightly hypointense appearance compared with the surrounding parenchyma. With this contrast agent the hepatobiliary phase image was acquired after 20 minutes

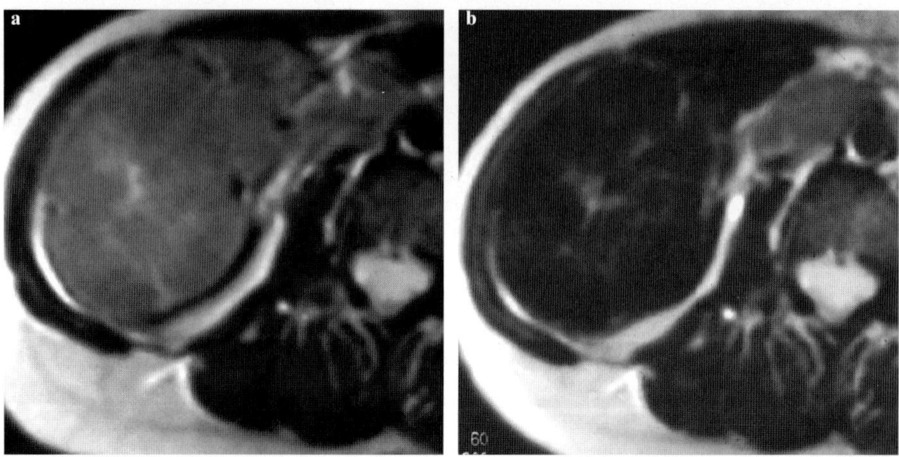

Fig. 24a,b. Focal nodular hyperplasia after SPIO. The unenhanced T2-weighted image (**a**) reveals a large lesion with a central hyperintense area corresponding to scar. On the T2-weighted image acquired after the administration of SPIO (**b**) the lesion shows significant signal drop compared with that seen on the pre-contrast image. The central scar is still seen as a hyperintense area

4.1.4 Hepatocellular Adenoma

The term hepatocellular adenoma (HCA) is used to describe a spectrum of lesions associated with different pathological and etiological factors that give rise to a variety of histological forms. A new classification of adenomas has been proposed, according to which anabolic steroid-associated HCA is considered separately from the classical form [58]. This is due to its distinct histological appearance which often resembles that of hepatocellular carcinoma. An additional separate form is liver adenomatosis (LA), which is characterized by the presence of more than 10 adenomas in an otherwise normal liver, with no history of glycogen storage disease or chronic anabolic steroid use. Typical HCA is defined as a tumor composed of hepatocytes arranged in cords that occasionally form bile. The tumor lacks portal tracts and a terminal hepatic vein [72]. Although the precise pathogenic mechanism of hepatic adenomas is still unknown, the use of estrogen-containing [129] or androgen-containing [111] steroid medications clearly increases their prevalence, number and size within the affected population and often within individual patients. Moreover, this causal relationship is related to dose and duration, with the greatest risk encountered in patients taking large doses of estrogen or androgen for prolonged periods of time [111]. In women who have never used oral contraceptives, the annual incidence of hepatic adenoma is about 1 per million. This increases to 30–40 per million in long-term users of oral contraceptives [93]. Withdrawal of estrogen derivates may result in regression of the HCA. Another risk group for HCA are patients affected by glycogenosis, in particular, type I glycogen storage disease [61]. In these patients, the adenomas are also more likely to be multiple and to undergo malignant transformation, although the latter is still quite rare [113]. HCA occur sporadically in patients without known predisposing factors and rarely in children and adult males. A recently recognized association is that of congenital or acquired abnormalities of the hepatic vasculature. Portal vein absence or occlusion [78] or portohepatic venous shunts [57] have been noted, particularly in patients with LA [40]. Although the adenomas in LA are histologically similar to other adenomas, they are not steroid dependent, but are multiple, progressive, symptomatic, and more likely to lead to impaired liver function, hemorrhage, and perhaps malignant degeneration [40]. An association with pregnancy has also been described, probably due to increased levels of endogenous steroid hormones [118].

Most patients with only one or few adenomas are asymptomatic and almost invariably have normal liver function and no elevation of serum "tumor markers", such as α-fetoprotein. Large adenomas may cause a sensation of right upper quadrant fullness or discomfort. However, the classic clinical manifestation of HCA is spontaneous rupture or hemorrhage, leading to acute abdominal pain, which may progress to hypotension and even death [62].

HCA are reported to be solitary in 70–80% of cases, but it is not unusual to encounter two or three adenomas in one patient, particularly at multiphasic CT or MR imaging [50, 86]. Patients with glycogen storage disease or LA, may have dozens of adenomas detected at CT or MR imaging and even more at close examination of resected specimens [30, 40, 96]. Individual adenomas vary in size from less than 1 cm to more than 15 cm. The typical steroid-related adenoma often comes to clinical attention when it reaches about 5 cm in diameter. Large and multiple adenomas are more prone to spontaneous hemorrhage [62]. The propensity to hemorrhage reflects the histological characteristics of adenomas in which the cord-like arrangement of cells structured in large plates are separated by dilated sinusoids. These sinusoids are equivalent to thin-walled capillaries. Because adenomas lack a portal-venous supply, they are perfused by arterial pressure deriving solely from peripheral arterial feeding vessels. The hypervascular nature of HCA is due principally to the extensive sinusoids and feeding arteries, and to the poor connective tissue support which also predisposes the lesion to hemorrhage. Because a tumor capsule is usually absent or incomplete, hemorrhage often spreads to the normal liver or abdominal cavity [72]. Kupffer cells are often found in adenomas but in reduced number and with little or no function, as reflected by the absent or diminished uptake of technetiom [Tc)-99m sulfur colloid [101]. A key histologic feature that helps distinguish HCA from FNH is the notable absence of bile ductules in adenomas [11]. Adenoma cells are generally larger than normal hepatocytes and contain large amounts of glycogen and lipid. Intra- and intercellular lipid may appear as macroscopic fat deposits within the tumor [50], and it is this accumulation of lipid that is responsible for the characteristic yellow appearance at the cut surface of adenoma. Evidence of lipid on CT or MR imaging can be helpful for the diagnosis of HCA.

Ultrasound typically reveals a large hypoechoic lesion with central anechoic areas that correspond to areas of internal hemorrhage, if present (Fig. 25) [134]. However, these findings are not specific for adenoma. Occasionally, adenomas undergo massive necrotic and hemorrhagic changes, with the result that the ultrasound appearance is that of a complex mass with large cystic components. Color Doppler ultrasound demonstrates peripheral arteries and veins, which correlate well with both gross and angiographic findings (Fig. 26). In addition color Doppler may identify intratumoral veins. This finding is absent in FNH and may be a useful discriminating feature for HCA [34].

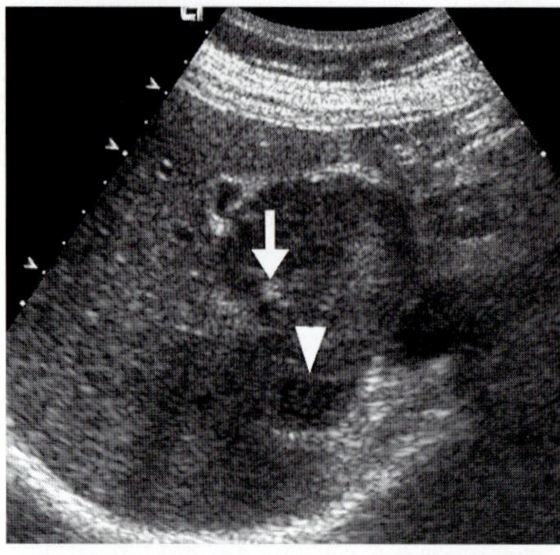

Fig. 25. Hepatocellular adenoma. On ultrasound, adenoma is often heterogeneous in echogenicity, with both hyperechoic (*arrow*) and hypoechoic (*arrowhead*) areas that correspond to areas of hemorrhage, necrosis and fatty infiltration

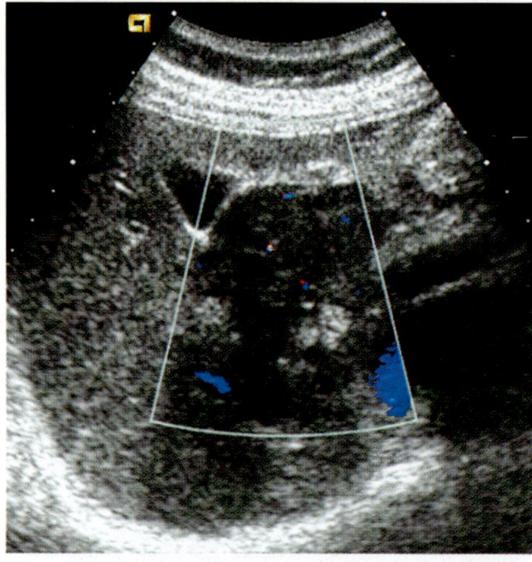

Fig. 26. Hepatocellular adenoma. Color Doppler ultrasound reveals the hypervascular intratumoral and peripheral vessels characterizing this lesion

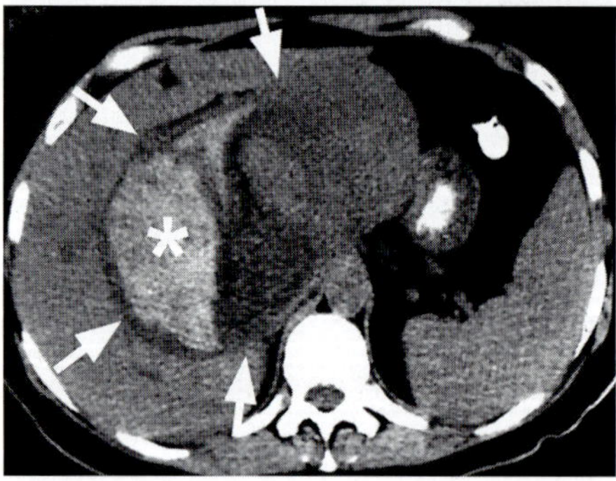

Fig. 27. Hemorrhagic hepatocellular adenoma. The pre-contrast CT scan reveals a large and inhomogeneous hypodense lesion (*arrows*) with a hyperdense component (*asterisk*) corresponding to acute hemorrhage

Adenomas are usually seen as hypodense masses on unenhanced CT images due to the presence of fat and glycogen within the tumor. However, hyperdense areas corresponding to fresh hemorrhage are frequently noted (Fig. 27). During dynamic bolus-enhanced CT imaging, small, non-complicated adenomas generally enhance rapidly and have increased attenuation relative to the normal liver (Fig. 28) [47]. However, the enhancement does not persist in adenomas because of arterio-venous shunting [100]. Large or complicated adenomas may be more heterogeneous than smaller lesions and thus the appearance on CT is not specific [47].

Adenomas frequently show heterogeneous hyperintensity on unenhanced T2-weighted images and heterogeneous hypointensity on unenhanced T1-weighted images, with areas of increased signal intensity indicating the presence of fat and hemorrhage and areas of reduced signal intensity indicating necrosis [86]. Sometimes, adenomas have a peripheral hypointense rim, corresponding to a fibrous capsule. In most cases, the rim is of low signal intensity on both T1- and T2-weighted images [4] (Fig. 29).

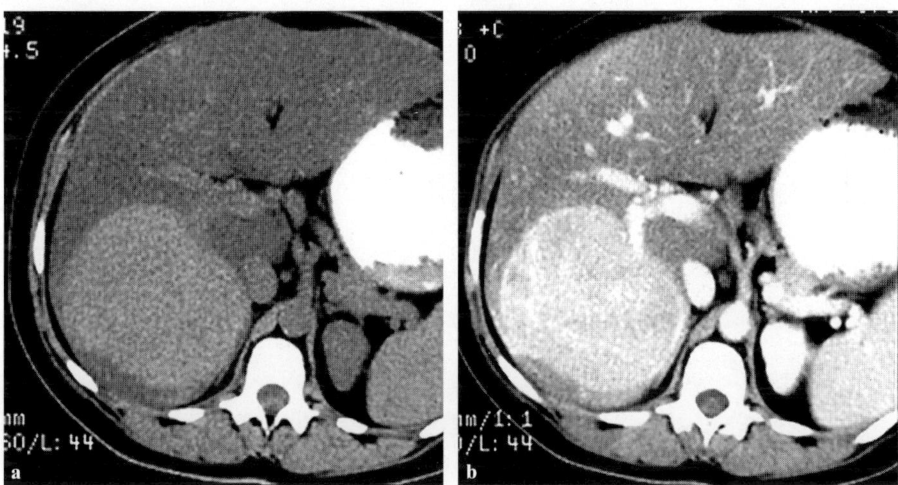

Fig. 28a,b. Non-complicated hepatocellular adenoma. On the pre-contrast CT scan (**a**), the mass appears homogeneously hyperdense compared to the surrounding liver tissue, demonstrating fatty changes. During the arterial phase after the administration of contrast medium (**b**), the density of the lesion markedly increases homogeneously

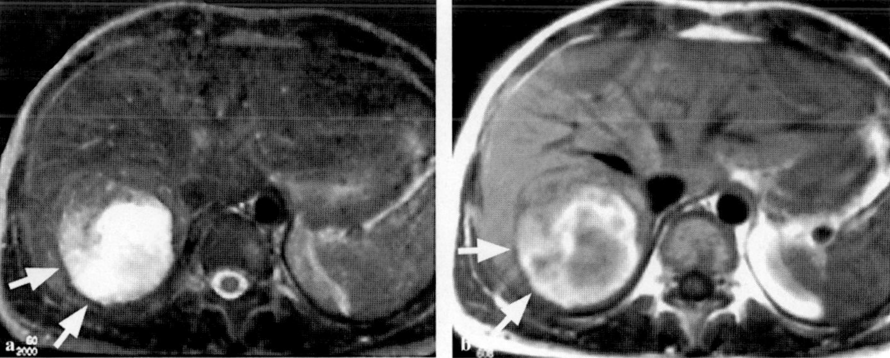

Fig. 29a,b. Complicated hepatocellular adenoma. Diffuse intratumoral hemorrhage within the hepatocellular adenoma appears heterogeneously hyperintense on the unenhanced SE T2-weighted image (**a**) and heterogeneously hypointense on the corresponding unenhanced SE T1-weighted image (**b**). A peripheral hypointense rim (*arrows*) representing a fibrous capsule is visible on both sequences

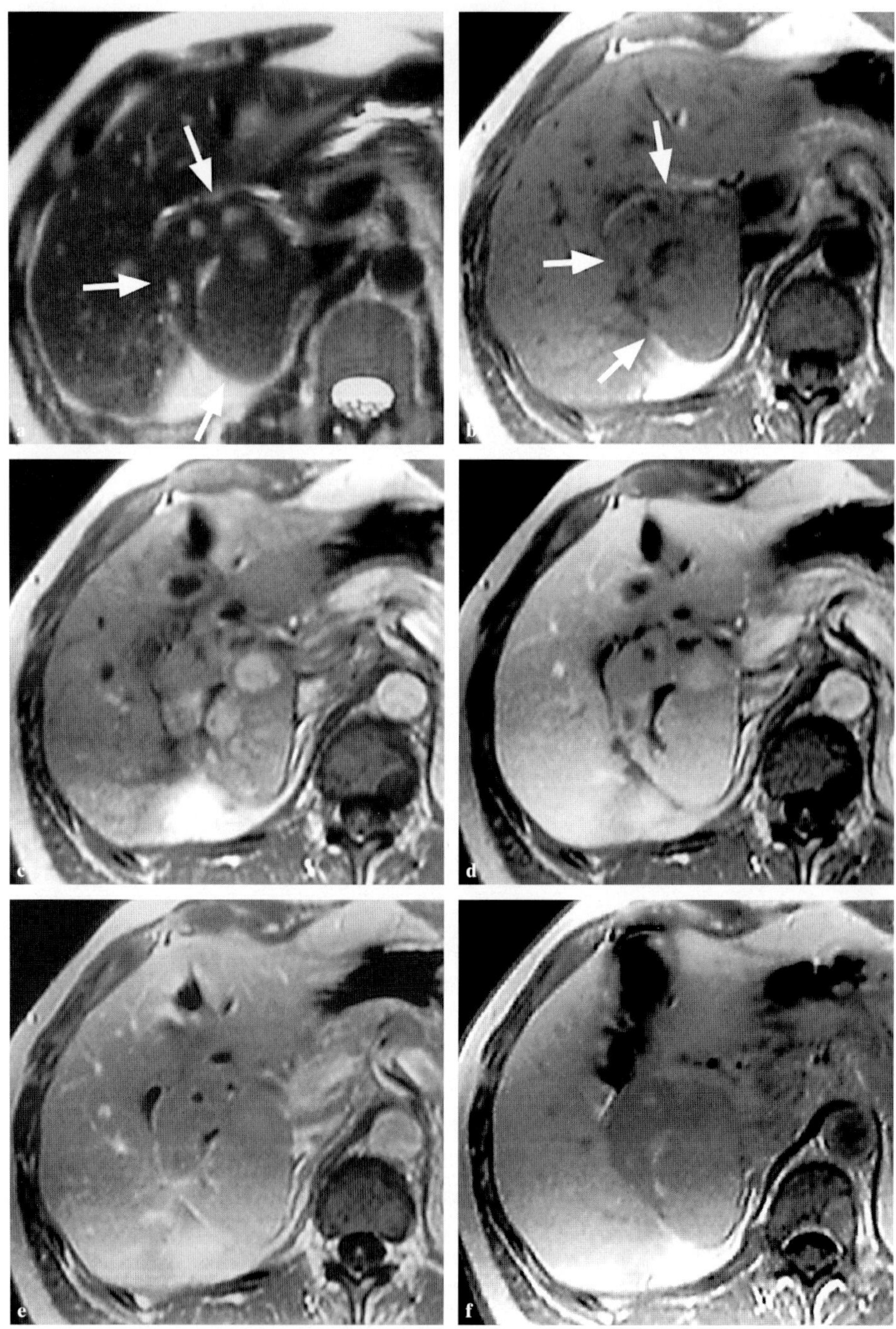

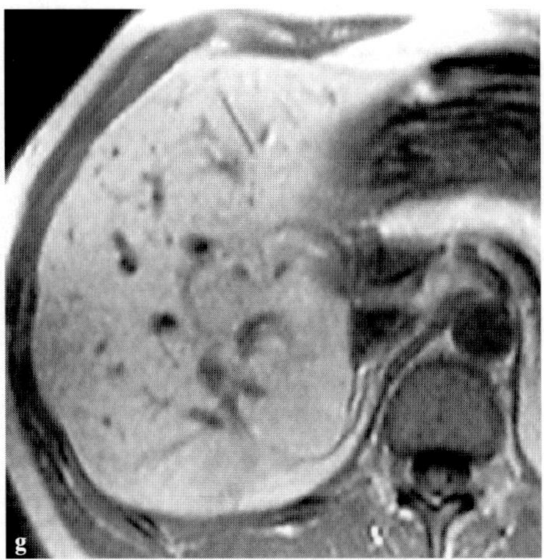

Fig. 30a-g. Hepatocellular adenoma: Gd-BOPTA versus Mn-DPDP. A lesion (*arrows*) appears isointense compared to surrounding liver tissue with intratumoral hyperintense areas on the HASTE T2-weighted image (**a**) and heterogeneously isointense on the pre-contrast T1-weighted image (**b**). During the arterial phase after the bolus injection of Gd-BOPTA (**c**), the lesion demonstrates heterogeneous enhancement. On the subsequent portal-venous and equilibrium phases (**d** and **e**, respectively) the lesion appears mainly isointense to the liver. In the liver-specific phase after administration of Gd-BOPTA (**f**) the lesion is seen as hypointense but shows some internal hyperintense peliotic areas. The hypointense appearance may be due to a decreased uptake of Gd-BOPTA into the hepatocytes in HCA as well as to the absence of bile ductules. On delayed phase images acquired after the administration of mangafodipir (Mn-DPDP) (**g**), the lesion demonstrates uptake of the contrast medium and appears isointense in comparison with the normal liver tissue. This may be explained by a non-specific uptake of free Mn^{++} in HCA

The presence of subcapsular feeding vessels and the hypervascular nature of adenomas results in their enhancement during the arterial phase of the dynamic series after injection of Gd-BOPTA or other gadolinium-based agents. On portal-venous and equilibrium phase images, adenomas generally appear isointense or slightly hyperintense, although focal heterogeneous hypointense areas may be seen if necrosis, calcification or fibrosis is present. Adenomas typically appear hypointense to the normal parenchyma on delayed, hepatobiliary phase images after Gd-BOPTA, due to the absence of biliary ducts (Figs. 30, 31). This criterion is useful for distinguishing non complicated HCA from FNH which generally appear isointense or slightly hyperintense. After the administration of Mn-DPDP hepatic adenomas usually resemble FNH in appearing iso- or slightly hyperintense to the normal liver (Figs. 30, 31). Thus, the differentiation of adenoma from FNH is more difficult with Mn-DPDP.

In some cases, adenomas may take up SPIO, resulting in decreased signal intensity on T2-weighted images. However the uptake of SPIO in adenoma is usually poor compared to that which occurs in FNH [124].

It has been noted that both FNH and HCA occur more often in patients who have coexistent vascular tumors, portal-venous absence or occlusion, or portohepatic venous shunts [31, 50]. It is possible that a focal disturbance of the hepatic blood supply may somehow facilitate the hyperplastic development of these two similar benign lesions [40].

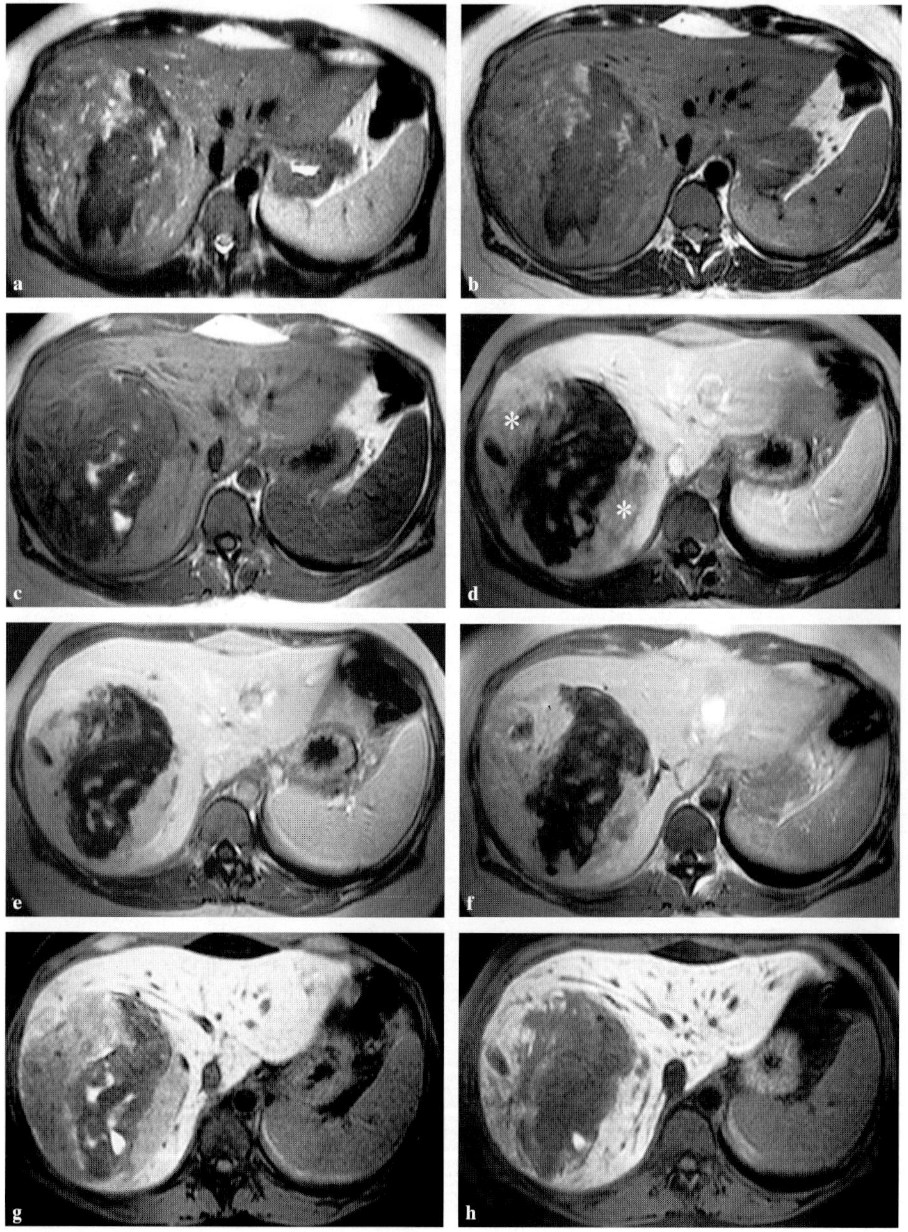

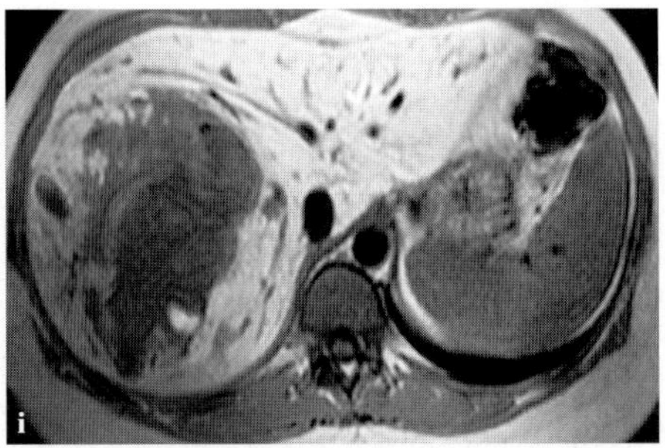

Fig. 31a-i. Complicated hepatocellular adenoma: Gd-BOPTA versus Mn-DPDP. Unenhanced HASTE T2-weighted (**a**) and Turbo SE T2-weighted images (**b**) reveal a large heterogeneous hyper-hypointense mass in the right lobe. This lesion is seen as heterogeneously hypointense on the unenhanced GE T1-weighted image (**c**). T1-weighted imaging during the arterial (**d**), portal-venous (**e**) and equilibrium (**f**) phases after the bolus injection of Gd-BOPTA, reveals enhancement only in the periphery of the lesion (*asterisks in* **d**); a large hypointense central area corresponding to intratumoral hemorrhage does not show any enhancement. On the delayed hepatobiliary phase image after the administration of Gd-BOPTA (**g**), the lesion appears hypointense. Conversely, the cellular peripheral component shows enhancement and appears isointense with the surrounding liver parenchyma on delayed phase images after mangafodipir (**h**, **i**)

Liver adenomatosis (LA) is characterized by the presence of multiple (>10) lesions of adenoma, by the absence of any correlation with steroid medication, by involvement in both men and women, and by abnormal increases in serum alkaline phosphatase and γ-glutamyltransferase levels [30]. The conditions that may predispose patients to LA are poorly understood, although congenital or acquired abnormalities of the hepatic vasculature, such as hepatic vein abnormalities and/or the congenital absence of a portal vein, may be involved [40].

Patients with LA are at increased risk for the development of HCC and should be monitored closely with CT or MR imaging as well as with serum α-fetoprotein and other tumor marker examinations [62, 96].

Clinically, patients with LA may be asymptomatic or have chronic or acute abdominal pain. The multiple adenomas in LA may have a variety of appearances, but the CT and MR characteristics of individual lesions are similar to those reported for sporadic or solitary adenomas (Fig. 32) [50, 86].

Management of LA remains difficult because there is no predictive sign of potential complications other than the size of the lesions. Liver resection is the preferred option because LA is essentially a benign disease that does not impair hepatocellular function. Liver transplantation remains a difficult decision, although it is sometimes the last option in progressive forms. Surgery is indicated for acute complications such as hemorrhage [16].

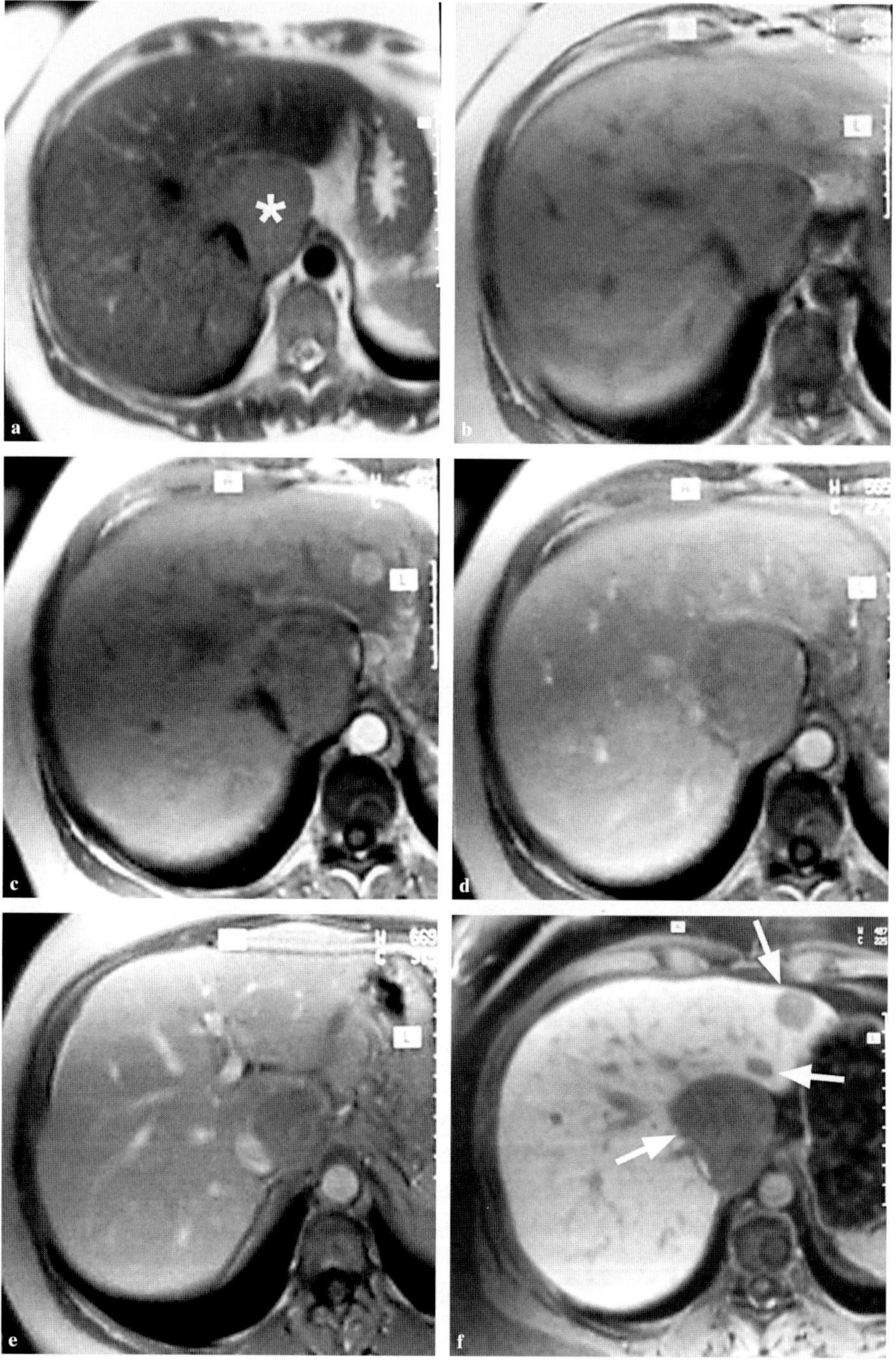

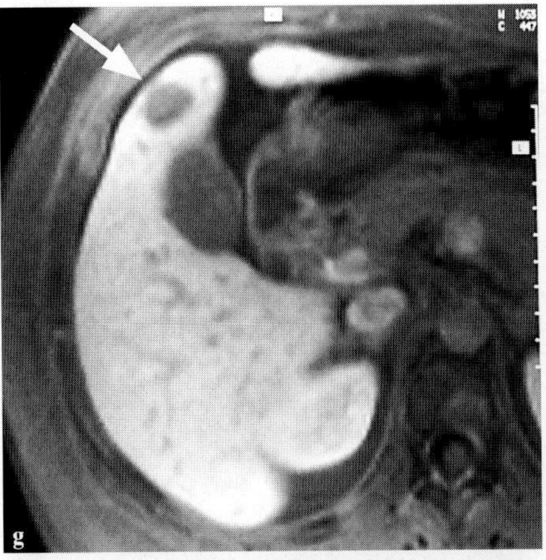

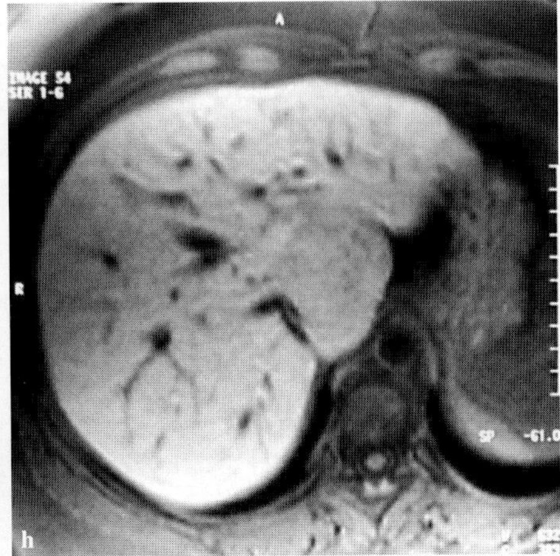

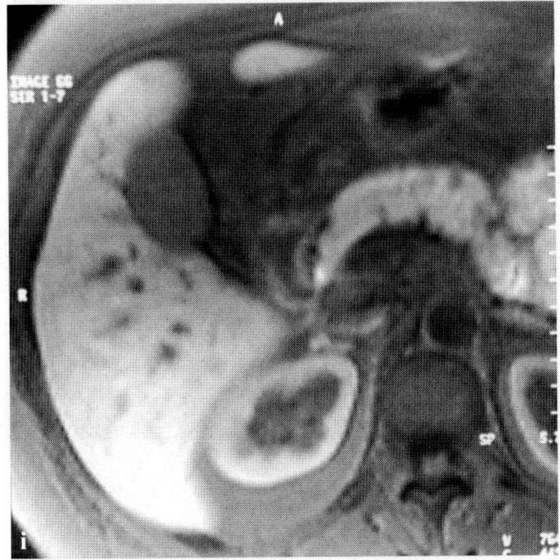

Fig. 32a-i. Liver adenomatosis: Gd-BOPTA versus Mn-DPDP. The HASTE T2-weighted image (**a**) reveals several large, slightly hyperintense nodules with the biggest (*asterisk*) located in the caudal lobe. These nodules appear isointense compared with the surrounding parenchyma on the unenhanced GE T1-weighted image (**b**). The lesions do not show significant enhancement on arterial phase images acquired after the bolus administration of Gd-BOPTA (**c**), whereas on the portal-venous (**d**) and equilibrium (**e**) phase images the lesions appear iso- to hypointense. On delayed phase images acquired after the administration of Gd-BOPTA (**f** and **g**), several hypointense nodules (*arrows*) are visible. Conversely, after mangafodipir administration, the lesions are isointense to the normal liver and not clearly delineated (**h** and **i**)

4.1.5   Nodular Regenerative Hyperplasia

Nodular regenerative hyperplasia (NRH) of the liver is a condition characterized by a diffuse micronodular transformation of the hepatic parenchyma without the formation of fibrous septa [127]. The nodules may vary in size between 0.1 and 1 cm but are usually smaller than 1 cm. Various systemic diseases and drugs are often associated with the appearance of NRH: myeloproliferative syndromes (polycytemia vera, chronic myelogeneous leukemia, and myeloid metaplasia); lymphoproliferative syndromes (Hodgkin's and non-Hodgkin's lymphoma, chronic lymphocytic leukemia, and plasma cell dysplasia); chronic vascular disorders (polyarteritis nodosa); rheumatological disorders (rheumatoid arthritis, Felty's syndrome, sclerodermia, calcinosis cutis, Raynaud's phenomenon, sclerodactyly and telangiectasia), lupus erythematosus; steroids and antineoplastic medication [24, 112, 130].

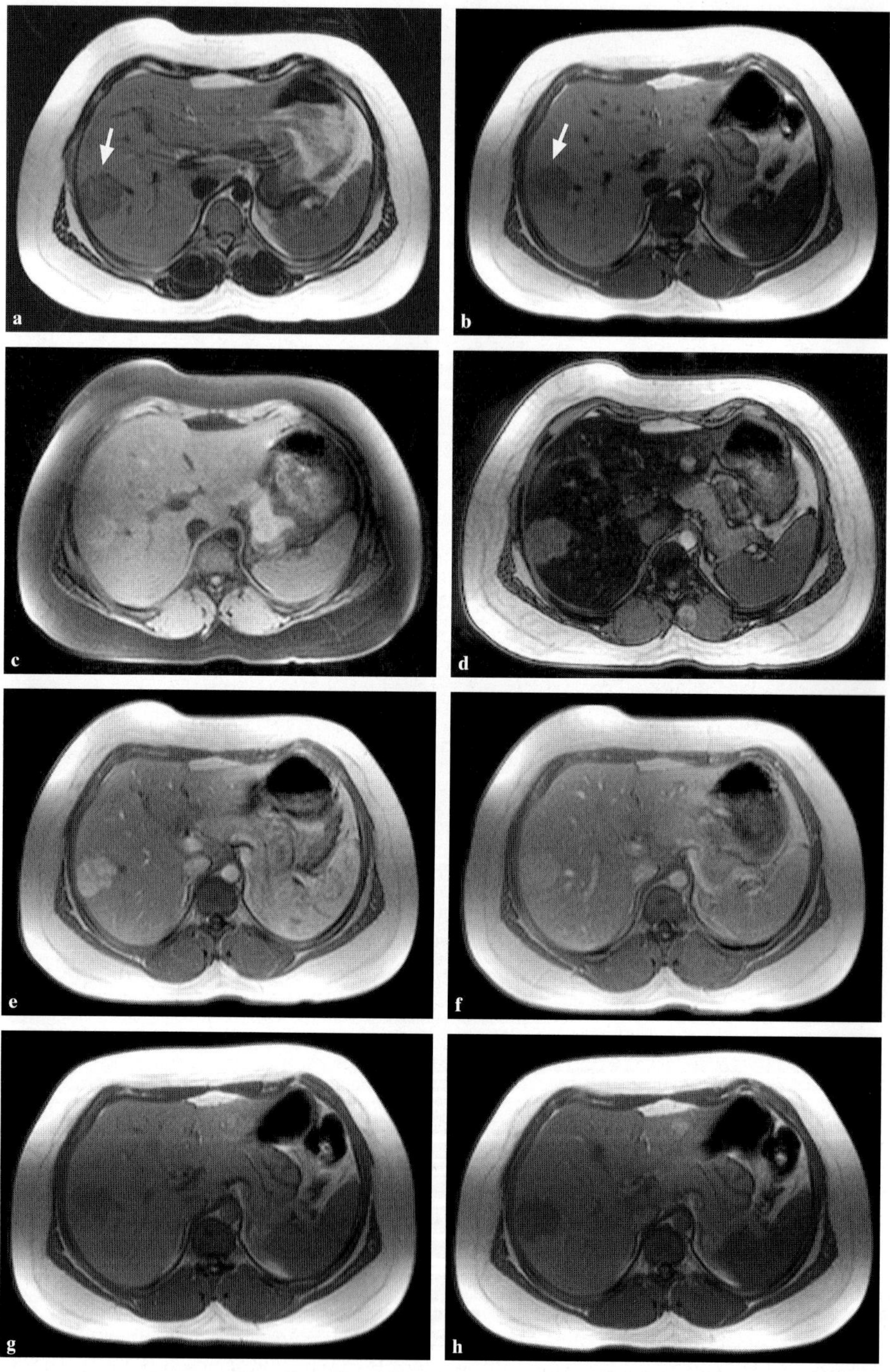

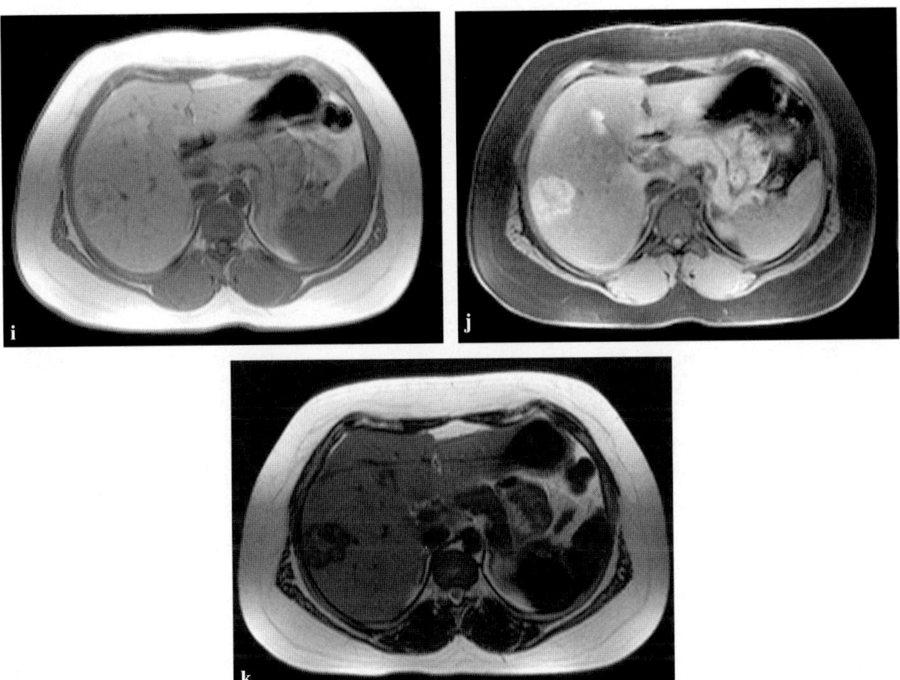

Fig. 33a-k. Nodular regenerative hyperplasia in a fatty liver: Gd-BOPTA versus USPIO. Due to diffuse fatty infiltration of the liver, the NRH nodule (*arrow*) in the right liver lobe appears hypointense on both T2w images (**a**) and T1w images (**b**). However, on fat suppressed T1w images (**c**), the lesion appears hyperintense. This is more apparent on opposed phase imaging (**d**), indicating diffuse fatty infiltration of the liver. On contrast enhanced imaging using Gd-BOPTA, a strong enhancement of the lesion in the arterial phase can be noted (**e**). The lesion appears slightly hyperintense in the portal-venous phase due to contrast medium pooling (**f**). Arterial phase imaging after the bolus injection of iron oxide (SHU 555A) suggests that the lesion is perfused (**g**). However, the lesion once again appears hypointense in the portal-venous phase (**h**). The lesion appears slightly hyperintense on T1w images acquired during the hepatobiliary phase after Gd-BOPTA (**i**). This is more obvious on T1w fs images acquired at the same time point (**j**) and is due to the fact that the NRH contains functioning hepatocytes that are able to take up Gd-BOPTA to a higher degree than the surrounding fatty liver tissue. This behavior clearly underlines the diagnosis of a benign lesion. On T2w images acquired after SHU 555 A injection (**k**) the lesion is even more hypointense as compared with unenhanced images (**a**). This indicates that the lesion contains functioning Kupffer cells

Disturbance of the hepatic microcirculation is believed to be the primary cause of NRH [127]. Several different combinations of vascular obliteration can lead to a variegated parenchyma with atrophy and secondary hyperplasia [128]. The particular pattern of obliteration determines the size and distribution of the nodules. The presence of uniform small nodules is usually produced by small portal vein obliteration. This commonly occurs because of inflammatory lesions in the small portal tracts, typically in early-stage primary biliary cirrhosis and various rheumatologic conditions. With these two examples, the primary lesion involves small ducts and small arteries, respectively, and the obliteration of the adjacent portal veins is a bystander effect. Because the tissue involvement is patchy, some small portal veins remain patent, giving a variegated pattern of patent and obliterated veins, which explains the presence of both atrophy and hyperplasia. Increased flow through the portal vein in the presence of splenomegaly may exacerbate nodule formation on those acini with a patent portal vein [9]. After thrombosis of large portal veins, there are often large contiguous regions of parenchyma near the hilum that retain portal flow and escape atrophy. This situation also leads to large regenerative nodules (macronodular hyperplasia, partial nodular transformation), a variant characterized by large nodules several centimeters in diameter near the large portal tracts and atrophy with small nodules in peripheral parts of the liver [51, 73, 108, 117]. In addition to this simple response to variegated portal vein flow, secondary arterial hyperemia and arterial growth may enhance the topographic variegation of blood flow. Arterial growth leads to large regenerative nodules that resemble FNH [114].

In non-cirrhotic conditions, the hepatic venules are usually normal despite severe portal vein disease. Nodular hyperplasia may result from primary outflow obstruction through either hepatic vein thrombosis or congestive heart failure [15]. In these situations, the nodules are less uniformly distributed and are accompanied by sinusoidal congestion and fibrous septation [114, 132].

NRH occurs in all ages with a mean age of 50 years, with no sex difference. It is rarely reported in childhood but when present, is usually associated with portal vascular abnormalities such as congenital portal vein absence [41]. It may also occur in the setting of diffuse fatty liver due to toxic or hormonal changes (Fig. 33).

The lesions may be found incidentally during surgery or imaging studies. Symptoms and signs, when present, can be divided into the following broad categories:

- symptoms of the underlying disease (Felty's syndrome, myeloproliferative disorders);
- manifestations of portal hypertension such as esophageal varices, splenomegaly and ascites;
- hepatic failure
- acute abdominal crisis following rupture of a large nodule with hemoperitoneum
- symptoms of hypersplenism.

Liver function tests are usually either normal or slightly altered. The most common abnormalities observed are elevation of alkaline phosphatase and γ-glutamyl-transferase (GGT).

In most ultrasound examinations, the hepatic parenchyma of patients with NRH appears normal and no nodules of NRH are visible. In a few cases, however, well-delineated hypoechoic or isoechoic nodules can be depicted (Fig. 34) [24, 85, 87, 120].

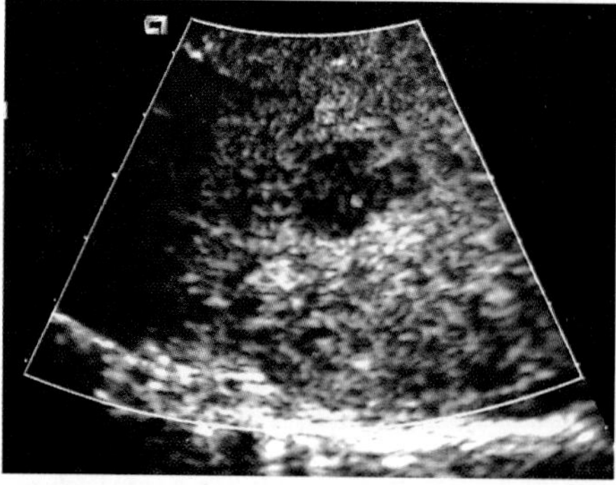

Fig. 34. Nodular regenerative hyperplasia. The ultrasound scan reveals a well demarcated homogeneous hypoechoic nodule. Color Doppler may show vascularity within the lesion

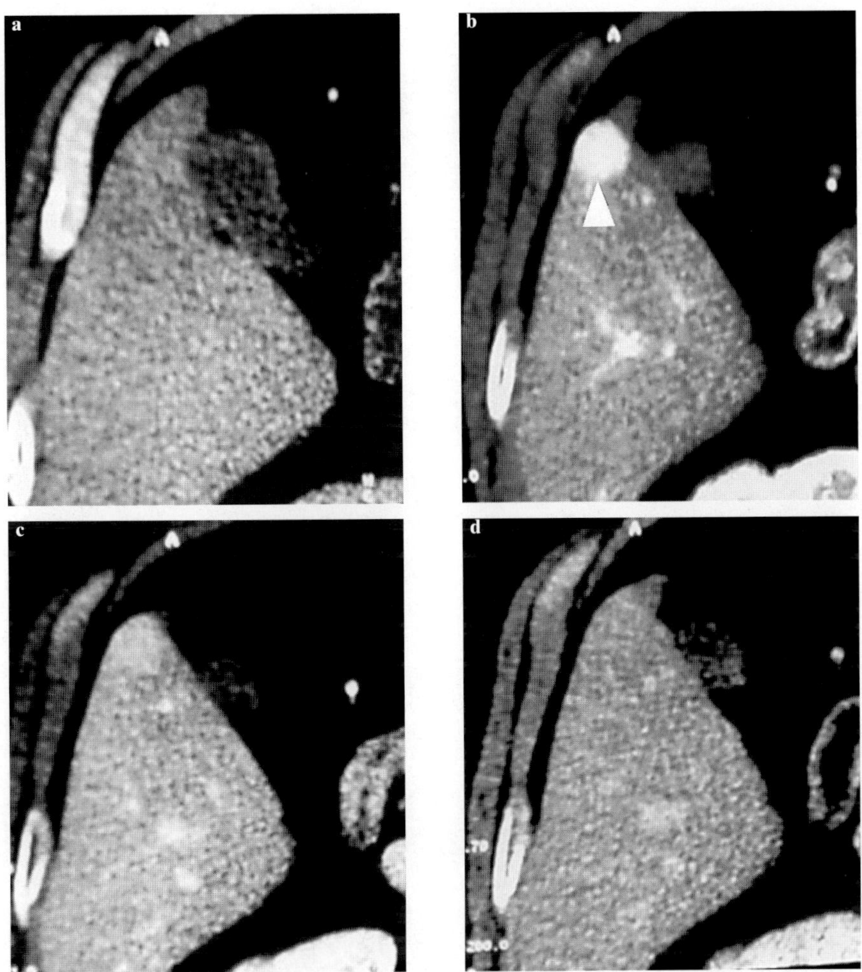

Fig. 35a-d. Nodular regenerative hyperplasia. Whereas the pre-contrast CT scan (**a**) appears normal, on arterial phase images acquired after the administration of contrast medium (**b**), the NRH nodule (*arrowhead*) enhances markedly and homogeneously. In the portal-venous (**c**) and equilibrium (**d**) phases, the nodule is seen as slightly hyperdense and isodense, respectively

Hyperechoic nodules have been reported on very rare occasions [19], while on other occasions, a diffusely heterogeneous hepatic parenchyma can be seen.

With CT imaging, approximately half of the cases appear normal, while the nodules in the remaining cases are typically hypoattenuating relative to the adjacent normal hepatic parenchyma [24, 87]. Rarely, spontaneously hyperattenuating nodules can be depicted [24]. Usually the nodules do not enhance after administration of contrast material, although hyperenhancing nodules with arterioportal shunting have been reported (Fig. 35) [14, 29].

On unenhanced T1-weighted MR images, the lesions are generally isointense or slightly hyperintense to the surrounding liver parenchyma, while on unenhanced T2-weighted images they appear isointense or slightly hypointense. A peripheral

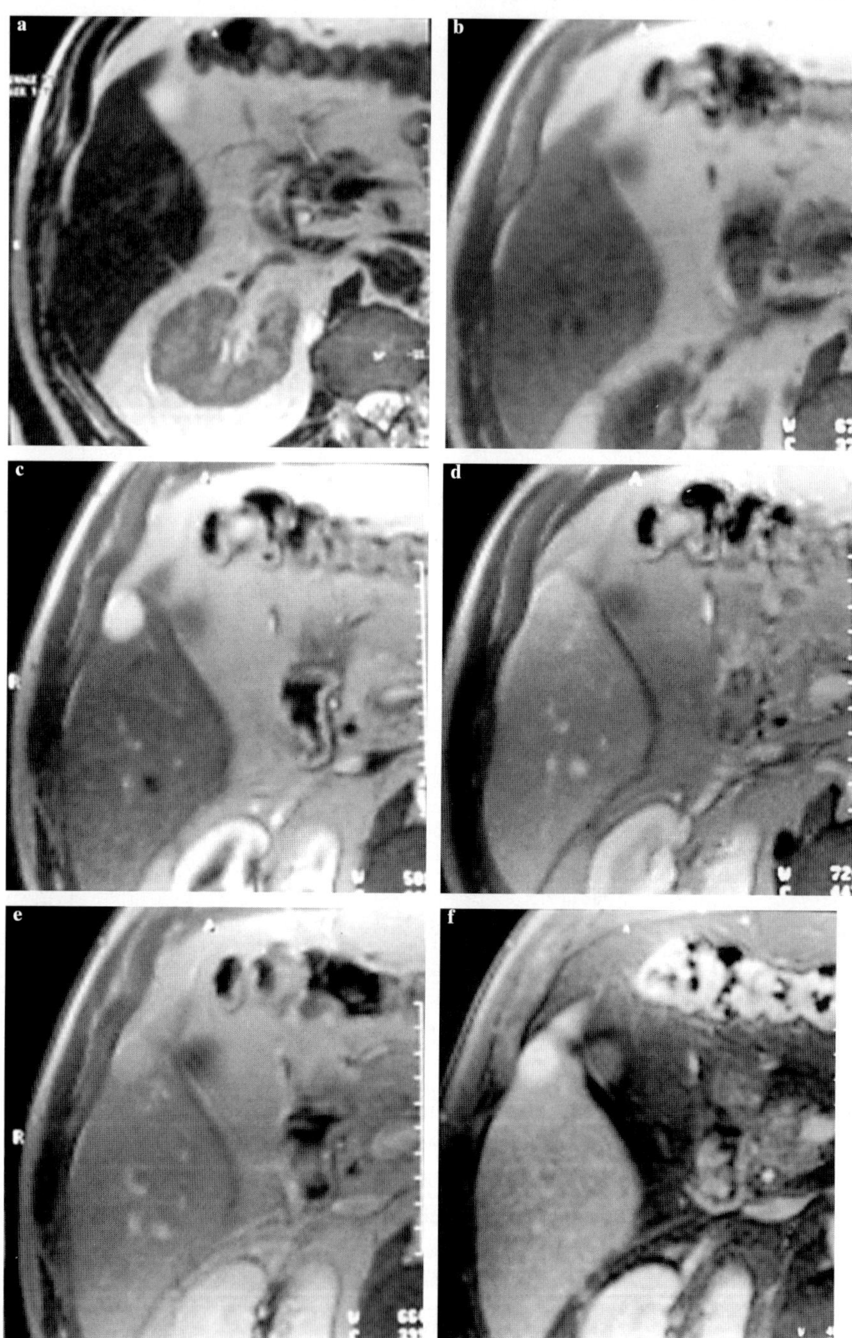

Fig. 36a-f. Nodular regenerative hyperplasia. The same case as shown in Fig. 35. The lesion is seen as isointense compared with the normal liver tissue on the pre-contrast T2- and T1-weighted images (**a** and **b**, respectively) and then highly hyperintense on arterial phase images after the bolus injection of Gd-BOPTA (**c**). The lesion retains a slightly hyperintense appearance during the subsequent portal-venous (**d**) and equilibrium (**e**) phases, and is seen as homogeneously hyperintense on the delayed, liver-specific phase image (**f**)

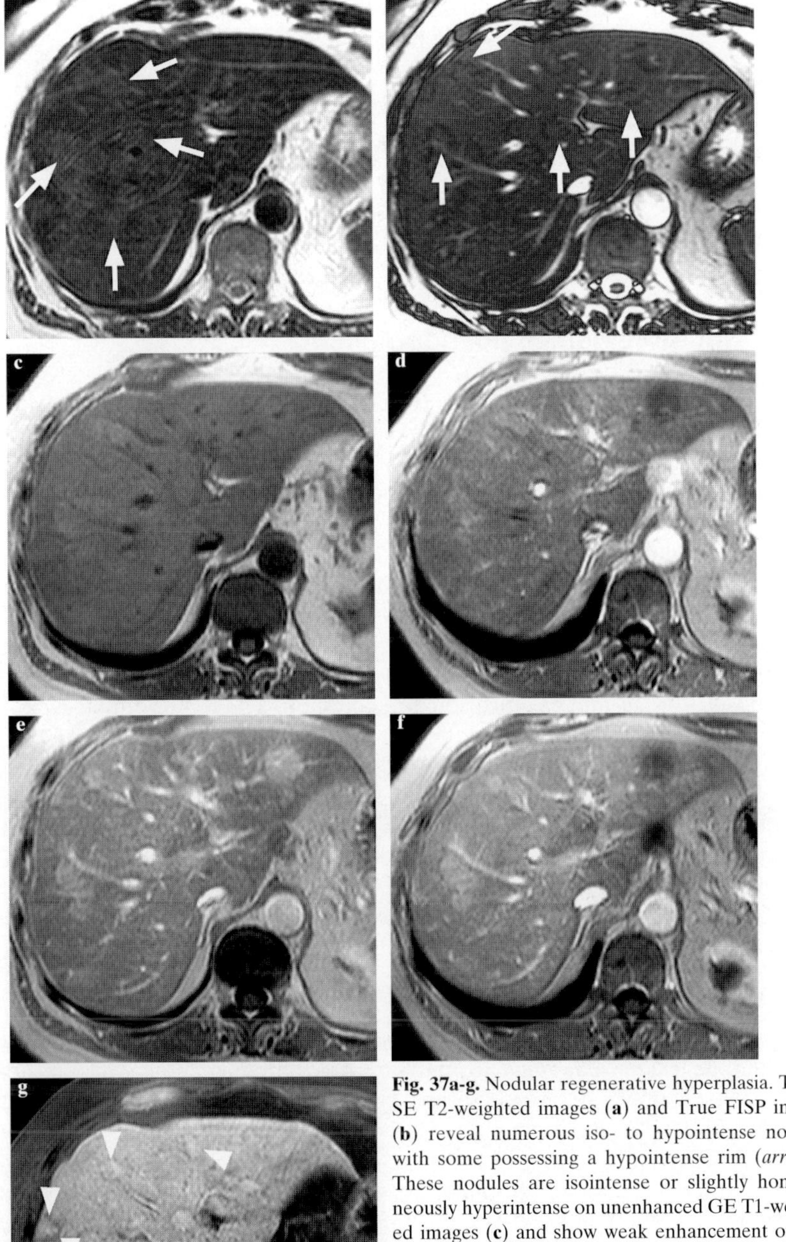

Fig. 37a-g. Nodular regenerative hyperplasia. Turbo SE T2-weighted images (**a**) and True FISP images (**b**) reveal numerous iso- to hypointense nodules with some possessing a hypointense rim (*arrows*). These nodules are isointense or slightly homogeneously hyperintense on unenhanced GE T1-weighted images (**c**) and show weak enhancement on T1-weighted arterial phase images acquired after Gd-BOPTA administration (**d**). The lesions remain slightly hyperintense on the subsequent portal-venous (**e**) and equilibrium (**f**) phase images. Delayed hepatobiliary phase images (**g**) reveal numerous hyperintense nodules with peripheral hypointense rims (*arrowheads*). The delayed hyperintensity after Gd-BOPTA reflects abnormal biliary system drainage hypointense rim is often visible in large lesions on T1-weighted images. This usually appears hyperintense on arterial phase images and isointense in the subsequent portal-venous and equilibrium phases. On delayed phase images after Gd-BOPTA administration, the lesions may appear isointense or hyperintense since they consist of benign hepatocytes with abnormal biliary system drainage (Fig. 36). The peripheral hypointense rim is better evaluated in this delayed phase and probably represents an ischemic perinodular area (Fig. 37) [14, 110].

After injection of iron oxide particles, the lesions usually show a significant uptake of contrast agents due to the presence of Kupffer cells.

4.1.6   Infantile Hemangioendothelioma

Infantile hemangioendothelioma (IHE) is the most common benign liver tumor in children. It is a vascular tumor deriving from endothelial cells that proliferate and form vascular channels. IHE is relatively common and accounts for 10–15% of all childhood hepatic tumors [25]. Ninety percent of IHE are discovered within the first 6 months of life and females are affected more than males.

IHE are usually multiple and diffuse; a solitary lesion is an uncommon variant [69]. The nodules vary from a few millimeters to 15 cm or more in size. They are round, red-brown and spongy or white-yellow with fibrotic predominance in mature cases [98]. Microscopically, IHEs represent a proliferation of small vascular channels lined by endothelial cells. Cavernous areas, as well as foci of hemorrhage, thrombosis, fibrosis and calcification, are common. The multinodular type may also involve other organs as well as the skin [58].

Clinical findings, if present, may include hepatomegaly, congestive heart failure, thrombocytopenia caused by the trapping of platelets by the tumor, and occasional rupture with hemoperitoneum [65]. In symptomatic cases treatment modalities include steroid administration, chemo/radiotherapy, embolization or ligation of the hepatic artery and resection.

The natural history of IHEs is benign, and lesions tend to regress gradually over a matter of months [84]. However, malignant transformation of IHE into angiosarcoma may occur on rare occasions.

The ultrasonographic features of IHE are varied. Typically, there is a complex liver mass with large, draining hepatic veins [133]. Single or multiple lesions may be seen, and the lesions may range from hypoechoic to hyperechoic. These lesions may involute slowly over a period of months and develop increased echogenicity [23, 84].

On unenhanced CT examinations, IHE appears as a hypodense mass with or without calcifications [89]. Early enhancement of the edge of the mass with variable delayed central enhancement is usually seen after administration of contrast agent [89].

Vascular channels and cyst-like components, which are usually well defined, determine the hypointensity of the lesions on unenhanced T1-weighted MR images. On T2-weighted images the lesions usually appear homogeneously hyperintense. After contrast agent administration, intense, peripheral enhancement or, less frequently, globular enhancement may be seen. Complete or incomplete filling-in during the portal-venous or equilibrium phases is also observed. On delayed phase images after Gd-BOPTA, IHE tend to be isointense or hypointense compared to the surrounding liver parenchyma (Fig. 38) [81, 89].

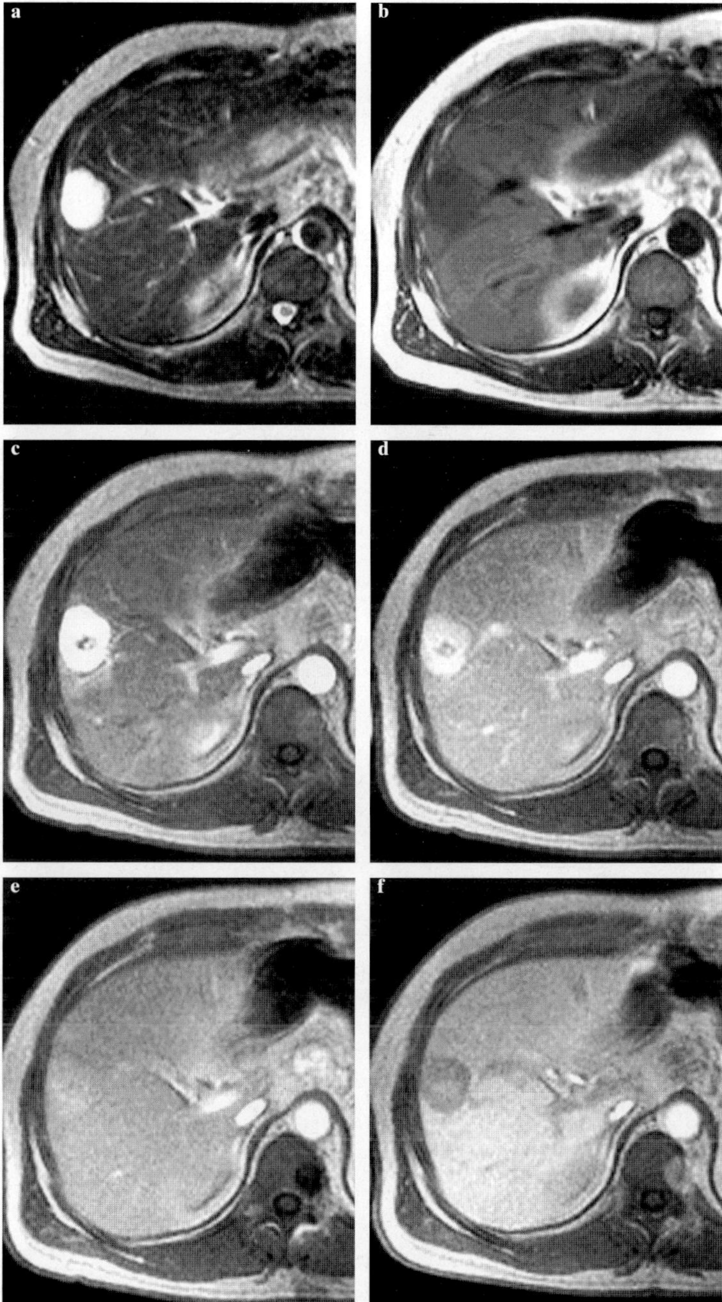

Fig. 38a-f. Infantile hemangioendothelioma. The nodule is homogeneously hyperintense compared to the adjacent liver tissue on the pre-contrast T2-weighted image (**a**), and is seen as hypointense on the pre-contrast T1-weighted image (**b**). Dynamic phase imaging after the administration of Gd-BOPTA reveals peripheral intense enhancement during the arterial phase (**c**), incomplete filling-in during the portal-venous phase (**d**) and complete filling-in during the equilibrium phase (**e**). The nodule is well-defined and hypointense with central contrast agent pooling on the delayed hepatobiliary phase image (**f**)

4.1.7   Cysts and Cystic Tumors

4.1.7.1   Cysts

Primary hepatic cysts should be distinguished from other cystic masses of the liver. A true cyst of the liver or a bile duct cyst is distinguished by the presence of an epithelial lining on the inner surface. A simple hepatic cyst, on the other hand, is defined as a single unilocular cyst and the wall is composed of a thin layer of fibrous tissue. If more than 10 cysts are seen, adult polycystic kidney liver disease should

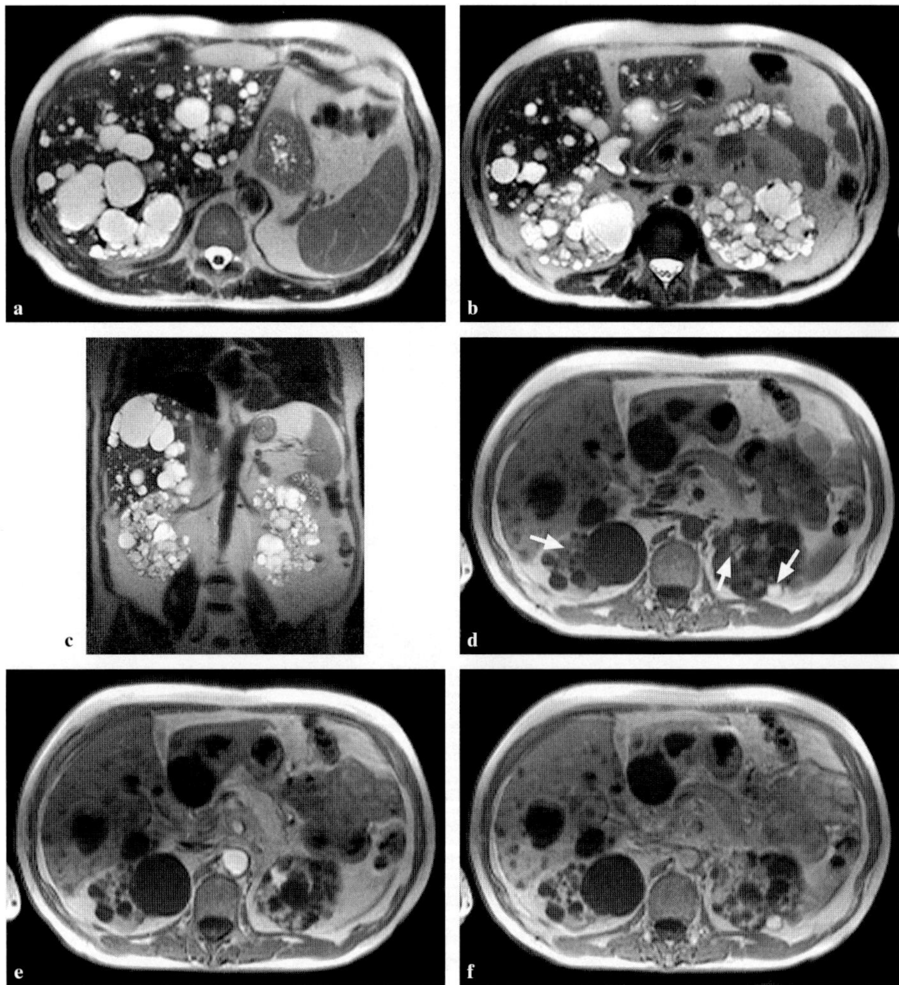

Fig. 39a-f. Polycystic liver and kidneys in adult polycystic kidney disease. Both the kidneys and the liver show multiple high signal intensity cysts on T2w images (**a-c**). On T1w images (**d**), the liver cysts appear hypointense, whereas some of the kidney cysts appear hyperintense due to hemorrhage (*arrows*). After contrast medium injection, homogenous enhancement of the liver parenchyma can be noted in both the arterial phase (**e**) and the portal-venous phase (**f**). The remaining kidney parenchyma also shows homogenous enhancement. Since the risk of developing renal cell carcinoma is increased in patients with polycystic kidney disease, a very precise evaluation of the renal cysts is necessary

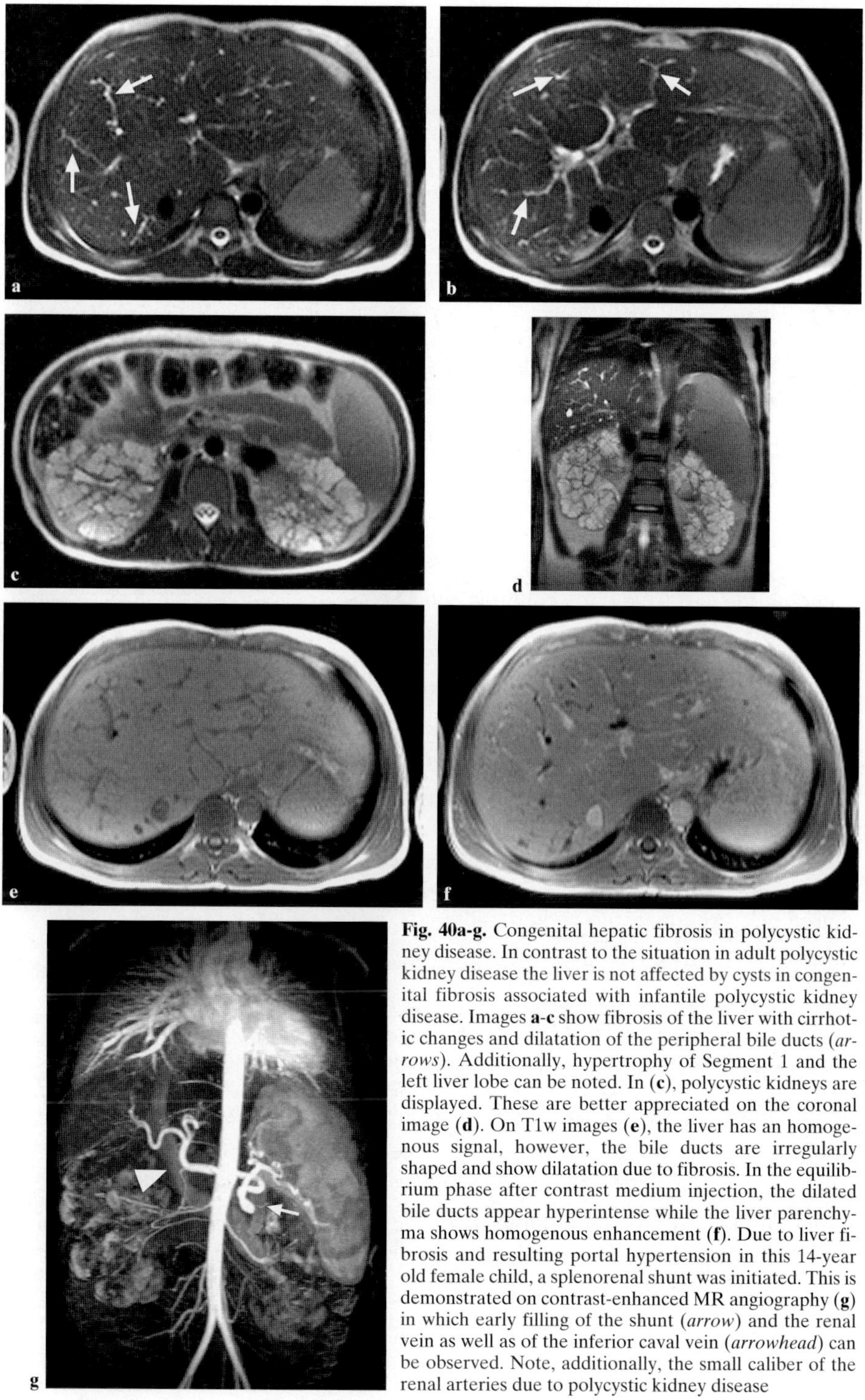

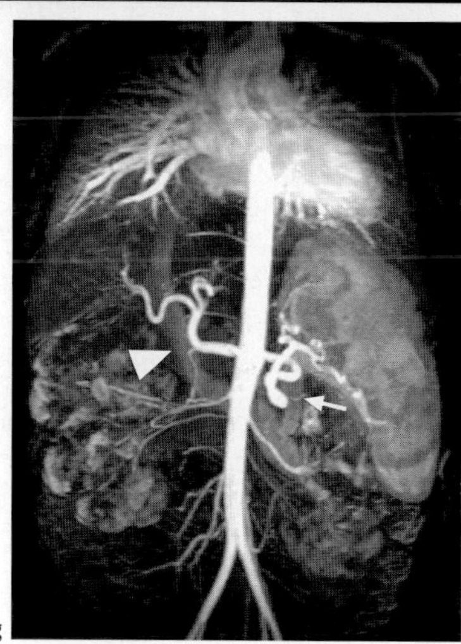

Fig. 40a-g. Congenital hepatic fibrosis in polycystic kidney disease. In contrast to the situation in adult polycystic kidney disease the liver is not affected by cysts in congenital fibrosis associated with infantile polycystic kidney disease. Images **a-c** show fibrosis of the liver with cirrhotic changes and dilatation of the peripheral bile ducts (*arrows*). Additionally, hypertrophy of Segment 1 and the left liver lobe can be noted. In (**c**), polycystic kidneys are displayed. These are better appreciated on the coronal image (**d**). On T1w images (**e**), the liver has an homogenous signal, however, the bile ducts are irregularly shaped and show dilatation due to fibrosis. In the equilibrium phase after contrast medium injection, the dilated bile ducts appear hyperintense while the liver parenchyma shows homogenous enhancement (**f**). Due to liver fibrosis and resulting portal hypertension in this 14-year old female child, a splenorenal shunt was initiated. This is demonstrated on contrast-enhanced MR angiography (**g**) in which early filling of the shunt (*arrow*) and the renal vein as well as of the inferior caval vein (*arrowhead*) can be observed. Note, additionally, the small caliber of the renal arteries due to polycystic kidney disease be considered (Fig. 39). The incidence of simple hepatic cyst is about 15% in autopsy series and is more common in women than in men. Cysts are usually discovered incidentally, although up to 20% have been reported in surgical series of patients who presented with symptoms caused by mass effect, such as abdominal pain, and jaundice [103].

On ultrasound, uncomplicated simple cysts present as anechoic, round, well-defined lesions with smooth borders, no septations and no mural calcifications. Moreover, there is no acoustic shadow. Similarly, on CT, uncomplicated hepatic cysts appear as well-defined water attenuation masses with smooth thin walls, no internal septa or solid nodules and no enhancement after administration of contrast material.

On T2-weighted MR images, simple uncomplicated cysts are extremely hyperintense and homogeneous. Conversely, on T1-weighted images they have an homogeneous hypointense appearance. The intensity of the cysts on T1-weighted images can vary, however, if protein and/or hemorrhage is present within the cyst fluid. These materials can shorten the T1 relaxivity leading to hyperintensity.

Congenital hepatic fibrosis is part of the spectrum of hepatic cystic disease, and is characterized by aberrant bile duct proliferation and periductal fibrosis. In typical congenital hepatic fibrosis, cysts are not visible due to their very small size (Fig. 40). In polycystic liver disease, numerous large and small cysts coexist with fibrosis. In cases of polycystic liver and/or kidney disease, the liver parenchyma surrounding the cyst frequently contains von Meyenburg complexes and increased fibrous tissue (Fig. 39) [58].

Hepatic involvement in patients with polycystic kidney disease occurs in approximately 30–50% of cases. Clinically, the majority of patients present in childhood, when congenital hepatic fibrosis predominates with bleeding, varices and other manifestations of portal hypertension. In patients with predominating polycystic liver disease, the lesions are usually identified incidentally. Approximately 70% of patients with polycystic liver disease also have adult polycystic kidney disease. Congenital hepatic fibrosis is also related to Caroli's disease. Cross-sectional images reveal multiple cysts in the liver which are often associated with multiple kidney cysts [10]. In this clinical setting, the cysts may have variable signal intensity, presumably caused by a proteinaceous content within the cysts, and/or intracystic hemorrhage.

4.1.7.2   Biliary Cystadenoma

Biliary cystadenoma is a rare cystic neoplasm, representing less than 5% of all intrahepatic cysts that arise from intra-and extra-hepatic bile ducts [53, 60]. This neoplasm may occur anywhere along the intra-or extra-hepatic bile ducts, although nearly all lesions are found at least partly or completely within the liver. Most lesions are > 10 cm in diameter at the time of diagnosis. Microscopically, biliary cystadenomas have a mucin-secreting columnar epithelium lining the cysts. The lining cells have a pale eosinophilic cytoplasm and basally oriented nuclei, typical of biliary-type epithelium. The epithelium is supported by a mesenchymal stroma. This is compact and cellular, and resembles the stroma of the ovary [26]. Biliary cystadenoma is regarded as a pre-malignant tumor. When malignancy develops, it is termed cystadenocarcinoma. *In situ* carcinoma with papillary growth into the cysts may be the only lesion present, although invasive adenocarcinoma may also be seen [26, 135].

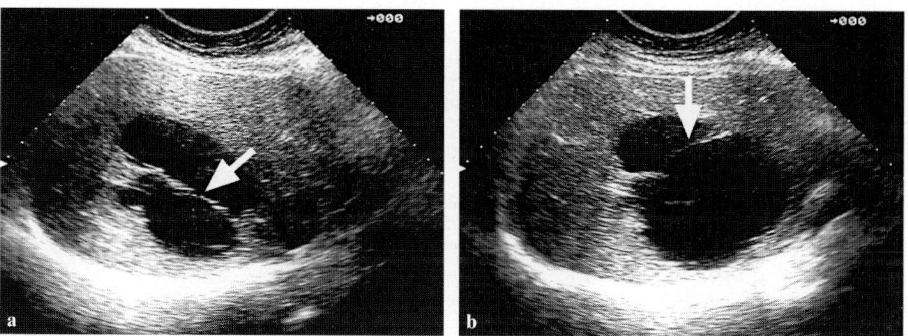

Fig. 41a,b. Biliary cystadenoma. Ultrasound reveals hypo- to anechoic lesions with thin septa (*arrows*)

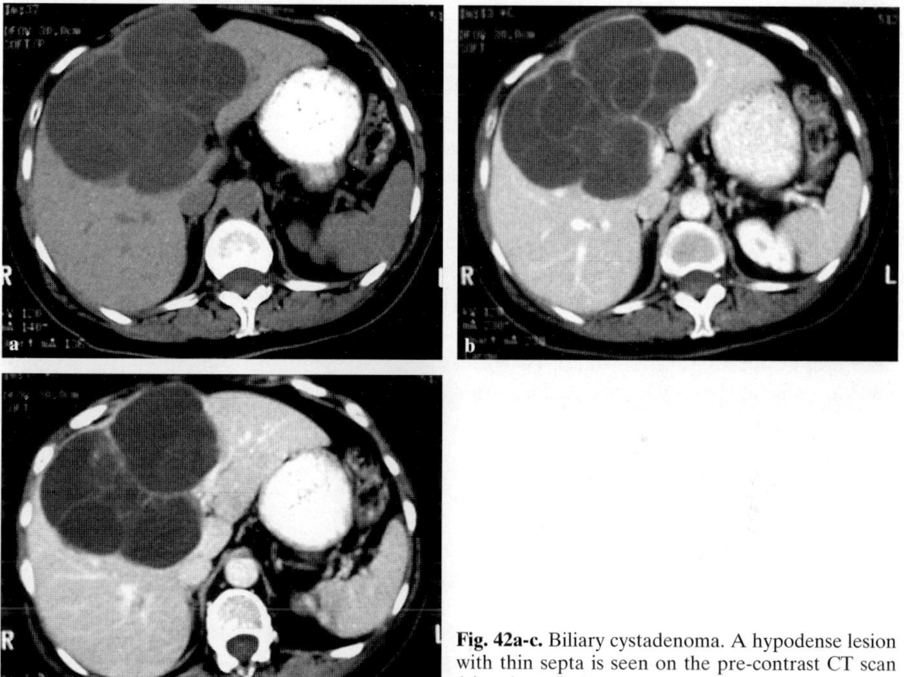

Fig. 42a-c. Biliary cystadenoma. A hypodense lesion with thin septa is seen on the pre-contrast CT scan (**a**). After administration of contrast medium (**b** and **c**) the septa show enhancement

Approximately 90% of these neoplasms occur in middle-aged women [17]. When present, the symptoms are those of a growing abdominal mass. Right upper quadrant abdominal pain, occasionally irradiating to the scapula, is the main symptom [27].

On ultrasound, biliary cystadenoma is seen as a hypoechoic, multiloculated, cystic-like lesion with intralesional septa (Fig. 41). Occasionally, mural nodules occur on the cystic walls of benign cystadenoma, but these are more common in cystadenocarcinoma, where they sometimes form a mass [59, 82].

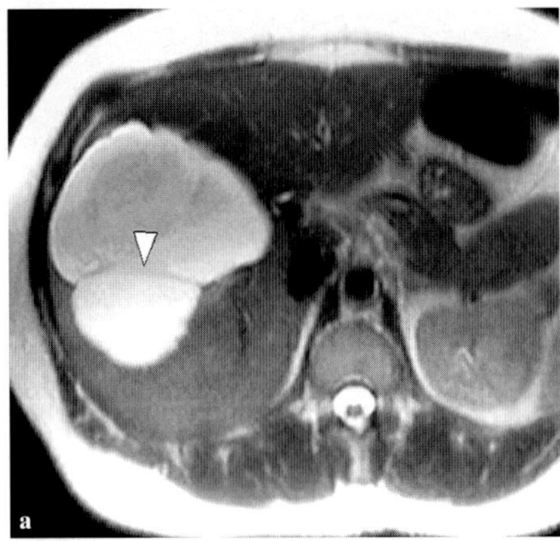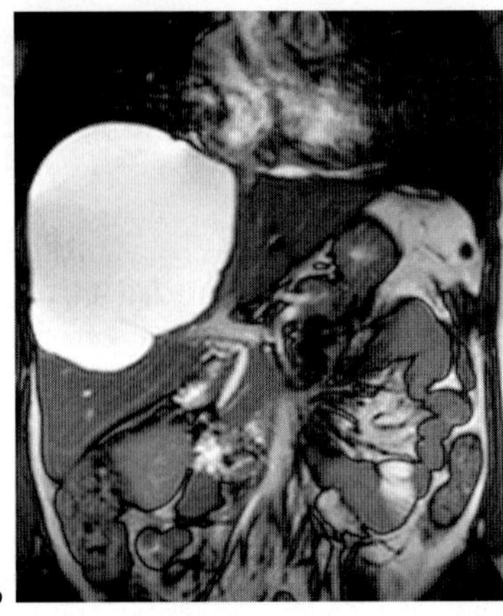

Fig. 43a,b. Biliary cystadenoma, HASTE T2-weighted images acquired in the axial plane (**a**) and True-FISP images acquired in the coronal plane (**b**) reveal large, lobulated cystic lesions in the right lobe. The lesions are homogeneously hyperintense due to the fluid component and thin septa are visible (*arrowhead*)

On CT, these tumors are large, low attenuating intrahepatic masses with lobulated margins and irregular walls with fibrous septa, which enhance following the intravenous administration of contrast material (Fig. 42) [1, 59, 77].

On MR imaging, biliary cystadenoma appears as a multiloculated septated mass, whose signal intensity on T1- and T2-weighted images depends on the composition of the cystic fluid, which may be serous, mucinous, bilious, hemorrhagic, or a combination of these fluids (Fig. 43). Low signal intensity within the wall on T2-weighted images may represent hemorrhage. The internal septa, mural nodules and papillary projection enhance following the intravenous administration of contrast material [17].

4.1.7.3   Mesenchymal Hamartoma

Mesenchymal hamartoma is a benign cystic developmental lesion and is not considered a true neoplasm. It is an uncommon lesion accounting for about 10% of all childhood liver tumors. It is a large, predominantly cystic mass frequently measuring 15 cm or more in diameter at the time of diagnosis. The tumors are generally well-defined and encapsulated or pedunculated. Cysts are present in 80% of cases [52]. On cut sections, mesenchymal hamartomas are either of mesenchymal predominance (solid appearance) or cystic predominance (multiloculated cystic appearance). Histologically, the tumor consists of the cystic remnants of portal triads, hepatocytes and fluid-filled mesenchyma [97]. Patients usually present with only an asymptomatic enlarging abdominal mass.

On ultrasound, a mesenchymal hamartoma has the appearance of a large cyst with internal septa (cystic appearance), or, less commonly, as a smaller cyst with thick septa (mesenchymal appearance).

On imaging, the tumor appears as a well-defined mass with central hypodense areas and internal septa. Both solid and cystic components may be distinguished, although calcifications have not been reported. Both the septa and the solid components enhance following the administration of contrast material [97].

The MR appearance of mesenchymal hamartoma depends on the predominance of the stromal and cystic components. For lesions with a stromal predominance, the signal intensity on T1-weighted images is lower than that of the normal liver, because of increased fibrosis. Conversely, if the cystic component predominates, the appearance is similar to that of other cystic masses with marked hyperintensity on T2-weighted images. Multiple septa traversing the tumor can be seen, indicating that the lesion is not a simple cyst [97]. The intensity of the different locules may vary, indicating different concentrations of proteinaceous material. After the injection of contrast medium, both the mesenchymal component and the septa enhance in a manner similar to that observed on CT.

4.1.7.4 Caroli's Disease

Caroli's disease is considered a congenital disorder. Proposed mechanisms for bile duct malformation include abnormal growth of the developing biliary epithelium and supporting connective tissue, and a lack of normal involution of the ductal plates that surround the portal tracts, resulting in epithelium-lined cysts surrounding the portal triads. Caroli's disease occurs with equal frequency in males and females. Two types of the disease have been described: the real, so-called "pure" type, and the more common type associated with congenital hepatic fibrosis. The "pure" type is characterized by segmental, saccular, communicating intrahepatic bile duct ectasia, and frequently also by stone formation, cholangitis and abscess formation. Liver involvement may be limited or diffuse. Biliary infection and stones account for the usual presenting symptoms of fever and abdominal pain. Cholangiocarcinoma develops in approximately 5 to 10 % of cases [70].

Caroli's disease associated with congenital hepatic fibrosis presents in childhood with abnormalities related to hepatic fibrosis and portal hypertension. Histologically, intrahepatic bile-duct ectasia and proliferation are associated with severe periportal fibroses. Cholangitis and biliary stone formation are usually absent, although death may occur due to liver failure or portal hypertension complications. Associated conditions include infantile polycystic kidney disease, choledochal cyst, and medullary sponge kidney.

For the pure form of Caroli's disease, cholangiography reveals multiple communicating sacculi of the intrahepatic biliary tree. Stones are common and appear as filling defects. Bile duct strictures and wall irregularities may occur as a consequence of recurrent cholangitis. A similar appearance may be observed with magnetic resonance cholangiopancreatography (MRCP).

On CT and ultrasound examinations, the sacculi appear as well-defined intrahepatic cystic water-density and anechoic areas, respectively. Demonstration of communication between sacculi and bile duct is important in distinguishing Caroli's disease from polycystic liver disease [70].

On MR, the sacculi appear as homogeneously hypointense areas on T1-weighted images and as homogeneously hyperintense areas on T2-weighted images. MRCP is a valid tool for demonstrating the communication between sacculi and bile ducts, which is positively demonstrated with Gd-BOPTA if the contrast agent is present within the sacculi and bile ducts during the hepatobiliary phase (Fig. 44).

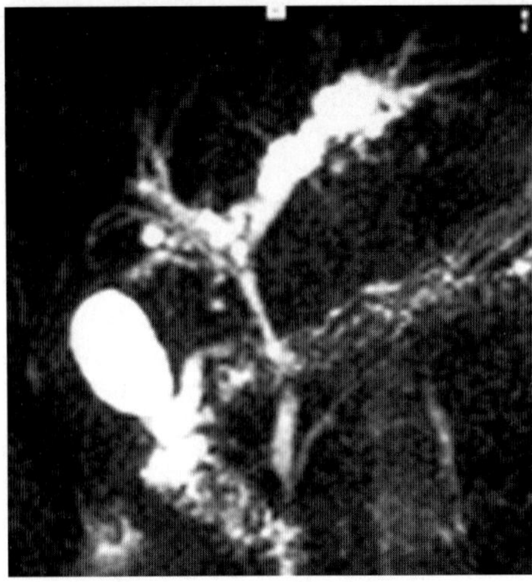

Fig. 44. Caroli's disease. MRCP demonstrates the communication between the sacculi and the biliary ducts in a patient with Caroli's disease

4.1.8   Miscellaneous Tumors

4.1.8.1   Lipomatous Tumors

Benign hepatic tumors composed of fat cells include lipoma, and combined tumors such as angiomyolipoma (fat and blood vessels), myelolipoma (fat and hematopoietic tissue) and angiomyelolipoma [35].

Grossly, lipomatous tumors are usually solitary, well circumscribed, and round, and occur in non-cirrhotic livers [36]. They contain variable proportions of adipose tissue and smooth muscle with thick-walled blood vessels. Flow cytometry shows a DNA-diploid pattern consistent with a benign lesion [119]. Hematopoietic foci may be present, and when prominent, the term myelolipoma [80] or angiomyelolipoma has been used.

Angiomyolipomas are rare, usually asymptomatic solitary tumors. However, these tumors occasionally bleed causing abdominal pain [48]. Liver angiomyolipomas usually range in size from 0.3–36 cm in diameter and occur predominantly in women [48]. Liver angiomyolipomas may occur in association with Bourneville-Pringle syndrome. In this clinical setting, the lesions are generally multiple, progressive, and symptomatic.

Angiomyolipomas are highly echogenic on US and indistinguishable from hemangiomas. Frequently, they present a mixed hyper-hypoechoic pattern on US [91].

Density measurements on unenhanced CT are characteristic of fat (–20 to –115 HU). Pure lipomas do not enhance, but variable enhancement occurs in lesions containing angiomatous elements (Fig. 45) [54, 91].

On MR imaging, the fatty component of angiomyolipoma leads to high signal intensity on both T1- and T2-weighted images [76]. Hepatocellular carcinomas containing fat deposits may have a similar appearance. The early phase of contrast-enhanced dynamic CT or MR imaging may be useful in discriminating between angiomyolipomas and hepatocellular carcinomas with fat, because the fatty areas of angiomyolipo-

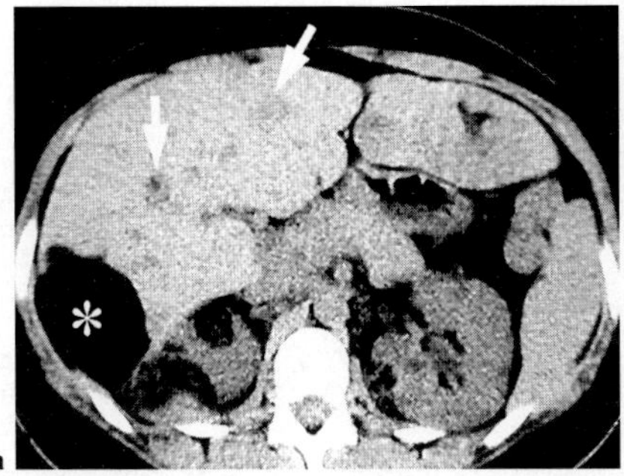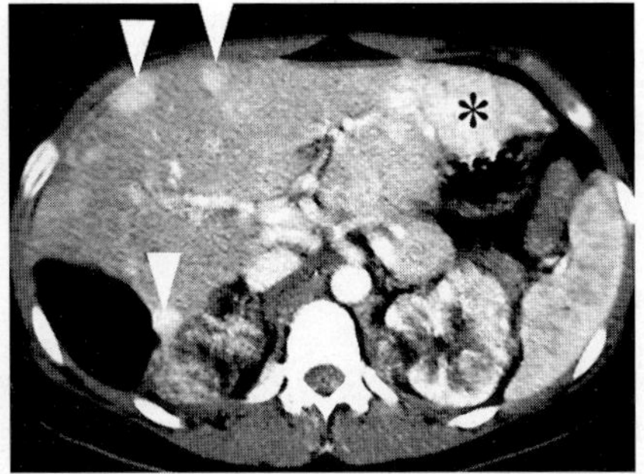

Fig. 45a,b. Lipomatous tumor in Bourneville Syndrome. Pre-contrast CT (**a**) reveals multiple hypodense lesions (*asterisks*) and mixed lesions (*arrows*). The hypodensity of the largest lesion reflects the abundant fatty content. After administration of contrast medium (**b**), some nodules enhance homogeneously (*arrowheads*) whereas others enhance heterogeneously (*asterisk*). Note the presence of angiomyolipomas in both kidneys as well

ma are well vascularized and enhance early [76]. Conversely, the areas of fatty change in hepatocellular carcinoma are relatively avascular, and enhancement is less obvious [76]. MR imaging with fat suppression is useful for the characterization of hepatic angiomyolipoma since lipid components show a typical signal drop with these sequences [49]. The lesions have high signal intensity on T1- and T2-weighted images and appear hypointense to the normal liver parenchyma on images obtained with fat suppression [49]. The appearance on contrast-enhanced MR imaging with gadolinium agents may mimic the pattern observed with hemangioma with peripheral nodular enhancement or irregular non-nodular vascular enhancement. However, arterial hyperintensity is also a common pattern of enhancement (Fig. 46).

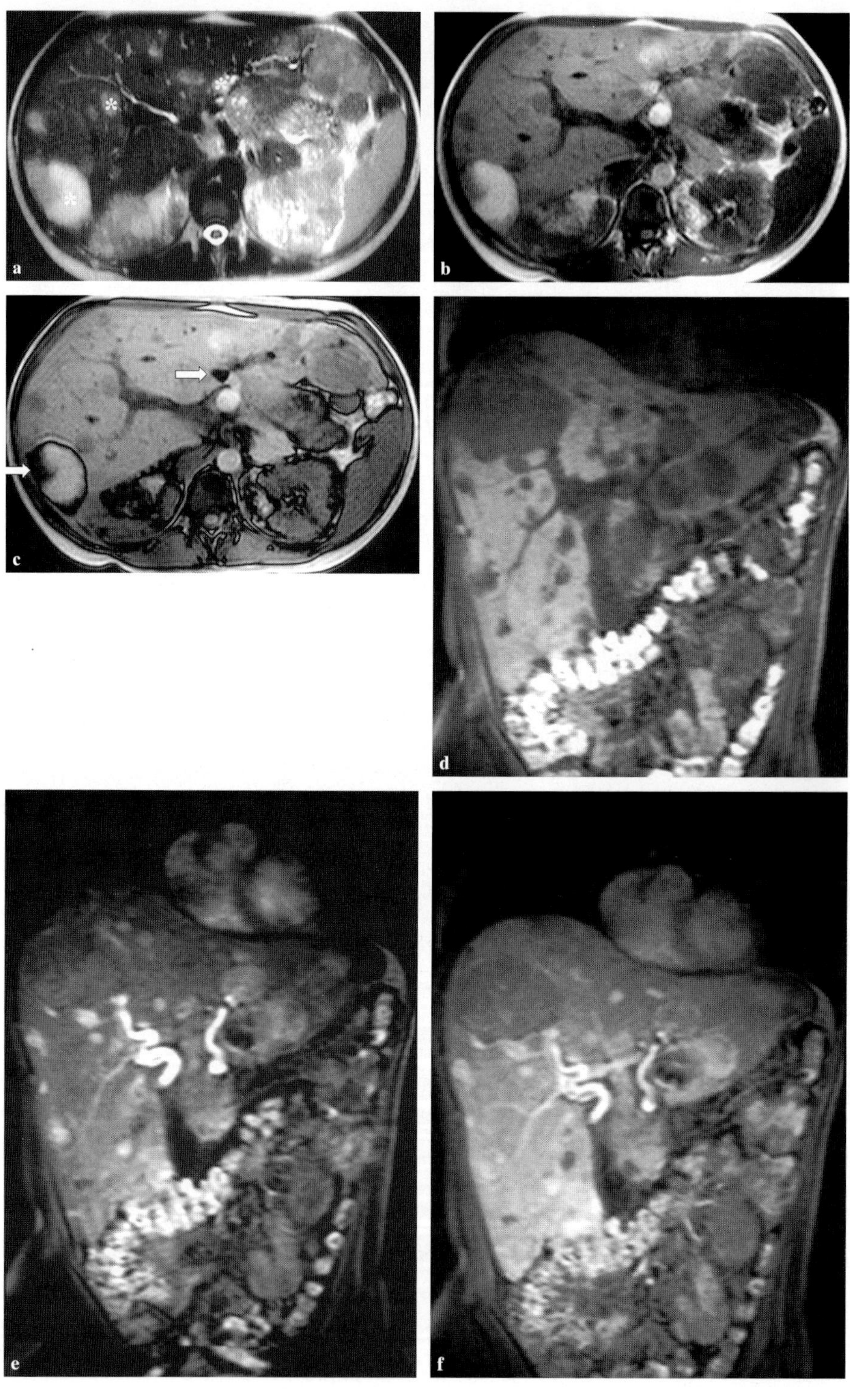

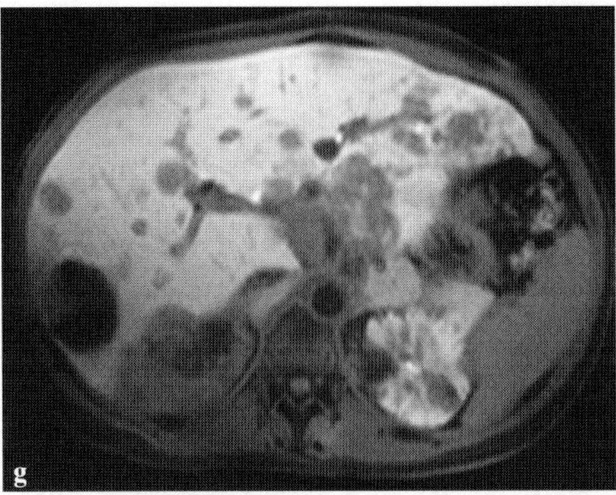

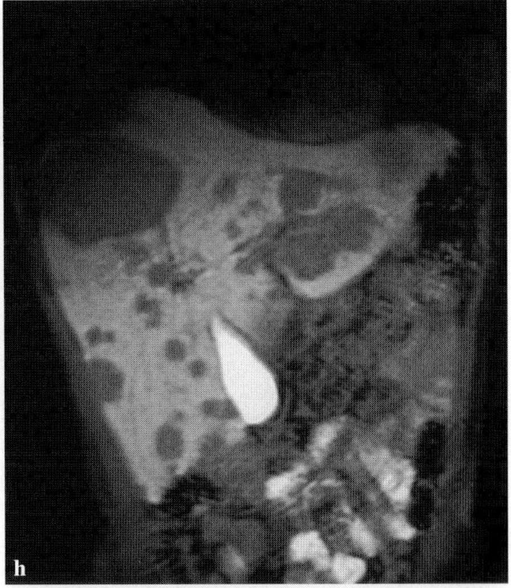

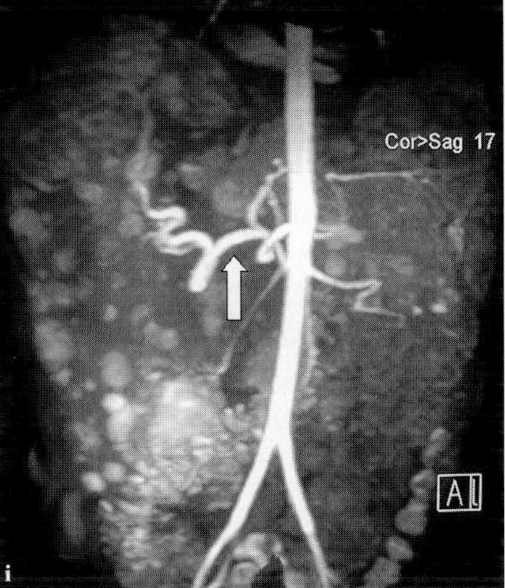

Fig. 46a-i. Lipomatous tumor. On the unenhanced HASTE T2-weighted image (**a**) numerous hyperintense lesions (*asterisks*) can be seen in the liver. On the unenhanced GE T1-weighted image (**b**) some of the lesions are hypointense. Several of these lesions (*arrows*) demonstrate a decrease of signal intensity on the T1-wighted out-of-phase images due to the fat component (**c**). On the unenhanced coronal VIBE sequence (**d**) the nodules are seen as mainly hypointense. Some lesions are seen as hypointense while others are hyperintense during the arterial phase after the administration of Gd-BOPTA (**e**). Numerous lesions remain hypointense on the portal-venous phase image (**f**). On GE T1-weighted axial (**g**) and coronal (**h**) fat suppressed images acquired during the delayed hepatobiliary phase, all of the lesions appear hypointense. MR angiography obtained with the VIBE sequence (**i**) reveals dilated and tortuous tripod celiac and hepatic arteries (*arrow*)

4.1.8.2   Leiomyoma

This extremely rare lesion is a well-circumscribed smooth muscle tumor arising in the liver [46]. Several cases of leiomyoma have been reported in adults and children infected with the human immunodeficiency virus, suggesting that there may be a clinical association between these two entities [75, 126].

Leiomyoma has non-specific radiological characteristics. On ultrasound, leiomyomas appear as solid or hypoechoic lesions with internal echoes [95, 126]. They have low attenuation relative to normal liver on unenhanced CT, but following contrast agent administration, may display two distinct enhancement patterns: either peripheral rim enhancement, similar to that seen for abscess, or homogeneous enhancement which sometimes may be delayed [75, 126].

Leiomyomas are hypointense relative to the liver on T1-weighted MR images and hyperintense on T2-weighted images [95, 126]. Enhancement patterns after contrast medium administration are similar to those described for CT imaging.

4.2   Secondary Benign Liver Lesions

4.2.1   Pyogenic Abscess

Abscesses of the liver may be caused by bacterial, amebic or fungal infections, which result in the localized collection of inflammatory cells, and destruction of surrounding parenchyma [92]. Hepatic abscesses can develop via several major routes [33]:

- the biliary route, due to ascending cholangitis, benign or malignant biliary obstruction and choledocholitiasis
- the portal vein route, due to pylephlebitis from appendicitis diverticulitis, proctitis, infected hemorrhoids, inflammatory bowel disease and others
- the hepatic artery route, subsequent to septicemia
- the direct extension route, from contiguous organ infections
- the traumatic route, from blunt or penetrating injuries.

Before the development of antibiotics, pylephlebitis of the portal vein through seeding from appendicitis diverticulitis was the most common cause of hepatic abscesses. Pyogenic abscesses today are most often associated with benign or malignant obstruction with cholangitis. Abscesses of biliary tract origin are multiple and frequently involve both hepatic lobes (Fig. 47). Abscesses of portal vein origin are often solitary and mainly localized in the right lobe.

The clinical symptoms of patients with hepatic abscesses include fever, malaise, right upper abdominal pain, nausea and vomiting. Tender hepatomegaly is the most common clinical sign and leukocytosis, elevated serum alkaline phosphatase and hypoalbuminemia are the most common laboratory abnormalities. The onset of symptoms may be acute (pyogenic abscesses) or prolonged (amebic abscesses) [33].

Ultrasound can detect hepatic abscesses as small as 1.5 cm with a sensitivity of 75% to 90%. Pyogenic hepatic abscesses are extremely variable in shape and echogenicity and may appear as anechoic (50%), hyperechoic (25%) or hypoechoic (25%) (Fig. 48). Septa and fluid-fluid internal necrosis are frequently seen while calcifications and gas may also be detected. Early lesions tend to be echogenic and poorly demarcated [45, 79].

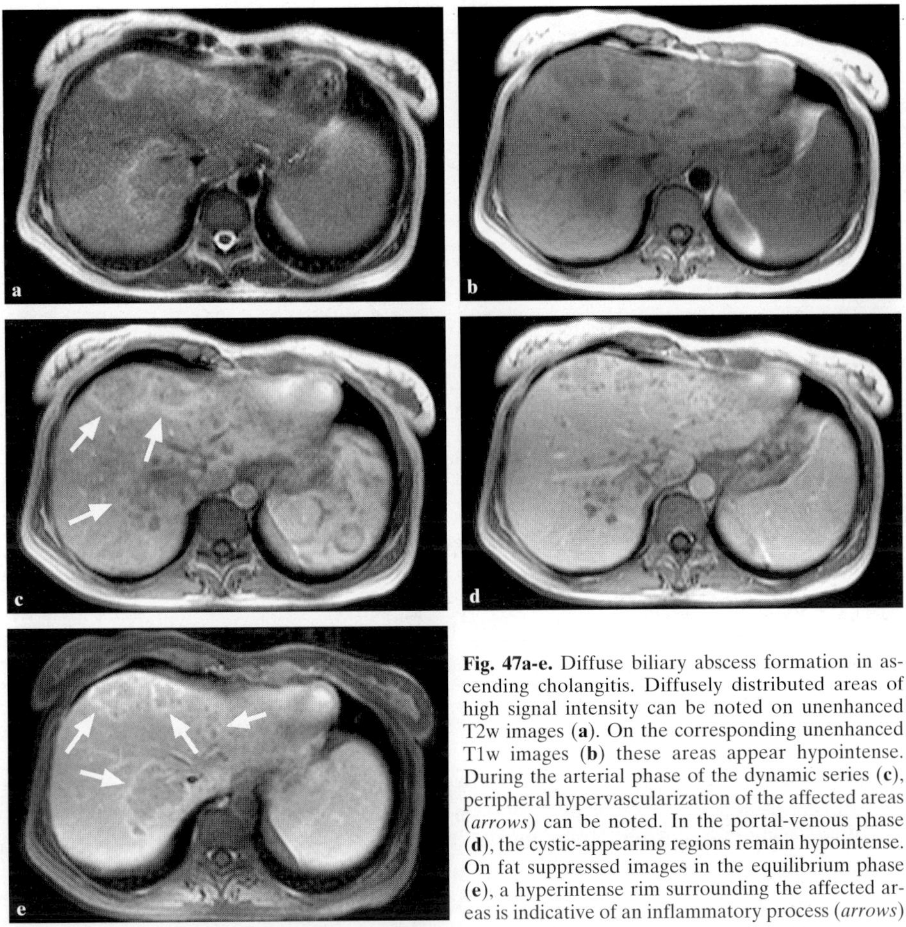

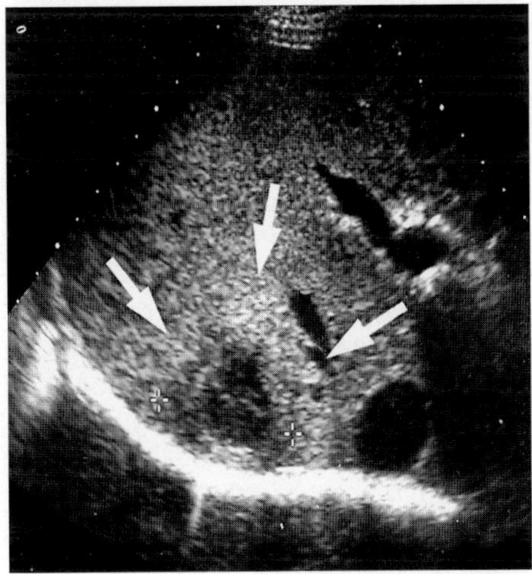

Fig. 47a-e. Diffuse biliary abscess formation in ascending cholangitis. Diffusely distributed areas of high signal intensity can be noted on unenhanced T2w images (**a**). On the corresponding unenhanced T1w images (**b**) these areas appear hypointense. During the arterial phase of the dynamic series (**c**), peripheral hypervascularization of the affected areas (*arrows*) can be noted. In the portal-venous phase (**d**), the cystic-appearing regions remain hypointense. On fat suppressed images in the equilibrium phase (**e**), a hyperintense rim surrounding the affected areas is indicative of an inflammatory process (*arrows*)

Fig. 48. Pyogenic abscess. Ultrasound reveals a heterogeneous hypo- to isoechoic lesion with ill-defined margins (*arrows*)

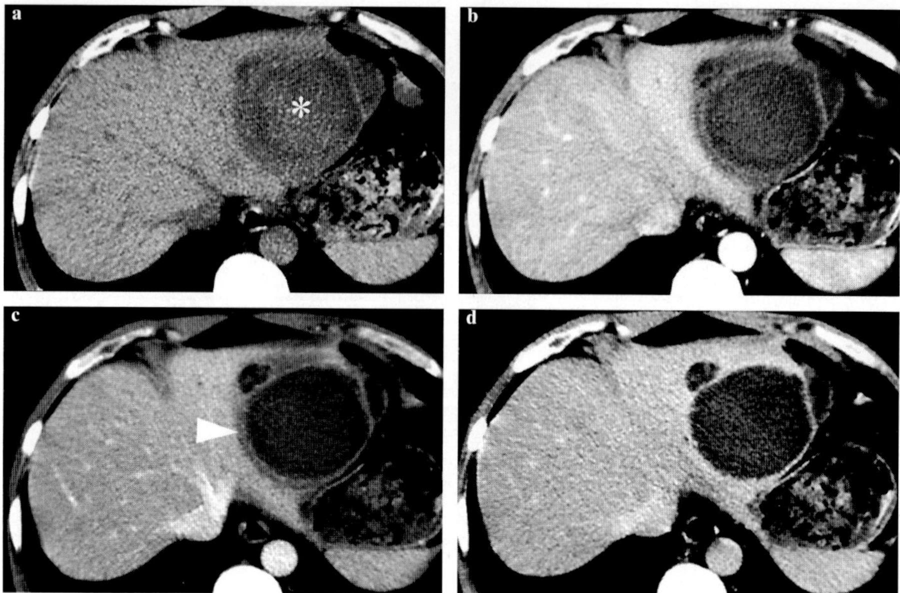

Fig. 49a-d. Pyogenic abscess. On the unenhanced CT scan (**a**), the abscess (*asterisk*) appears as a heterogeneously iso- to hypodense lesion. Peripheral rim enhancement is seen on arterial phase images after the administration of contrast medium (**b**). This is seen better in the portal-venous (**c**) and equilibrium (**d**) phases due to peripheral edema (*arrowhead in c*)

CT is a valid method for detecting hepatic abscesses with high sensitivity. On CT, hepatic abscesses appear as hypodense lesions with an internal pattern of varying density compared with liver tissue. The lesions generally appear as rounded masses that show minimal contrast enhancement. Most abscesses have a peripheral rim that enhances. The "cluster" sign is suggestive for abscess and represents smaller lesions surrounding a large abscess. Another CT sign, the "double target", is seen with early abscesses and represents a hypodense lesion surrounded by a hyperdense rim and an outer low-density region (Fig. 49). The presence of central gas, as either air bubbles or an air-fluid level, is a specific sign of pyogenic hepatic abscess, but is present in fewer than 20% of cases [6, 99].

Abscesses appear as areas of decreased signal intensity on T1-weighted MR images and increased signal intensity on T2-weighted images. Perilesional edema, characterized by high signal intensity on T2-weighted images, is seen in one third of cases. The abscess cavity may appear with homogeneous or heterogeneous intensity. After administration of contrast material, abscesses typically show rim enhancement followed by a slower increase in signal intensity at the center of the lesion (Fig. 50). Small lesions may enhance homogeneously in a manner similar to that seen with small hemangiomas [5].

Persistent reduced signal intensity of peripheral edema may be seen on delayed phase images after administration of contrast media with hepatobiliary properties (Fig. 50g). Similarly, decreased signal intensity after SPIO administration may be indicative of peripheral edema due to the high content of Kupffer cells and macrophages.

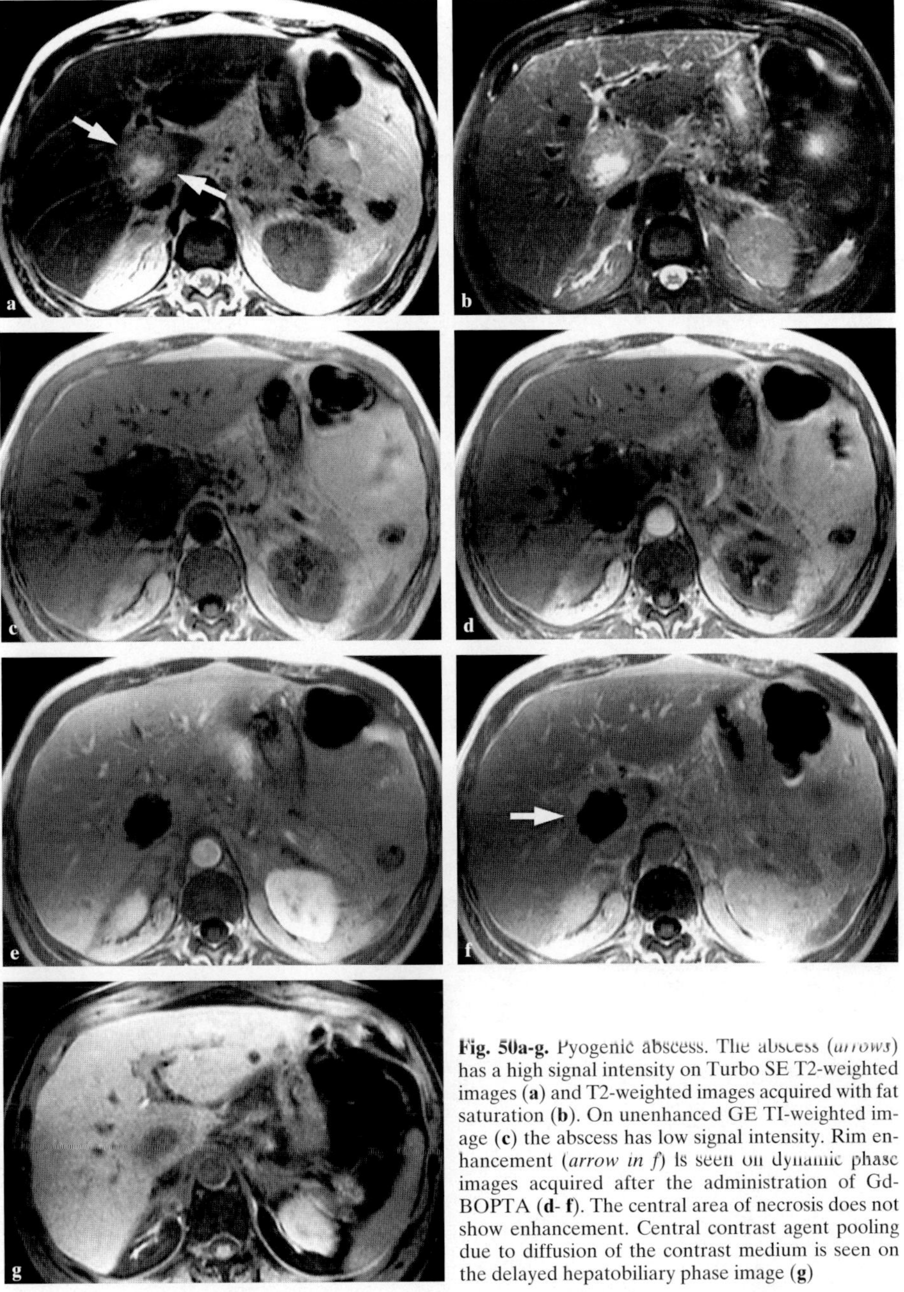

Fig. 50a-g. Pyogenic abscess. The abscess (*arrows*) has a high signal intensity on Turbo SE T2-weighted images (**a**) and T2-weighted images acquired with fat saturation (**b**). On unenhanced GE TI-weighted image (**c**) the abscess has low signal intensity. Rim enhancement (*arrow in f*) is seen on dynamic phase images acquired after the administration of Gd-BOPTA (**d-f**). The central area of necrosis does not show enhancement. Central contrast agent pooling due to diffusion of the contrast medium is seen on the delayed hepatobiliary phase image (**g**)

4.2.2   Amebic Abscess

Amebiasis, caused by the parasite *Entamoeba histolytica*, is an endemic disease in tropical areas, such as Mexico, Central and South America, Africa and Asia. Amebic liver abscess occurs after infestation of colonic mucosa by the parasite, which lodges in the portal system. The liver can be invaded in one of three ways:
- via the portal vein, (most common)
- through lymphatics
- via direct extension through the colon wall into the peritoneum and then through the liver capsule.

Amebic liver abscess is the most common extraintestinal manifestation. Most patients with amebic liver abscesses present with a tender liver and right upper abdominal pain. Amebae are not found in the stool of most patients with an amebic liver abscess. Because the clinical features and findings of stool examinations for amebae are usually not specific or negative, serologic tests are necessary in suspected amebic abscesses. Such tests are positive in about 90% of patients [94].

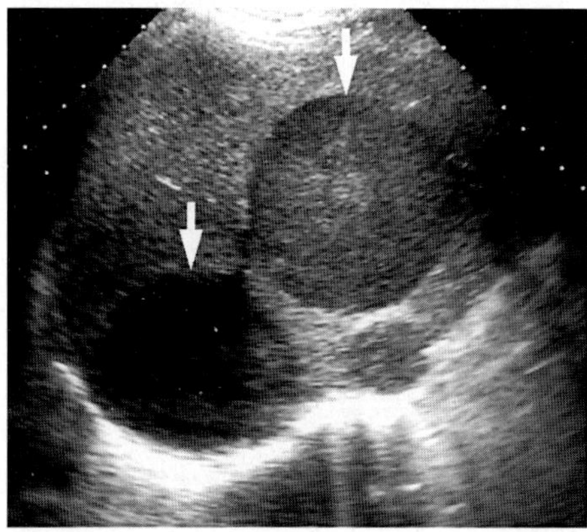

Fig. 51. Amebic abscess. The ultrasound scan reveals two large lesions with different echogenicity (*arrows*)

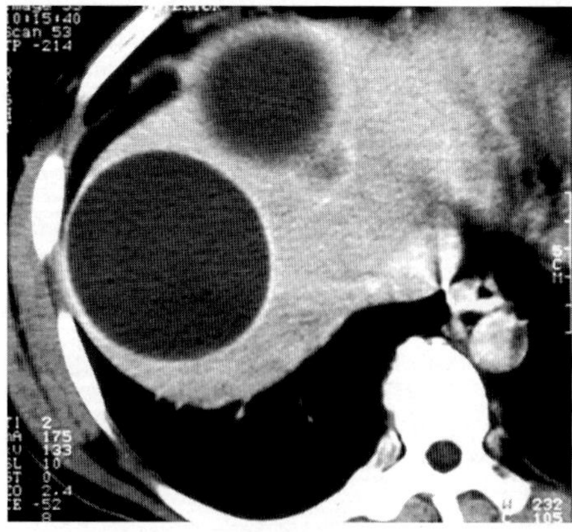

Fig. 52. Amebic abscess. The CT scan reveals hypodense lesions with a thin hyperdense peripheral rim. The hypodense appearance is due to the high liquid content

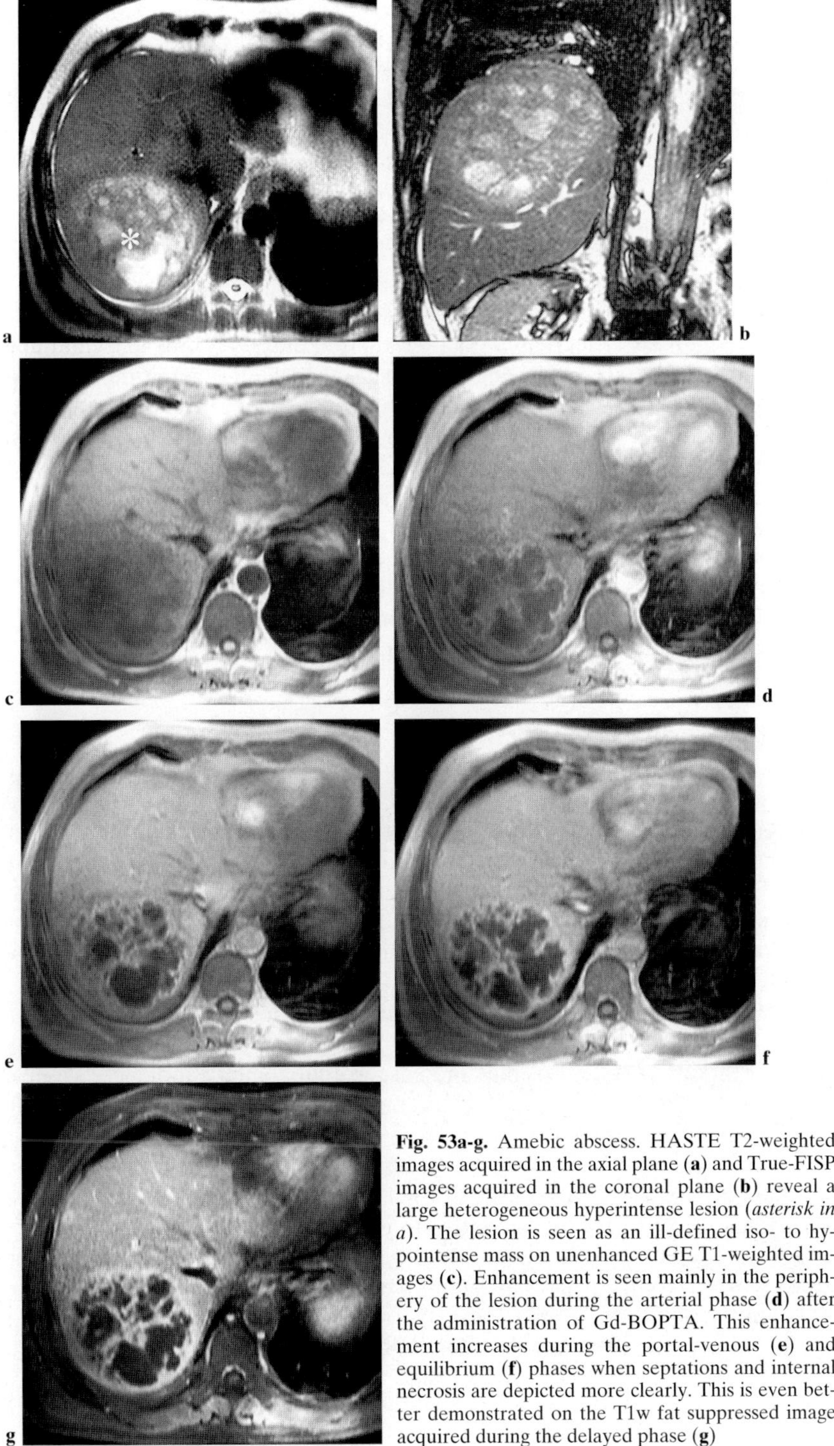

Fig. 53a-g. Amebic abscess. HASTE T2-weighted images acquired in the axial plane (**a**) and True-FISP images acquired in the coronal plane (**b**) reveal a large heterogeneous hyperintense lesion (*asterisk in a*). The lesion is seen as an ill-defined iso- to hypointense mass on unenhanced GE T1-weighted images (**c**). Enhancement is seen mainly in the periphery of the lesion during the arterial phase (**d**) after the administration of Gd-BOPTA. This enhancement increases during the portal-venous (**e**) and equilibrium (**f**) phases when septations and internal necrosis are depicted more clearly. This is even better demonstrated on the T1w fat suppressed image acquired during the delayed phase (**g**)

On ultrasound studies, amebic abscesses are usually large, round, sharply defined, hypoechoic masses with fine, low-level internal echoes at high gain setting (Fig. 51) [32, 71].

The CT appearance of amebic abscess is non-specific and variable; the lesion is usually round or oval and demonstrates peripheral hypodensity. A slightly hyperdense peripheral rim can be seen on unenhanced scans, which generally shows marked enhancement after administration of contrast material (Fig. 52). Lesions may appear as unilocular or multilocular masses, with internal debris and nodularity at the margins [121].

Amebic abscesses are well-defined structures with rim-like areas of varying signal intensity on both T1- and T2-weighted MR images. Within the abscess cavity, the signal intensity is decreased on T1-weighted images compared with the normal hepatic parenchyma. On T2-weighted images the lesion is hyperintense with an homogeneous or heterogeneous appearance and is often surrounded by areas of even higher signal intensity that correspond to edema within the normal liver tissue. No enhancement is seen in the central necrotic area after contrast medium administration, whereas heterogeneous enhancement can be observed at the periphery of the lesion which corresponds to inflammatory tissue. Persistent enhancement on late hepatobiliary phase images can be observed when contrast agents with hepatobiliary properties are used (Fig. 53). MR also offers the advantage of multiplanar capabilities to clearly depict the extension of the lesion and is helpful in follow-up studies to evaluate response under therapy.

4.2.3. Candidiasis Infection

Hepatic candidiasis is relatively frequent in immuno-compromised patients and is found in more than 50% of patients with acute leukemia or lymphoma. On ultrasound scans, three major patterns of candidiasis are seen:
- "wheel within a wheel", in which a peripheral zone surrounds an inner echogenic area
- "Bull's eye", a lesion with a hyperechoic center surrounded by a hypoechoic rim
- Uniformly hypoechoic, which is the most common appearance, attributable to progressive fibrosis.

After therapy, the lesions may increase in echogenicity and decrease in size, although in some cases sonographic inhomogeneity of the liver may persist for several years after treatment [37].

On CT, the lesions are generally multiple, small round hypodense areas on both pre-and post-contrast images. Calcifications can often be seen within the lesions [109].

On MR imaging, candida lesions are generally hyperintense on fat-suppressed images and have variable signal intensity on conventional T1-weighted spin-echo images. After contrast medium administration, more lesions are detected, which are mainly round, ill-defined focal hypointense areas. Frequently, percutaneous needle biopsy is needed to achieve a definitive diagnosis [106].

4.2.4   Echinococcal Cysts

Hydatid disease is caused by the parasite *Echinococcus granulosus*. The disease is mainly present in rural areas where dogs are used for herding livestock, especially sheep, and occurs frequently in Mediterranean countries, in Australia and in South America. The wall of the hydatid cyst is composed of two layers: the endocyst (a germinal layer), and the ectocyst (a proteinaceous membrane). A dense fibrous capsule containing collagen, the pericyst, is formed by the host.

Echinococcal cysts usually develop in the liver (75% of cases), but may occur in any part of the body. The lesions are often asymptomatic for many years and are discovered incidentally on ultrasound or CT scans. Hydatidosis can also be detected by serological tests. Classic symptoms of hepatic hydatid cyst include upper abdominal pain and hepatomegaly [3, 64].

Treatment consists of antiparasitic drug therapy and, on occasion, surgical removal of the cyst. If left untreated, a hepatic hydatid cyst may rupture into surrounding structures such as the liver parenchyma, biliary system, peritoneum, GI tract, or pleura. Hydatic cyst rupture is the major complication of echinococcal disease [3, 20, 99].

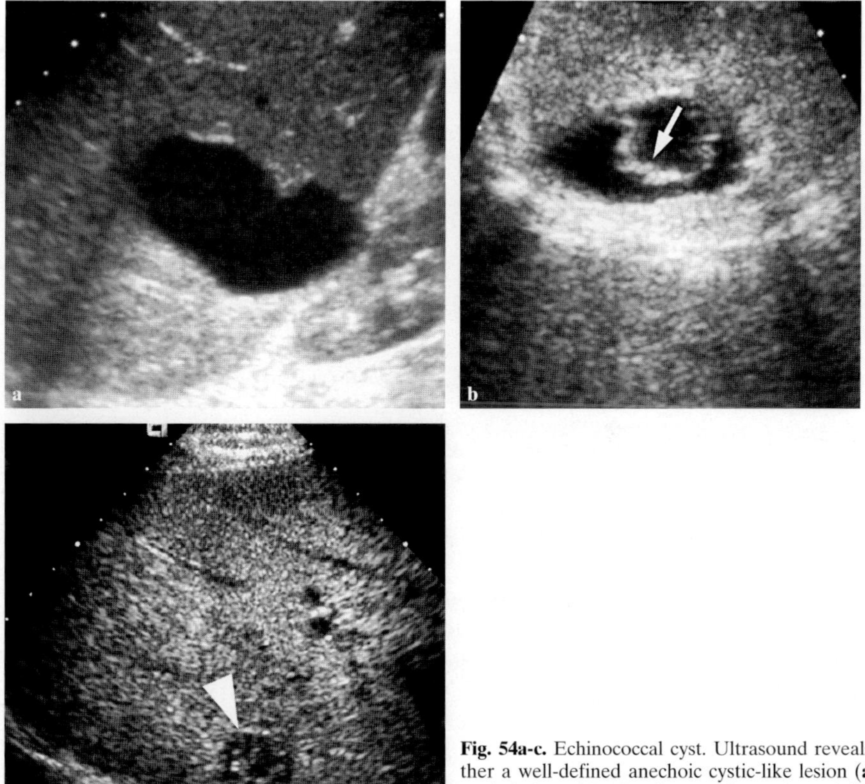

Fig. 54a-c. Echinococcal cyst. Ultrasound reveals either a well-defined anechoic cystic-like lesion (**a**), a cystic-lesion with a floating membrane (*arrow*) (**b**), or a dense and inhomogeneous nodule (*arrowhead*) (**c**)

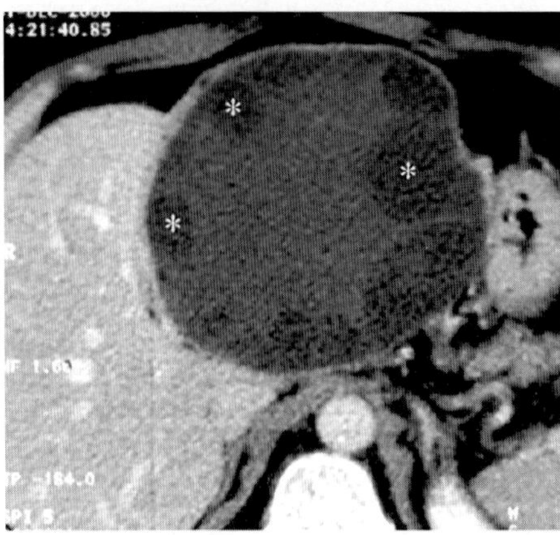

Fig. 55. Echinococcal cyst. CT scans after contrast medium administration reveal a large well-delineated cystic lesion. Peripheral round areas of lower density (*asterisks*) are indicative of daughter cysts

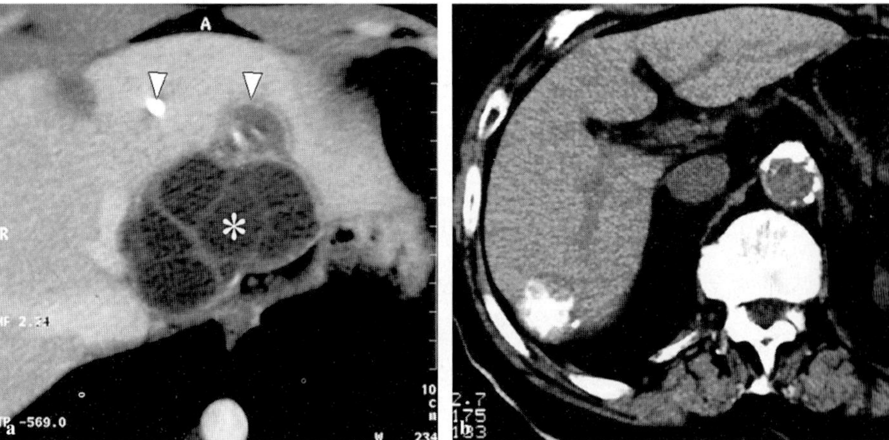

Fig. 56a,b. Echinococcal cyst. The CT scan after contrast medium administration (**a**) reveals a multilocular well-defined cystic lesion with thick hyperdense walls and septa (*asterisk*). Additional nodules with a heterogeneous appearance and gross calcifications (*arrowheads*) can be seen around the bigger lesion. The almost complete replacement of the lesion by central calcification is a sign of death of the cyst (**b**)

On abdominal plain film, curvilinear or ring-like calcifications can be seen in the right upper abdominal quadrant in about 20–30% of cases. However, calcifications do not necessarily indicate death of the parasite.

The appearance of hydatic cyst on ultrasound is variable and depends on the stage of evolution and maturity. The lesion may appear as a well-defined anechoic cyst, as an anechoic cyst except for hydatid sand, as a multiseptate cyst with daughter cysts, as a cyst with a floating membrane, or finally, as a density-calcified mass [20, 44, 99] (Fig. 54). Ultrasound has also been used to monitor the efficacy of medical antihydatid therapy. Positive responses include cyst size reduction, membrane detachment, increased echogenicity and mural calcification [7].

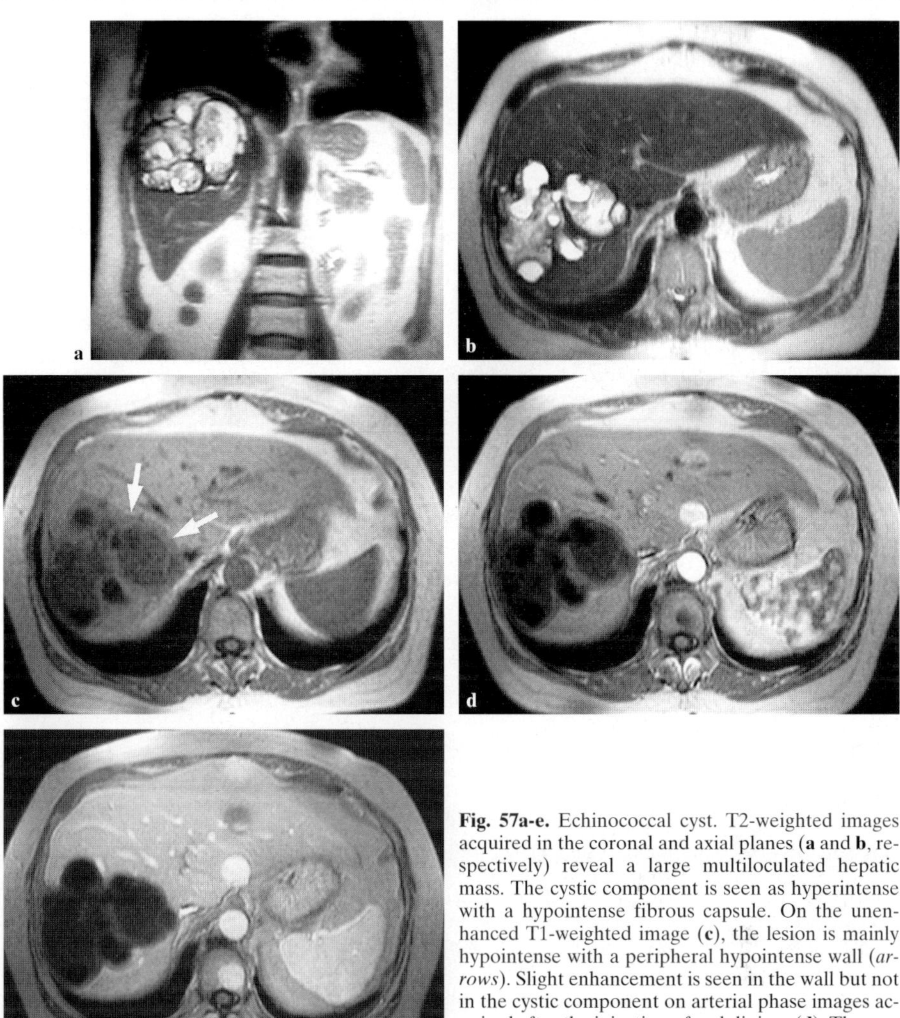

Fig. 57a-e. Echinococcal cyst. T2-weighted images acquired in the coronal and axial planes (**a** and **b**, respectively) reveal a large multiloculated hepatic mass. The cystic component is seen as hyperintense with a hypointense fibrous capsule. On the unenhanced T1-weighted image (**c**), the lesion is mainly hypointense with a peripheral hypointense wall (*arrows*). Slight enhancement is seen in the wall but not in the cystic component on arterial phase images acquired after the injection of gadolinium (**d**). The cystic mass remains hypointense on the subsequent portal-venous phase image (**e**)

On CT scans, hydatid disease appears as unilocular or multilocular well-defined cysts. Daughter cysts are seen as areas of lower density and are usually oriented towards the periphery of the lesion (Fig. 55). Daughter cysts can also float in the lumen of the mother cyst. Curvilinear ring-like calcifications or grossly diffuse calcifications are also common features. The peripheral walls may show enhancement after contrast medium administration (Fig. 56) [77, 99].

On MR imaging, the cystic component of echinococcal disease is similar to that of other cysts, with long T1 and T2 relaxation times. A low intensity rim around the cyst is present in most cases and is more conspicuous on T2- than T1-weighted sequences. This rim corresponds to the pericyst which is rich in collagen and has a

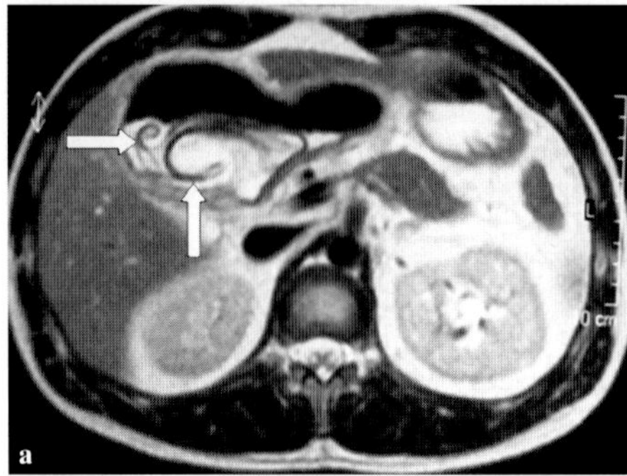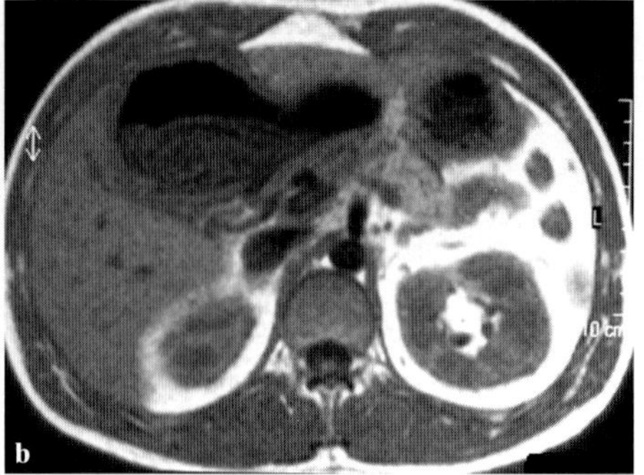

Fig. 58a,b. Complicated echinococcal cyst. The T2- and T1-weighted images (**a** and **b**, respectively) reveal air within the upper portion of the echinococcal cyst and fluid level in the lower portion (duodenal fistula). A floating hypointense membrane can also be recognized (*arrows*)

short T2 relaxation time [3]. The rim and a multiloculated or multicystic appearance are distinctive features (Fig. 57). Floating membranes have low signal intensity on both T1- and T2- weighted images (Fig. 58). Small cystic extensions from the main lesion are seen as peripheral areas of increased signal on T2-weighted images and probably represent the active portions of the disease [55, 115, 125].

References

1. Agildere AM, Haliloglu M, Akhan O. Biliary cystoadenoma and cystoadenocarcinoma. AJR 1991; 156:1113.
2. Aibe H, Hondo H, Kuroiwa T, Yoshimitsu K, Irie H, Tajima T, Shinozaki K, Asayama Y, Taguchi K, Masuda K. Sclerosed hemangioma of the liver. Abdom Imaging 2001; 26:496-499.
3. Allen DA. Focal infection processes. Section 6, chapter 10. pp 228-233. In Abdominal Magnetic Resonance Imaging. Ros. P.R:, Bidgood W.D.. Mosby (eds). 1993.
4. Arrive L, Flejou JF, Vilgrain V, Belghiti J, Najmark D, Zins M, Menu Y, Tubiana JM, Nahum H. Hepatic adenoma: MR findings in 51 pathologically proved lesions. Radiology 1994; 193:507-512.
5. Balci NC, Semelka RC, Noone TC, Siegelman ES, de Beeck BO, Brown JJ, Lee MG. Pyogenic hepatic abscess: MR findings on T1 and T2 weighted and serial Gadolinium-enhanced gradient-echo images. J Magn Reson Imaging 1999; 9:285-290.
6. Barreda R. Ros PR. Diagnostic imaging if liver abscess, Crit. Rev. Diagn Imaging 1992;33:29-58.
7. Bezzi M, Teggi A, De Rosa F, Capozzi A, Tucci G, Bonifacino A, Angelini L. Abdominal hydatid disease: US findings during medical treatment. Radiology 1987; 162:91-95.
8. Bioulac-Sage P, Balabaud C, Wanlees IR. Diagnosis of focal nodular hyperplasia. Not so easy. The Am J Surg Pathol 2001; 25 (10):1322-1325.
9. Blendis LM, Parkinson MC, Shilkin KB, Williams R. Nodular regenerative hyperplasia of the liver in Felty's sindrome. Q J Med 1974; 43:25-32.
10. Bosniak MA, Ambos MA. Policystic kidney disease. Semin Roentgenol 1975; 10:133-143.
11. Boulahdour H, Cherqui D, Charlotte F, Rahmouni A, Dhumeaux D, Zafrani ES, Meignan M. The hot spot hepatobiliary scan in focal nodular hyperplasia. J.Nucl. Med. 1993; 34:2105-2110.
12. Brancatelli G, Federle MP, Grazioli L, Blachar A, Peterson MS, Thaete L. Focal nodular hyperplasia: CT findings with emphasis on multiphasic helical CT in 78 patients. Radiology 2001; 219:61-68.
13. Brancatelli G, Federle MP, Blachar A, Grazioli L. Hemangioma in the Cirrhotic Liver: Diagnosis and Natural Hystory. Radiology 2001; 219:69-74.
14. Brancatelli G, Federle MP, Grazioli L, Golfieri R, Lencioni R. Large regenerative nodules in Budd-Chiari syndrome and other vascular disorders of the liver: CT and MR imaging findings with clinico-pathologic correlation. AJR 2002; 178:877-883.

15. Brancatelli G, Federle MP, Grazioli L, Golfieri R, Lencioni R. Benign regenerative nodules in Budd-Chiari syndrome and other vascular disorders of the liver: radiologic-pathologic and clnical correlation. Radiographics 2002; 22:847-862.

16. Brophy CM, Bock JF, West AB, McKhann CF. Liver cell adenoma: diagnosis and tratment of a rare hepatic neoplastic process. Am. J. Gastroenterol 1989; 84(4):429-432.

17. Buetow PC, Buck JL, Pantongrag-Brown L, Ros PR, Devaney K, Goodman ZD, Cruess DF. Biliary cystoadenoma and cystoadenocarcinoma: clinical-imaging-pathologic correlation with emphasis on the importance of ovarian stroma. Radiology 1995; 196:805-810.

18. Buetow PC, Pantongrag-Brown L, Buck JL, Ros PR, Goodman ZD. Focal nodular hyperplasia of the liver: radiologic-pathologic correlation. Radiographics 1996 Mar;16(2):369-88

19. Buffet C., Altman C. Regenerative nodular hyperplasia (in French). Gastroenterol Clin Biol 1994; 18:123-132.

20. Caremani M, Benci A, Maestrini R, Rossi G, Menchetti D. Abdominal cystic hydatid disease: classification and sonographic appearance and response to treatment. J Clin Ultrasound 1996; 24:491-500.

21. Choi BI, Kim TK, Han JK, Chung JW, Park JH, Han MC. Power versus conventional color Doppler sonography: comparision in the depiction of vasculature in liver tumors. Radiology 1996; 200:55-58.

22. Conter RL, Longmire WPJ. Recurrent hepatic hemangiomas. Possible association with estrogen theraphy. Ann.Surg. 1988; 207:115-119.

23. Dachman AH, Lichtenstein JE, Friedman AC, Hartman DS. Infantile hemangioendothelioma of the liver: a radiologic-pathologic-clinical correlation. AJR 1983; 140:1091-1096.

24. Dachman AH, Ros PR, Goodman ZD, Olmsted WW, Ishak KG. Nodular regenerative hyperplasia of the liver: clinical and radiologic observation. AJR 1987; 148:717-722.

25. Dehner LP. Hepatic tumors in the pediatric age group: a distinctive clinicopathologic spectrum. Perspect Pediatr pathol 1978; 4:217-268.

26. Devaney K, Goodman ZD, Ishak KG. Hepatobiliary cystoadenoma and cystoadenocarcinoma: a light microscopic and immunohistochemical study of 70 cases. Am J Surg Pathol 1994; 18:1078-1091.

27. Edmonson HA. Benign epithelial tumours and tumour-like lesions of the liver. In Okuda K, Peters R.L. (eds). Hepatocellular carcinoma. Wiley, New York, pp 309-330.

28. Edmonson HA. Tumors of the liver and intrahepatic bile ducts. In atlas tumorpathology, First series. Washington D.C: Armed Forces Institute of Pathology, 1958.

29. Feng WJ, Takayasu K, Konda C, Yamazaki S, Sakamoto M, Hirohashi S, Takenaka T. CT of nodular hyperplasia of the liver in non-Hodgkin lymphoma. J Comput Assisi Tomogr. 1991; 15:1031-1034.

30. Flejou JF, Barge J, Menu Y, Degott C, Bismuth H, Potet F, Benhamou JP. Liver adenomatosis: an entity distinct from liver adenoma?. Gastroenterology 1985; 89:1132-1138.

31. Friedman LS, Gang DL, Hedberg SE, Isselbacher KJ. Simultaneous occurrence of hepatic adenoma and focal nodular hyperplasia: report of a case and review of the literature. Hepatology 1984; 4:536.

32. Fujihara T, Nagai Y, Kubo T, Seki S, Satake K. Amebic liver abscess. J Gastroenterol 1996; 31:659-633.

33. Goldman IS, Farber BF, Brandborg LL. Bacterial and miscellaneous infections of the liver. In Zakim D, Boyer T.D. (eds): Hepatology (3th ed). Philadelphia: W.B. Sauders 1996, pp 1232-1242.

34. Golli M, Van Nhieu JT, Mathieu D, Zafrani ES, Cherqui D, Dhumeaux D, Vasile N, Rahmouni A. Hepatocellular adenoma: color Doppler US and pathologic correlation. Radiology 1994; 190:741-744.

35. Goodman ZD. Benign tumors of the liver: In Okuda K, Ishak K.G. (eds): Neoplasms of the liver. Tokyo: Springer-Verlag, 1987, pp 105-125.

36. Goodman ZD, Ishak KG. Angiomyolipoma of the liver. Am J Surg Pathol 1984; 8:745-750.

37. Gorg C, Weide R, Schwerk WB, Koppler H, Havemann K. Ultrasound evaluation of hepatic and splenic macroabscesses in the immunocompromized patients: sonographic patterns, differential diagnosis and follow-up. J Clin Ultrasound 1994; 22:525-529.

38. Grandin C, Van Beers BE, Robert A, Gigot JF, Geubel A, Pringot J. Benign hepatocellular tumors: MRI after superparamagnetic iron oxide administration. J Comput Assist Tomogr 19:412-418, 1995.

39. Grangier C, Tourniaire J, Mentha G, Schiau R, Howarth N, Chachuat A, Grossholz M, Terrier F. Enhancement of liver hemangiomas on T1-weighted MR SE images by Superparamagnetic Iron Oxide Particles. JCAT 18 (6):888-896, 1994.

40. Grazioli L, Federle MP, Ichikawa T, Balzano E, Nalesnik M, Madariaga J. Liver adenomatosis: clinical, pathologic, and imaging findings in 15 patients.Radiology 2000; 216:395-402.

41. Grazioli L, Alberti D, Olivetti L, Rigamonti W, Codazzi F, Matricardi L, Fugazzola C, Chiesa A. Congenital absence of portal vein with nodular regenerative hyperplasia of the liver. Eur. Radiol. 2000; 10:820-825.

42. Grazioli L, Morana G, Federle MP, Brancatelli G, Testoni M, Kirchin MA, Menni K, Olivetti L, Nicoli N, Procacci C. Focal nodular hyperplasia: morphologic and functional information from MR imaging with gadobenate dimeglumine. Radiology 2001 Dec;221(3):731-9

43. Groshar D, Ben-Haim S, Gips S, Hardoff R, Jerushalmi J, Parmett S, Israel O, Front D. Spectrum of scintigraphic appearance of liver hemangiomas. Clin Nucl Med 1992 Apr;17(4):294-9

44. Gurses N, Sungur R, Gurses N, Ozkan K. Ultrasound diagnosis of liver hydatid disease. Acta Radiol. 1987; 28:161-163

45. Halvorsen RA, Korobkin M, Foster WL, Silverman PM, Thompson WM. The variable CT appearance of hepatic abscesses. AJR Am J Roentgenol 1984 May;142(5):941-6
46. Hawkins EP, Jordan GL, McGavran MH. Primary leiomyioma of the liver. Successful treatment by lobectomy and presentation of criteria for diagnosis. Am J Surg Pathol 1980; 4:301-304.
47. Heiken JP. Liver. In Lee JKT, sagal SS, Stanley RJ, et al (eds): Computed body tomography with MRI correlation (3rd ed). Philadelphia: Lippincott-Raven, 1998, pp 701-778.
48. Hoffman AL, Emre S, Verham RP, Petrovic LM, Eguchi S, Silverman JL, Geller SA, Schwartz ME, Miller CM, Makowka L. Hepatic angiomyolipoma: two cases reports of caudate-based lesions and review of the literature. Liver Transplant Surg 1997; 3:46-53.
49. Hooper LD, Mergo PJ, Ros PR. Multiple hepatorenal angiomyolipomas: diagnosis with fat suppression, gadolinoum.enhanced MRI. Abdom Imaging 1994; 19:549-551.
50. Ichikawa T, Federle MP, Grazioli L, Nalesnik M. Hepatocellular adenoma: multiphasic CT and histopathologic findings in 25 patients. Radiology 2000 Mar;214(3):861-8.
51. International Working Party. Terminology of nodular hepatocellular lesions. Hepatology 1995; 22:983-993.
52. Ishak KG, Rabin L. Benign tumors of the liver. Med Clin North Am. 1975; 59:995-1013.
53. Ishak KG, Willis GW, Cummins SD, Bullock AA. Biliary cystoadenoma and cystoadenocarcinoma. Report of 14 cases and review of the literature. Cancer 1977; 39:322-338
54. Jacobs J, Birnbaum B. Computed tomography imaging of focal hepatic lesions. Semin Roentgenol 1995; 30:308-323
55. Kalovidouris A, Gouliamos A, Vlachos L, Papadopoulos A, Voros D, Pentea S, Papavasiliou C. MRI of abdominal hydatid disease. Abdom Imaging 1994; 19:489-494.
56. Karhunen PJ. Begingn hepatic tumors and tumors-like conditions in men. J Clin Pathol. 1986; 39:183-188.
57. Kawakatsu M, Vilgrain V, Belghiti J, Flejou JF, Nahum H. Association of multiple liver cell adenomas with spontaneous intrahepatic portohepatic shunt. Abdom Imaging 1994 Sep-Oct;19(5):438-40
58. Kew MC: Hepatic tumors and cysts. In Feldman M, Scharschmidt BF, Sleisenger MH (eds): Sleisenger and Fordtran's Gastrointestinal and Liver disease (6th ed.). Philadelphia: WB Saunders, 1998, pp 1364-1387
59. Korobkin M, Stephens DH, Lee JK, Stanley RJ, Fishman EK, Francis IR, Alpern MB, Rynties M. Biliary cystoadenoma and cystoadenocarcinoma: CT and sonographic findings. AJR 1989; 153:507-511.
60. Kim K, Choi J, Park Y, Lee W, Kim B. Biliary cystoadenoma of the liver. J Hepatobiliary Pancreat Surg 1998;5:348-352.
61. Labrune P, Trioche P, Duvaltier I, Chevalier P, Odievre M. Hepatocellular adenomas in glycogen storaged disease type I and III: a series of 43 patients and review of the literature. J Pediatr. Gastrienterol. Nutr. 1997; 24:276-279
62. Leese T, Farges O, Bismuth H. Liver cell adenomas: a 12 years surgical experience from a specialist hepato-biliary unit. Ann.Surg. 1988; 208:558-564.
63. Leslie DF, Johnson CD, Johnson CM, Ilstrup DM, Harmsen WS. Distinction between cavernous hemangiomas of the liver and hepatic metastases on CT: value of contrast enhancement patterns. AJR Am J Roentgenol 1995 Mar;164(3):625-9
64. Leval D.B.: Hydatid disease: biology, pathology, imaging and classification. Clin Raidiol. 1998; 53:863-874.
65. Levick CB, Rubie J. Hemangioendothelioma of the liver simulating congenital heart disease in infants. Arch Dis Child 1953; 28:49-51
66. Lloyd RL, Lyons EA, Levi CS, Bristowe JR, Schollenberg J. The sonographic appearance of peliosis hepatis.. J Ultrasound Med 1982 Sep;1(7):293-4
67. Mathieu D, Vilgrain V, Mahfouz AE, Anglade MC, Vullierme MP, Denys A. Benign liver tumors. Magn Reson Imaging Clin N Am 1997; 5:255-258.
68. McFarland EG, Mayo-Smith WW, Saini S, Hahn PF, Goldberg MA, Lee MJ. Hepatic hemangiomas and malignant tumors: improved differentiation with heavily T2-weighted conventional spin-echo MR imaging. Radiology 1994 Oct;193(1):43-7
69. McLean RH, Moller JH, Warwick WJ. Multinodular haemangiomatosis if the liver in infancy. Pediatrics 1972; 49:563-573
70. Millar WJ, Sechtin AJ, Campbell WL, Pieters PC. Imaging findings in Caroli's disease. AJR 1995; 165:333-337
71. Missalek W. Ultrasonography in the diagnosis of amoebic liver abscesses and its complications. Trop Doct 1992; 22:59-63.
72. Molina EG and Schiff ER. Benign solid lesion of the liver chapter 53, pag 1254-1257 Schiff's. Diseases of the liver. (8th edition) Vol.II. Lippincott-Raven 1999.
73. Moreno-Merlo F, Wanless IR, Shimamatsu K, Sherman M, Greig P, Chiasson D. The role of granulomatous phlebitis and thrombosis in the pathogenesis of cirrhosis and portal hypertension in sarcoidosis. Hepatology 1997; 26:554-560
74. Mortele KJ, Stubbe J, Praet M, Van Langenhove P, De Bock G, Kunnen M. Intratumoral steatosis in focal nodular hyperplasia coinciding with diffuse hepatic steatosis: CT and MRI findings with histologic correlation. Abdom Imaging 2000 Mar-Apr;25(2):179-81
75. Mueller BU, Butler KM, Higham MC, Husson RN, Montrella KA, Pizzo PA, Feuerstein IM, Manju-

nath K. Smooth muscle tumors in children with human immunodeficiency virus infection. Pediatrics 1992; 90:460-463

76. Murakami T, Nakamura H, Hori S, Nakanishi K, Mitani T, Kozuka T, Kimura Y, Monden M, Wakasa K, Sakurai M. Angiomyolipoma of the liver. Ultrasound, CT, MR imaging and angiography. Acta Radiol. 1993; 34:392-394

77. Murphy BJ, Casillas J, Ros PR, Morillo G, Albores-Saavedra J, Rolfes DB. The CT appearance of cystic masses of the liver. Radiographics 1989; 9:307-322

78. Nakasaki H, Tanaka Y, Ohta M, Kanemoto T, Mitomi T, Iwata Y, Ozawa A. Congenital absence of the portal vein. Ann Surg 1989 Aug;210(2):190-3

79. Newlin N, Silver TM, Stuck KJ, Sandler MA. Ultrasonic features of pyogenic liver abscesses. Radiology 1991; 139:155-159

80. Nishizaki T, Kanematsu T, Matsumata T, Yasunaga C, Kakizoe S, Sugimachi K. Myelolipoma of the liver. Cancer 1989; 63:930-934

81. O'Neil J, Ros PR. Knowing hepatic pathology aids MRI of liver tumors. Diagn Imaging 1989; 19:58-67

82. Okamura T, Murakami S, Nishioka Y, Hirayama R, Mishima Y, Awazu R. Biliary cystoadenoma of the extrahepatic bile ducts: report of a case and review of the literature. Jpn J Surg 1987; 17:281-288

83. Paley MR, Mergo PJ, Ros PR. Characterization of focal liver lesions with SPIO-enhanced T2WI: patterns of signal intensity and liver lesion contrast change. Radiology 1997;205:455-456

84. Pardes JG, Bryan PJ, Gauderer MW. Sponteneous regression of infantile hemangioendotheliomatosis of the liver. J Ultrasound Med 1982; 1:349-353

85. Patriarche C, Pelletier G, Attali P, Ladouch-Badre A, Fabre M, Roche A, Etienne JP. Ultrasonography, angiography, computed tomography and magnetic resonance in nodular regenerative hyperplasia of the liver: report a pseudo-tumoral case. Radiat Med 1988; 6:111-114.

86. Paulson EK, McClellan JS, Washington K, Spritzer CE, Meyers WC, Baker ME. Hepatic adenoma: MR characteristics and correlation with pathologic findings. AJR Am J Roentgenol 1994 Jul;163(1):113-6

87. Pelletier G, Roche A, Boccaccio F, Patriarche C, Ink O, Fabre M, Etienne JP. Imaging of nodular regenerative hyperplasia of the liver. Study of 9 cases. Gastroenterol Clin Biol 1988 Oct;12(10):687-90

88. Pliskin M. Peliosis hepatis. Radiology 1975; 114:29-30.

89. Pobiel R.S., Bisset G.S. III: Pictorial essay: imaging of liver tumors in the infant and child. Pediatr Radiol. 1995; 25:495-506.

90. Popescu I, Ciurea S, Brasoveanu V, Hrehoret D, Boeti P, Georgescu S, Tulbure D. Liver hemangioma revisited: current surgical indications, technical aspects, results. Hepatogastroenterology 2001 May-Jun;48(39):770-6

91. Prayer LM, Schurawitzti HJ, Wimberger DM. Case report: lipoma of the liver: ultrasound, CT and MR imsging. Clin Radiol 1992; 45:353-354

92. Rals PW. Focal inflammatory diseases of the liver. Radiol Clin North Am 1998; 36:377-389

93. Reddy KR, Schiff E. Approach to a liver lesion. Semin Liver Dis. 1993; 13:423-435.

94. Reed S.L.: Amebiasis: an update. Clin Infect Dis. 1992 ; 14 :385-393

95. Reinertson TE, Fortune JB, Peters JC, Pagnotta I, Balint JA. Primary leiomyoma of the liver. A case report and review of the literature. Dig Dis Sci 1992 Apr;37(4):622-7

96. Ribeiro A, Burgart LJ, Nagorney DM, Gores GJ. Management of liver adenomatosis: results with a conservative surgical approach. Liver Transpl Surg 1998 Sep;4(5):388-98

97. Ros PR, Goodman ZD, Ishak KG, Dachman AH, Olmsted WW, Hartman DS, Lichtenstein JE. Mesenchymal hamartoma of the liver: radiologic-pathologic correlation. Radiology 1986; 158:619-624

98. Ros PR, Rasmussen JF, Li KCP. Radiology of malignant and benign liver tumors. Curr Probl Diagn Radiol 1989; 18:95-155.

99. Ros PR, Helena M, Taylor HM., et al.: Focal hepatic infections. Chapter 86 in Gore –Levine. Textbook of gastrointestinal radiology, second edition. :pp 1569-1589.

100. Ros PR: Computed tomography-pathologic correlation in hepatic tumors. In Ferrucci JT, Mathieu DG (eds): Advances in hepatobiliary Radiology. St. Louis: CV Mosby, 1990, pp 75-108.

101. Rubin R, Lichtenstein G. Hepatic scintigraphy in the evaluation of solitary solid liver masses. J Nucl Med. 1993; 34:697-705

102. Saini S, Edelman RR, Sharma P, Li W, Mayo-Smith W, Slater GJ, Eisenberg PJ, Hahn PF. Blood-pool MR contrast material for detection and characterization of focal hepatic lesions: initial clinical experience with ultrasmall superparamagnetic iron oxide (AMI-227). AJR Am J Roentgenol 1995 May;164(5):1147-52

103. Sanfelippo PM, Beahrs OH, Weiland LK. Cystic diseases of the liver. Ann Surg 1974; 179:922-925.

104. Schima W, Saini S, Echeverri JA, Hahn PF, Harisinghani M, Mueller PR. Focal liver lesions: characterization with conventional spin-echo T2.-weighted MR imaging. Radiology 1997;202(2):389-394,.

105. Semelka RC, Sofka CM. Hepatic hemangiomas. Magn Reson Imaging Clin N Am 1997 May;5(2):241-53

106. Semelka RC, Kelekis NL, Sallah S, Worawattanakul S, Ascher SM. Hepatosplenic fungal disease: diagnostic accuracy and spectrum of appearance of MR imaging. AJR 1997; 169:1311-1316

107. Shamsi K, De Schepper A, Degryse H, Deckers F. Focal nodular hyperplasia of the liver: radiologic findings. Abdom Imaging 1993;18(1):32-8
108. Sherlock S, Feldman CA, Moran B, Scheuer PJ. Partial nodular transformation of the liver with portal hypertension. Am J Med. 1966; 40:195-203
109. Shirkhoda A.: CT findings in hepatosplenic and renal candidiasis. J Comput Assist Tomogr. 1987; 11:795-798.
110. Siegelman ES, Outwater EK, Furth EE, Rubin R. MR imaging of hepatic nodular regenerative hyperplasia. J Magn Reson Imaging 1995; 5:730-732
111. Soe KL, Soe M, Gluud S. Liver pathology associated with the use of anabolic-androgenic steroids. Liver 1992; 12:73-79
112. Stromeyer FW, Ishak KG. Nodular transformation (nodular "regenerative" hyperplasia) of the liver. A clinicopathological study of 30 cases. Hum Pathol 1981; 12:60-71.
113. Talente GM, Coleman RA, Alter C, Baker L, Brown BI, Cannon RA, Chen YT, Crigler JF Jr, Ferreira P, Haworth JC, et al. Glycogen storage disease in adults. Ann. Intern. Med. 1994; 120:218-226
114. Tanaka M, Wanless IR. Pathology of the liver in Budd-Chiari syndrome: portal vein thrombosis and the histogenesis of venocentric cirrhosis, veno-portal cirrhosis, and large regenerative nodules. Hepatology 1998; 27:488-496
115. Taourel P, Marty-Ane B, Charasset S, Mattei M, Devred P, Bruel JM. Hydatid cyst of the liver: comparison of CT and MRI. J Comput Assist Tomogr 1993; 17:80-85
116. Taylor KJ, Ramos I, Morse SS, Fortune KL, Hammers L, Taylor CR. Focal liver masses: differential diagnosis with pulsed Doppler US. Radiology 1987 Sep;164(3):643-7
117. Terayama N, Terada T, Hoso M, Nakanuma Y. Partial nodular transformation of the liver with portal vein thrombosis. A report of two autopsy cases. J Clin Gastroenterol. 1995; 20:71-76
118. Terkivatan T, de Wilt JH, de Man RA, Ijzermans JN. Management of hepatocellular adenoma during pregnancy. Liver 2000; 20:186-187
119. Terris B, Flejou JF, Picot R, Belghiti J, Henin D. Hepatic angiomyolipoma. A report of four cases with immunohistochemical and DNA-flow cytometric studies. Arch Pathol Lab Med 1996 Jan;120(1):68-72
120. Trauner M, Stepan KM, Resch M, Ebner F, Pristautz H, Klimpfinger M. Diagnostic problems in nodular regenerative hyperplasia (nodular transformation) of the liver. Z Gastroenterol 1992; 30:187-194
121. Verhaegen F, Poey C, Lebras Y, Iscain P, Guiot S, Lyonnet P, Duparc B. X-ray computed tomographic tests in the diagnosis and treatment of amebic liver abscesses. J Radiol 1996 Jan;77(1):23-8
122. Vignaux O, Legmann P, de Pinieux G, Chaussade S, Spaulding C, Couturier D, Bonnin A. Hemorrhagic necrosis due to peliosis hepatis: imaging findings and pathological correlation. Eur Radiol 1999;9(3):454-6
123. Vilgrain V, Boulos L, Vullierme MP, Denys A, Terris B, Menu Y. Imaging of typical hemangioma of the liver with pathologic correlation. Radiographics 2000; 20:379-397.
124. Vogl TJ, Hammerstingl R, Schwarz W, Mack MG, Muller PK, Pegios W, Keck H, Eibl-Eibesfeldt A, Hoelzl J, Woessmer B, Bergman C, Felix R. Superparamagnetic iron oxide-enhanced versus gadolinium-enhanced MR imaging for differential diagnosis of focal liver lesions. Radiology 1996; 198:881-887
125. von Sinner W, te Strake L, Clark D, Sharif H. MR imaging in the hydatid disease. AJR 1991; 157:741-745.
126. Wachsberg RH, Cho KC, Adekosan A. Two leiomyomas of the liver in an adult with AIDS: CT and MR appearance. J Comput Assist Tomogr 1994; 18:156-157
127. Wanless IR. Micronodular transformation (nodular regenerative hyplerplasia) of the liver: a report of 64 cases among 2500 autopsies a dna new classificaiotn of benign hepatocellular nodules. Hepatology 1990; 11:787-797.
128. Wanless IR. Noncirrhotic portal hypertension: recent concepts. Prog Liver Dis. 1996; 14:265-278.
129. Walness I, Medline A. Role of estrogens as promoters of hepatic neoplasia. Lab. Invest. 1982; 46:313-320.
130. Wanless IR, Solt LC, Kortan P, Deck JH, Gardiner GW, Prokipchuk EJ. Nodular regenerative hyperplasia of the liver asociated with macroglobulinemia. Am J Med 1982; 170:1203-1209.
131. Wanless IR, Mawdsley C, Adams R. On the pathogenesis of focal nodular hyperplasia of the liver. Hepatology 1985 Nov-Dec;5(6):1194-200
132. Wanless IR, Liu JJ, Butany J. Role of thrombosis in the pathogenesis of congestive hepatic fibrosis (cardiac cirrhosis). Hepatology 1995; 21:1232-1237.
133. Weiner SN, Parulekar SG. Scintigraphy and ultrasonography of hepatic hemangioma. Radiology 1979; 132:149-153
134. Welch TJ, Sheedy PF, Johnson CM. Radiographic characteristics of benign liver tumors: focal nodular hyperplasia and hepatic adenoma. Radiographics 1985;5:673-682
135. Wheeler DA, Edmonson HA. Cystoadenoma with mesenchymal stroma (CMS) I the liver and bile ducts. A clinicopathologic study of 17 cases, 4 with malignant change. Cancer 1985; 56:1434-1445
136. Yamashita Y, Ogata I, Urata J, Takahashi M. Cavernous hemangioma of the liver: pathologic correlation with dynamic CT findings. Radiology 1997 Apr;203(1):121-5
137. Yanoff M., Rawson A. Peliosis hepatis: an anatomic study with demonstration of two varieties. Arch Pathol 1964; 77:159-165.

5   Imaging of Malignant Focal Liver Lesions

Contents

5.1   Primary Malignant Liver Lesions

5.1.1   Hepatocellular Carcinoma

Hepatocellular carcinoma (HCC) is the most common primary hepatic malignancy and one of the most prevalent visceral malignances worldwide [31]. HCC often occurs in patients with liver cirrhosis for which the cause is known (e.g. chronic viral hepatitis or alcoholism) [47]. However, whereas in Asia HCC occurs almost exclusively in patients with chronic liver damage from hepatitis, in North America many patients develop HCC without cirrhosis or known risk factors [100]. In these latter patients it is possible that steroid hormones may play a role in carcinogenesis, as tumors occurring in non-cirrhotic livers have been associated with the use of exogeneous steroids such as anabolic steroids and oral contraceptives, as well as with genetic factors [70]. Environmental and dietary factors are known to play major etiological roles, while aflatoxins, nitrosamines, and other chemical carcinogens have also been implicated in non-cirrhotic HCC [25, 32].

HCC is much more common among males than females. In high-incidence countries, the male-to-female ratio may be as high as 7 or 8 : 1, while in the United States, it is approximately 2 : 1 [75]. The occurrence of HCC increases progressively with age, although again this varies by country. Thus, in high-incidence countries, the mean age at diagnosis is in the third decade of life, while in low-incidence countries, it occurs 2 to 3 decades later. HCC is also known to occur in

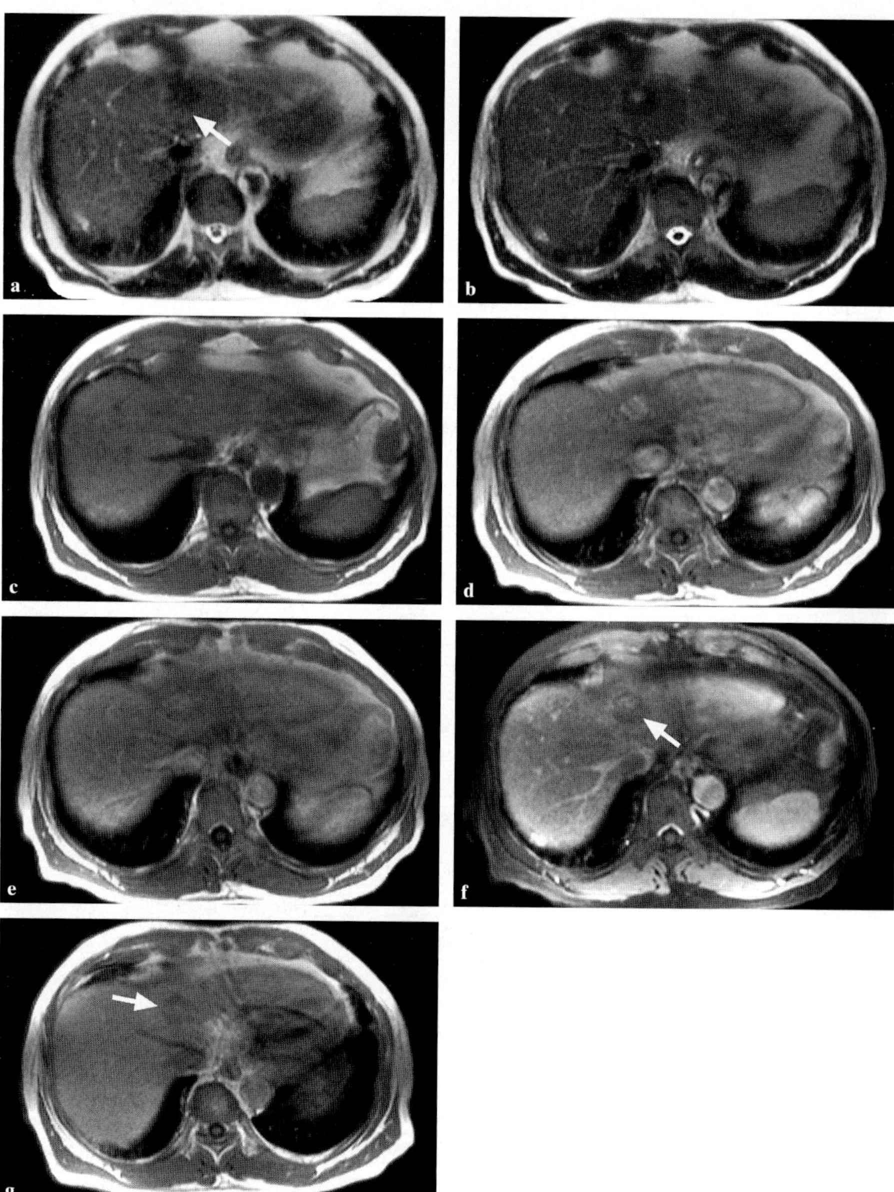

Fig. 1a-g. Hepatocellular carcinoma developing in a pre-existing regenerative nodule. In a first study, performed 6 months prior to later tests, a hypointense lesion (*arrow*) in the left liver lobe can be noted on the unenhanced T2w image (**a**). The 54-year old male patient with chronic hepatitis C had normal AFP levels at this time. Six months later a significant increase of AFP levels was noted, resulting in the initiation of a follow-up study. The unenhanced T2w scan (**b**) shows some hyperintense areas inside the previously noted regenerative nodule. On the corresponding unenhanced T1w image (**c**), these areas are hyperintense as well. On dynamic imaging after the bolus injection of Gd-BOPTA, the lesion shows strong hypervascularization during the arterial phase (**d**) and some peripheral wash-out in the portal-venous phase (**e**). This wash-out is more obvious on T1w fs images in the equilibrium phase (**f**) (*arrow*). In the hepatobiliary phase 1 h after the administration of Gd-BOPTA the lesion appears hypointense (**g**) (*arrow*), thereby indicating a lesion with nonfunctioning hepatocytes that are unable to take up Gd-BOPTA and excrete it into the bile. This case exemplifies the multi-step development of a well-differentiated HCC from a large regenerative nodule childhood, in patients as young as 4 years of age. Most childhood cases are associated with HBV infection or metabolic diseases, such as tyrosinemia [64].

Chronic liver disease including liver cirrhosis, is one of the most important factors in hepatocellular carcinogenesis. This is characterized by the development of a spectrum of nodules ranging from benign regenerative nodules to overt HCCs (Fig. 1). In carcinogenesis of the cirrhotic liver, the first step in the development of an overt HCC may be the formation of a benign regenerative nodule which then develops in a multistep fashion through the intermediate phases of ordinary low-grade dysplastic nodule (LGDN), high-grade dysplastic nodule (HGDN), and early HCC [22, 121]. Since dysplastic nodules containing malignant foci and early well-differentiated HCCs contain a great deal of fat, it has been postulated that fat deposition in dysplastic nodules is related to malignancy [69]. Dysplastic nodules containing foci of HCC (Fig. 1) are generally considered to be pre-malignant lesions.

Microscopically, HCC is composed of malignant hepatocytes that attempt to differentiate themselves into normal liver structures, mimicking hepatocyte growth, but are unable to form normal hepatic acini. Tumor cells, in well-differentiated HCCs, are difficult to distinguish from normal hepatocytes or hepatocytes in hepatocellular adenoma. Malignant hepatocytes may even produce bile. In other cases, there are microscopic variations, with HCC containing fat, tumoral secretions (large amounts of watery material), fibrosis, necrosis and amorphous calcification [99]. The most frequent patterns of HCC is the trabecular pattern, in which the tumor cells grow in thick cords that attempt to recapitulate the cell-plate pattern seen in normal liver tissue. The trabeculae are separated by vascular spaces with very little or no supporting connective tissue. Sometimes tumor secretions are in the center of the trabeculae, giving the tumor a pseudoglandular pattern. If the trabeculae grow together, they produce a solid pattern [96].

Macroscopically, there are also several patterns of growth. HCC is denominated single or massive when there is a solitary small or large mass, with or without a capsule. Multiple separate nodules characterize multifocal HCC, the second most common pattern. The least common pattern of diffuse or cirrhotomimetic growth is composed of multiple small tumoral foci distributed throughout the liver, mimicking nodules of cirrhosis. HCC is named encapsulated when it is completely surrounded by a fibrous capsule. Encapsulated HCC has better prognosis due to greater resectability. In general vascular invasion of intrahepatic and perihepatic vessels is common in HCC [33, 116].

The symptoms associated with HCC include malaise, fever, abdominal pain, and weight loss, while jaundice is rare [116]. Often the neoplasm is detected in asymptomatic patients, and the liver function tests are normal or slightly altered except for the elevation of α-fetoprotein levels. The α-fetoprotein values are high in more than 50% of cases and generally exceed 1000 ng/ml, however, alpha-fetoprotein values are not very useful for screening of patients with an increased risk of developing HCC. Proteins produced by HCC may give rise to numerous para-neoplastic syndromes, such as erythrocytosis, hypercalcaemia, hypoglycaemia and hirsutism [64]. Several investigators [100, 146] have consistently reported that HCC occurring in the noncirrhotic liver has different features: patients are younger, they are more likely to present with symptoms, have a single or dominant mass, and have a decreased mortality if liver resection is performed [129].

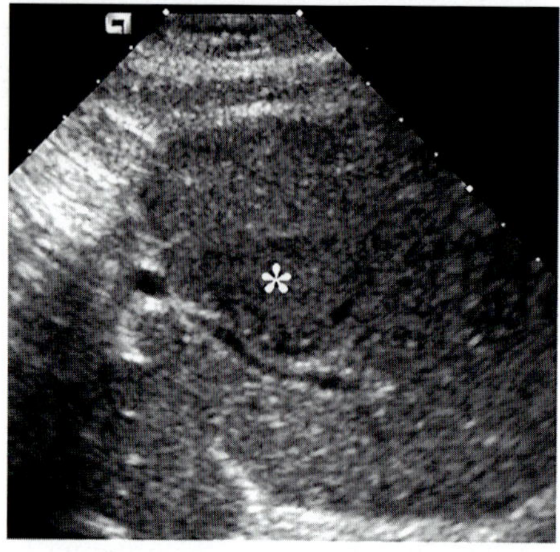

Fig. 2. Well-differentiated hepatocellular carcinoma. Ultrasound reveals a well-defined, homogeneous, and hypoechoic lesion (*asterisk*)

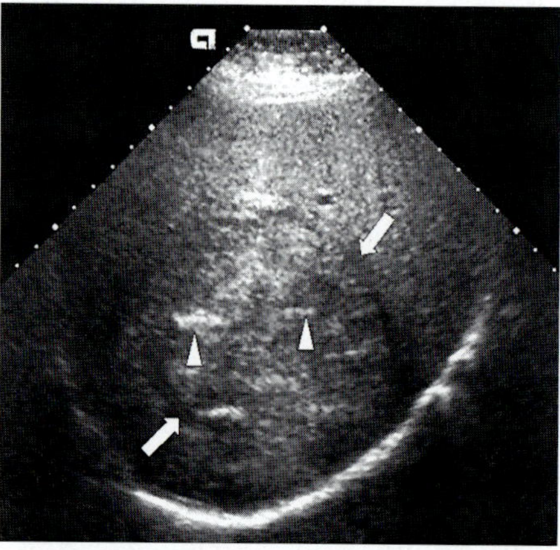

Fig. 3. Moderately differentiated hepatocellular carcinoma. On ultrasound, the lesion is heterogeneous with hypoechoic and hyperechoic areas (*arrowheads*). A thin, hypoechoic rim which corresponds to a pseudocapsule delimitates the lesion (*arrows*)

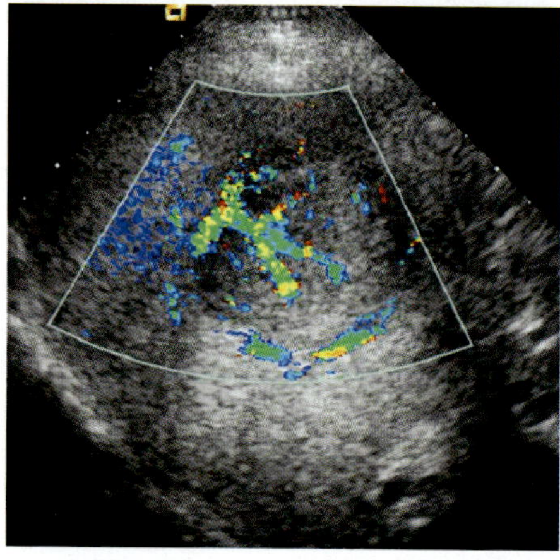

Fig. 4. Hepatocellular carcinoma. Color Doppler ultrasound reveals internal vascularization and a peritumoral hypervascular rim that gives the characteristic basket pattern. The vessels course from the periphery through the center

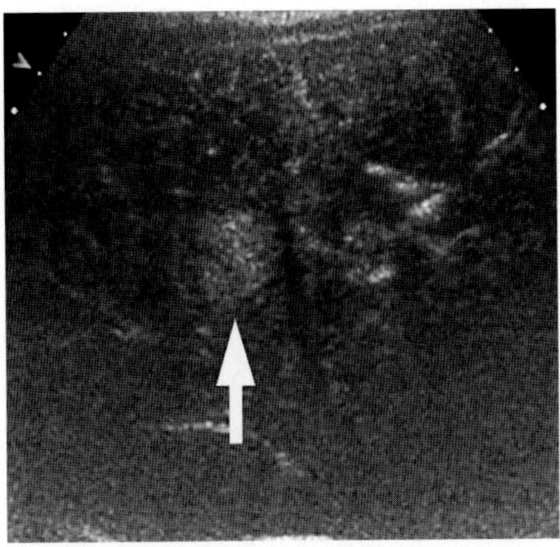

Fig. 5. Hepatocellular carcinoma on contrast-enhanced ultrasound. During the arterial phase, after the bolus injection of Sonovue®, the lesion shows intense and homogeneous enhancement, and becomes hyperechoic (*arrow*). Hyperechogenicity reflects the hypervascular nature of the tumor

Ultrasound is considered a screening method for patients at risk of hepatocellular carcinoma, often enabling neoplasms smaller than 2–3 cm (the so-called "small HCC"), to be demonstrated, even if α-fetoprotein levels are still normal. On ultrasound scans, the echogenicity of HCC neoplasms varies with the size of the lesion. Thus, nodules smaller than 3 cm are usually well-defined, hypoechoic, and homogeneous, with posterior acoustic enhancement (Fig. 2). Conversely, lesions larger than 3 cm are often heterogeneous, with a mosaic or mixed pattern arising from a combination of areas of necrosis, hemorrhage, fatty degeneration and interstitial fibrosis (Fig. 3) [21]. When visible, the capsule in encapsulated HCC, usually appears as a thin, hypoechoic band [69]. Color Doppler ultrasound frequently reveals a "basket" pattern which is indicative of hypervascularity and tumor shunting (Fig. 4). Power Doppler ultrasound is often considered superior to color Doppler ultrasound for the depiction of vascular flow because of its high sensitivity to slow flow, lack of any angle dependency, and absence of aliasing [79]. Recently various harmonic imaging techniques, such as tissue harmonic imaging, harmonic power Doppler US, and color coded harmonic angiography, have been developed and used, even in combination with contrast media, to improve the characterization of HCC (Fig. 5) [20, 61, 65].

On computed tomography (CT) scans, the appearance of HCC depends largely on tumor size and the histologic tumor grade, with low sensitivity for the detection of small neoplasms that are difficult to differentiate from unopacified vessels [50]. Unenhanced CT usually reveals a hypodense nodule. Occasionally, central areas of lower attenuation corresponding to tumor necrosis can be seen [66]. Since small HCCs have a proportionately greater arterial blood supply, they often demonstrate hyperattenuation on early arterial phase images and rapid washout in the subsequent portal-venous phase (Fig. 6) [102]. In larger lesions, the portal vein may also contribute significantly to the blood supply of the HCC, enabling its visualization on portal-venous phase images as well [58]. However, because large tumors may contain areas of hemorrhage or necrosis, they may be seen as either hyper- or hypoattenuating compared with the surrounding liver tissue during the arterial phase of hepatic enhancement and hypoattenuating in portal-venous phase (Fig. 7). Nodular HCCs are seen to possess a peripheral capsule in about

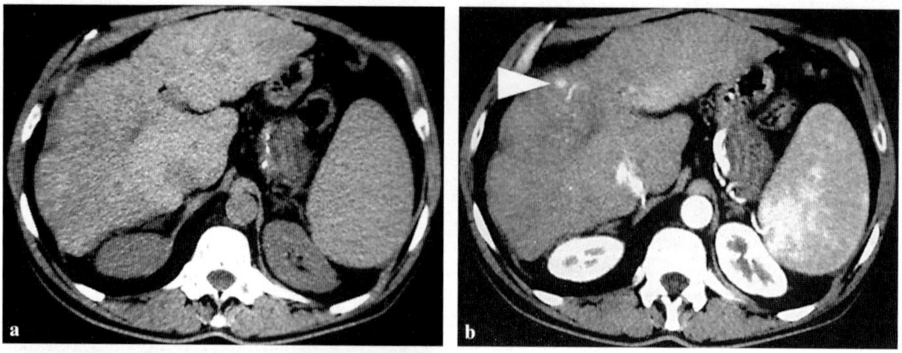

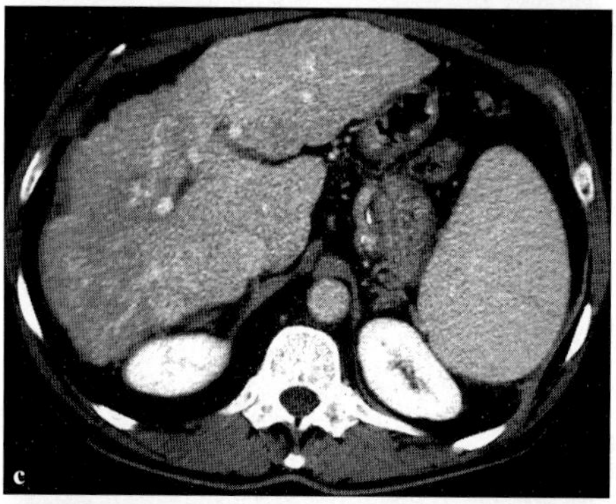

Fig. 6a-c. Small hepatocellular carcinoma. On unenhanced CT scans (**a**), the hepatic parenchyma appears heterogeneous due to cirrhosis. A hypervascular nodule (*arrowhead*) can be seen on the arterial phase after the administration of contrast material (**b**), but is no longer seen in the portal-venous phase (**c**)

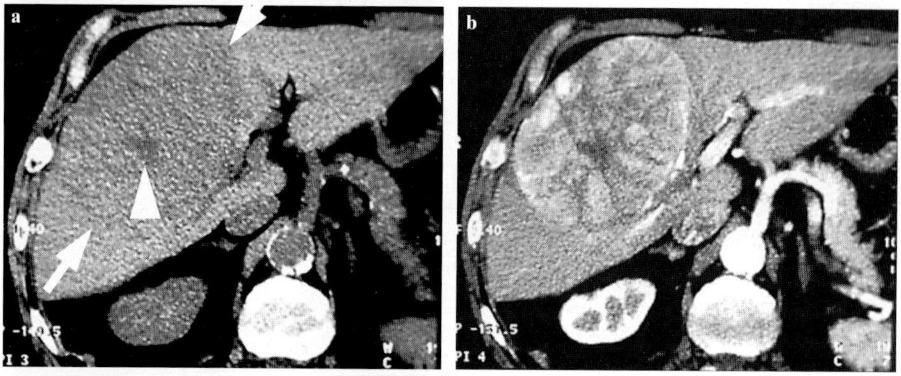

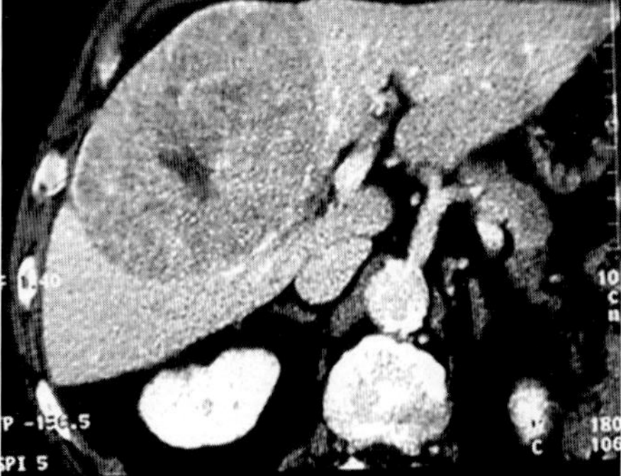

Fig. 7a-c. Hepatocellular carcinoma. On the unenhanced CT scan (**a**) a large HCC (*arrows*) appears as a well-defined hypodense nodule with a central area of lower attenuation, which corresponds to tumor necrosis (*arrowhead*). After administration of contrast medium, the nodule is seen as heterogeneously hyperattenuating during the arterial phase (**b**), becoming hypoattenuating compared to the surrounding parenchyma in the portal-venous phase (**c**)

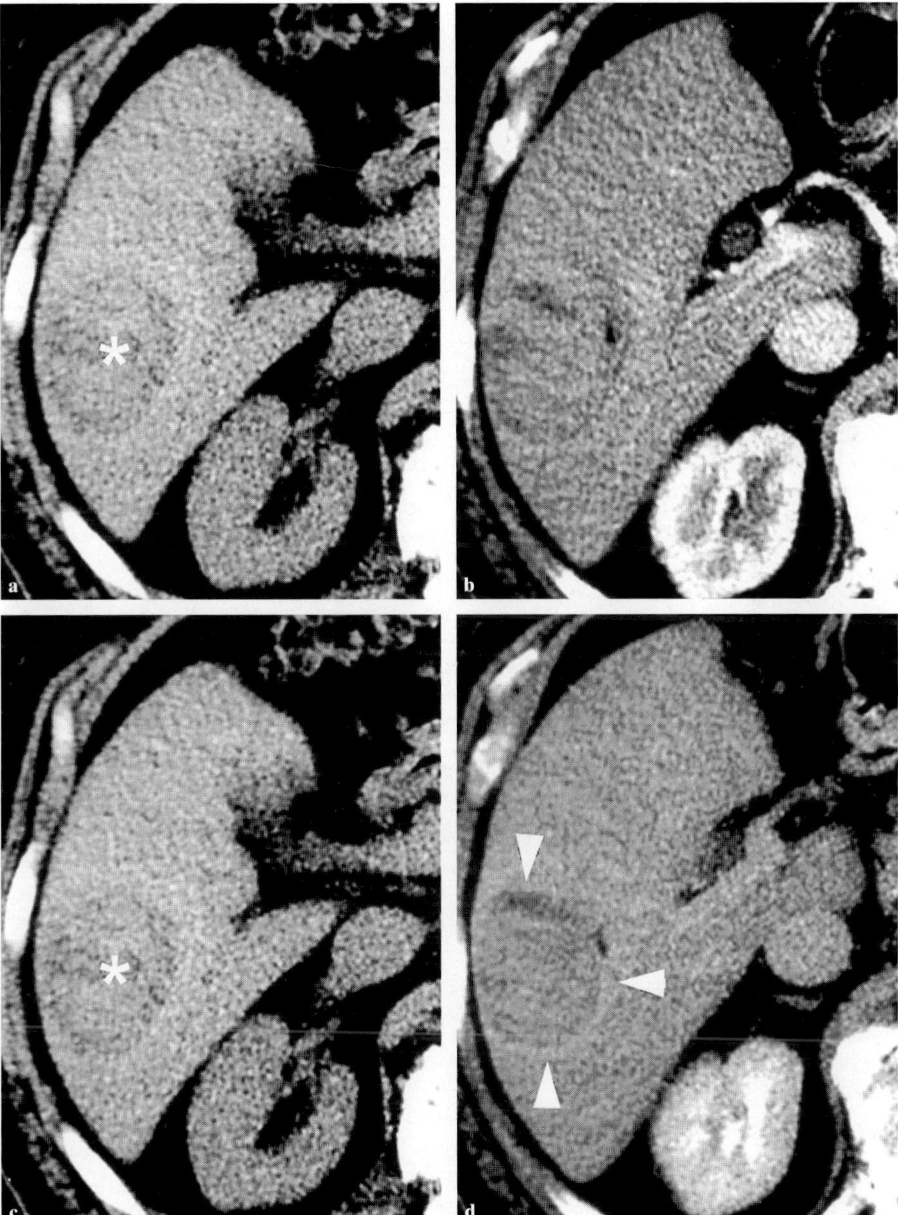

Fig. 8a-d. Encapsulated hepatocellular carcinoma. The unenhanced CT scan (**a**) shows a well-defined hypodense nodule (*asterisk*). The lesion shows poor enhancement during the arterial phase (**b**) and is seen as hypodense in the portal-venous (**c**) and equilibrium (**d**) phases. A peripheral hyperintense rim (*arrowheads*) can be seen mainly in the equilibrium phase

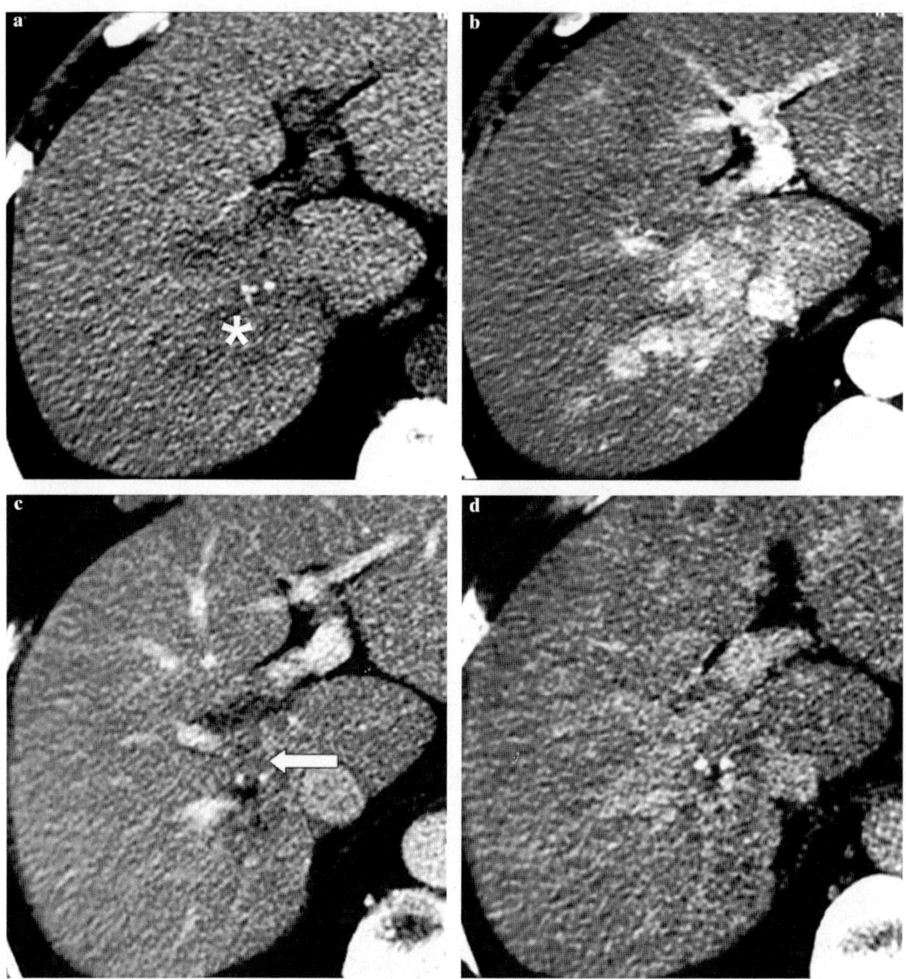

Fig. 9a-d. Non-encapsulated hepatocellular carcinoma. On the unenhanced CT scan (**a**), the nodule (*asterisk*) is seen as an ill-defined hypodense mass. The lesion enhances markedly during the arterial phase after the administration of contrast material (**b**) and subsequently shows right portal vein infiltration (*arrow*) in the portal-venous phase (**c**). During the equilibrium phase (**d**), the lesion becomes inhomogeneously isodense

50–80% of cases (Fig. 8) [42, 66, 95, 109]. Non-encapsulated tumors frequently appear as ill-defined, irregular, often hypervascular masses, showing a variable degree of vascular or bile duct infiltration (Fig. 9).

The role of CT in the detection of dysplastic nodules in the cirrhotic liver has been evaluated in several studies [48, 82]. However, these studies indicate that dysplastic nodules are usually isoattenuating to the adjacent liver parenchyma and thus cannot be seen on CT scans because the blood supply to those nodules is similar to that of the normal liver parenchyma.

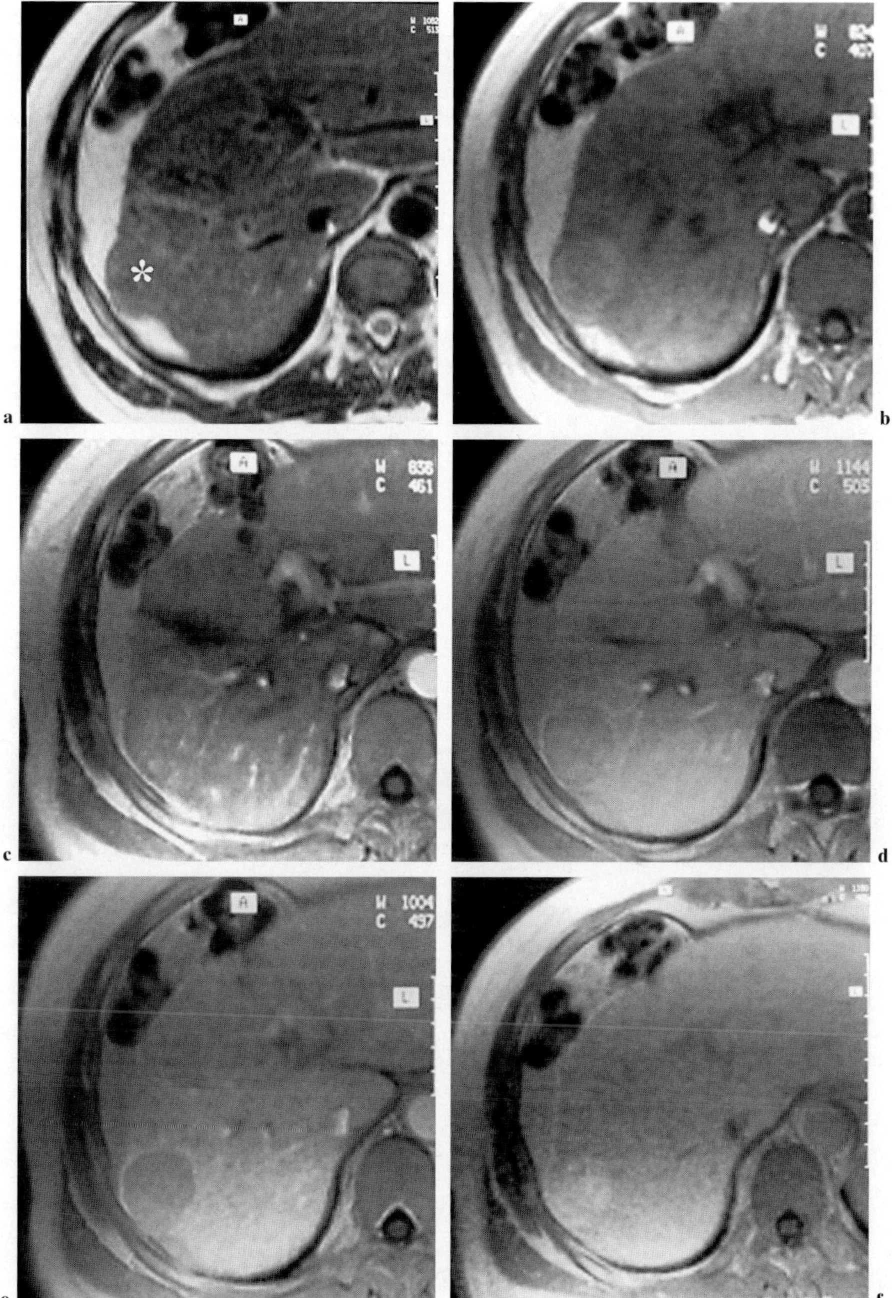

Fig. 10a-f. Dysplastic nodule. On the unenhanced T2-weighted image (**a**), the lesion (*asterisk*) is seen as isointense against the normal parenchyma, while on the corresponding T1-weighted image (**b**) it is seen as hyperintense. The lesion does not show significant enhancement on images acquired during the arterial phase after Gd-BOPTA administration (**c**), but reveals a thin enhancing peripheral rim during the portal-venous and equilibrium phases (**d** and **e**, respectively). In the delayed hepatobiliary phase (**f**), the dysplastic nodule demonstrates uptake of Gd-BOPTA

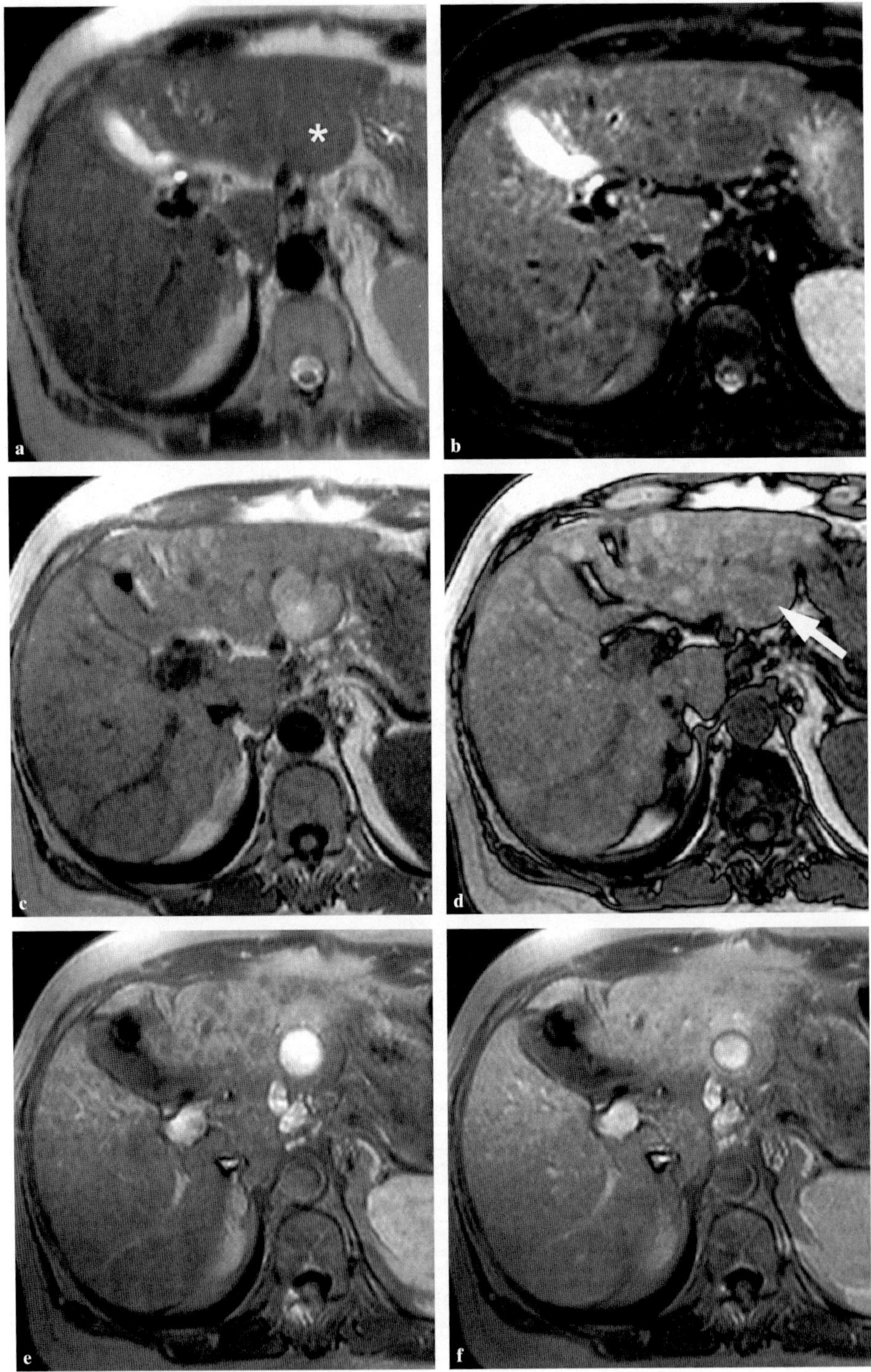

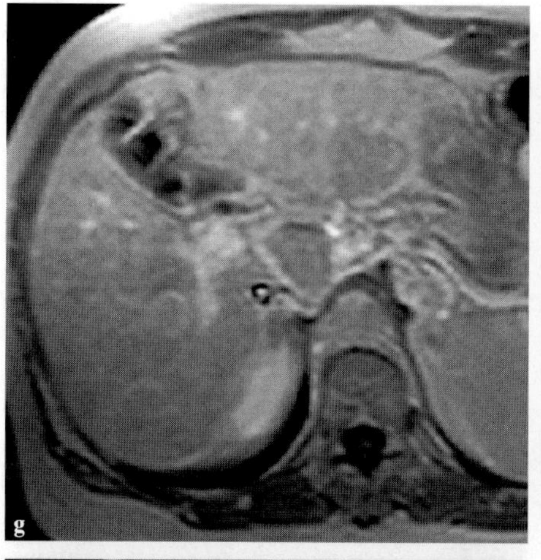

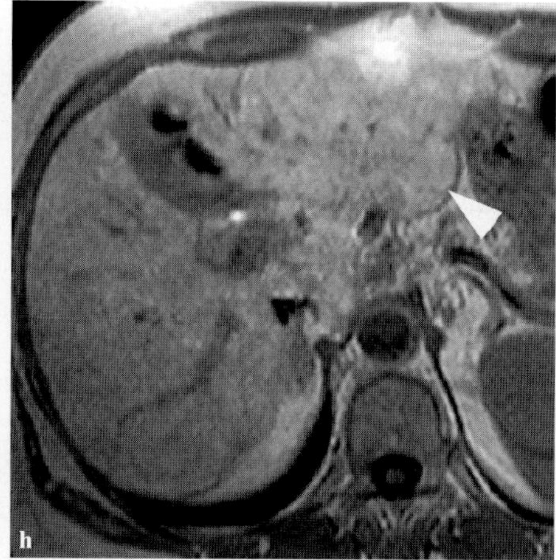

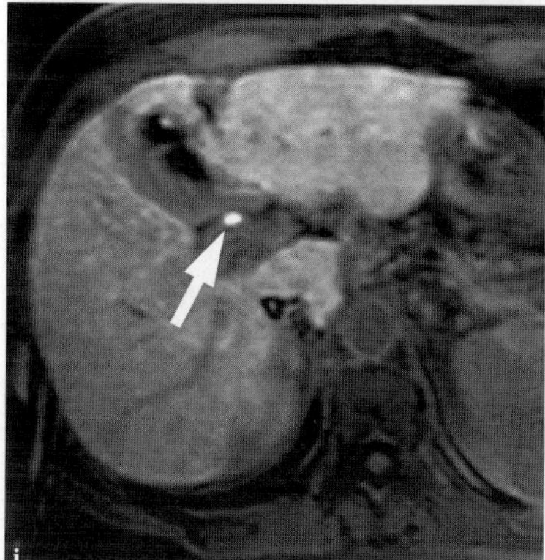

Fig. 11a-i. Dysplastic nodule in cirrhotic liver. On HASTE T2-weighted images (**a**), liver parenchyma appears heterogeneous with a large isointense nodule (*asterisk*). On fat-saturated T2-weighted images (**b**), many hypointense nodules are detected with variable signal intensity. On GE T1-weighted in- and out-of-phase images (**c, d**), the biggest lesion shows a signal drop on the "out-of-phase" image due to fatty infiltration (*arrow*). Dynamic evaluation does not reveal significant enhancement of the nodules (**e-g**). On hepatobiliary phase GE T1-weighted images with and without fat suppression acquired 1 h after injection of Gd-BOPTA (**h, i**), many nodules show uptake of the contrast agent. In particular the biggest nodule in the left liver lobe appears isointense (*arrowhead in* **h**). Note the high signal intensity in the common bile duct due to the excretion of Gd-BOP-TA (*arrowhead in* **i**)

On magnetic resonance (MR) imaging, dysplastic nodules are usually hyperintense on T1-weighted images, and iso- to hypointense on T2-weighted images. Conversely, HCCs are often hyperintense on T2-weighted images, and hypointense on T1-weighted images. However, an accurate distinction between dysplastic nodules and HCCs cannot usually be made on the basis of signal intensity characteristics on unenhanced MR, because of the overlapping signal intensities from multiple nodules [23, 71, 94].

Dysplastic nodules, particularly LGDN, do not usually show significant arterial enhancement after the bolus injection of gadolinium contrast agents. In the case of HGDN, arterial enhancement can be seen in a greater number of lesions, possibly because of neoangiogenesis. Delayed phase images acquired after the

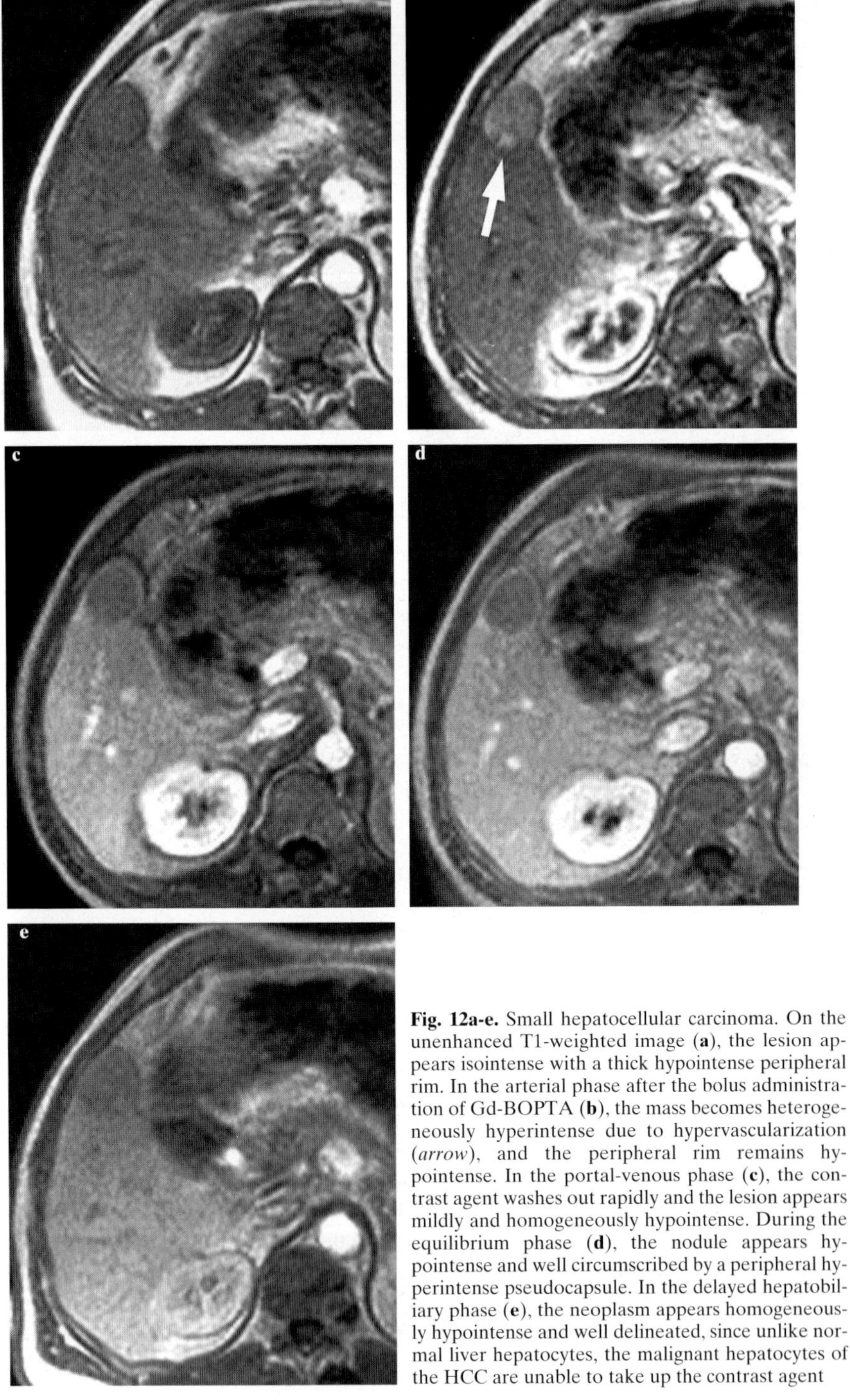

Fig. 12a-e. Small hepatocellular carcinoma. On the unenhanced T1-weighted image (**a**), the lesion appears isointense with a thick hypointense peripheral rim. In the arterial phase after the bolus administration of Gd-BOPTA (**b**), the mass becomes heterogeneously hyperintense due to hypervascularization (*arrow*), and the peripheral rim remains hypointense. In the portal-venous phase (**c**), the contrast agent washes out rapidly and the lesion appears mildly and homogeneously hypointense. During the equilibrium phase (**d**), the nodule appears hypointense and well circumscribed by a peripheral hyperintense pseudocapsule. In the delayed hepatobiliary phase (**e**), the neoplasm appears homogeneously hypointense and well delineated, since unlike normal liver hepatocytes, the malignant hepatocytes of the HCC are unable to take up the contrast agent administration of hepatobiliary contrast agents frequently reveal isointensity between the dysplastic nodules and the surrounding parenchyma (Fig. 10, Fig. 11). Since dysplastic nodules contain identical or slightly increased numbers of Kupffer cells compared to the normal liver parenchyma, they are not readily seen on T2-weighted fast spin echo imaging after the administration of superparamagnetic iron oxide (SPIO) contrast material [83].

Contrast-enhanced dynamic MR imaging is important for the detection and characterization of HCCs. Generally, most hypervascular HCCs are homogeneously hyperintense to the liver in the arterial phase, and hypointense in the portal-venous and equilibrium phases. Tumors smaller than 3 cm in diameter tend to have an homogeneous appearance (Fig. 12), and in about 20% of cases are visible mainly in the arterial phase (Fig. 13). Irregular mosaic-like or peripheral enhancement is usually seen in larger neoplasms, depending on the internal architecture [107, 150, 154].

In moderately differentiated trabecular or pseudo-glandular HCCs, a peak of enhancement is usually seen during the arterial phase followed by a rapid decrease during the subsequent portal-venous and equilibrium phases. Gradually increasing enhancement over time is found in poorly differentiated scirrhous HCCs, whereas minimal or no contrast enhancement is seen in small, well-differentiated neoplasms. Sometimes a mixture of variable differentiated areas may be found in large HCCs (Fig. 14).

Dynamic MR imaging is also helpful for the assessment of HCC pseudocapsule (see Fig. 10 and 12). When present, HCC pseudocapsules usually enhance prominently in the portal-venous phase (Fig. 15). Thereafter, enhancement persists with signs of washout into the equilibrium phase. This is due to the slow flow in the blood vessels which are present in the abundant fibrous granulation tissue [42]. Heterogeneous delayed retention of gadolinium in the equilibrium phase is not specific for HCC characterization and may correspond to abundant fibrous stroma, as in scirrhous HCCs [38, 107].

On T1-weighted images acquired during the delayed liver-specific phase after Gd-BOPTA administration, well-differentiated and moderately-differentiated HCCs may show superior signal enhancement ratios compared to poorly differentiated HCCs (see Fig. 14) [43, 86]. This is likely to be a consequence of the first two neoplastic forms retaining sufficient residual hepatocytic activity to take up Gd-BOPTA. These forms may also produce bile, which correlates with the degree of contrast enhancement as well. On the other hand, fewer than 20% of HCC appear iso-or hyperintense on hepatobiliary phase images after administration of liver-specific contrast media (Fig. 16), most poorly differentiated (Fig. 17) and large HCCs are usually hypointense to the normal liver on delayed, hepatobilliary phase images (see also Fig. 15).

Regarding SPIO agents, these are helpful for the detection of small HCCs in cirrhotic livers. A report on the relationship between the degree of SPIO uptake and the number of Kupffer cells in HCCs and dysplastic nodules revealed that the ratio between the number of Kupffer cells in tumorous versus non-tumorous tissue decreased as the degree of cellular differentiation decreased [54]. Thus, the ratio of the signal intensity of the neoplastic lesion compared with that of the non-neoplastic area on SPIO-enhanced imaging correlated well with the number of Kupffer cells present (Fig. 18; Fig. 14).

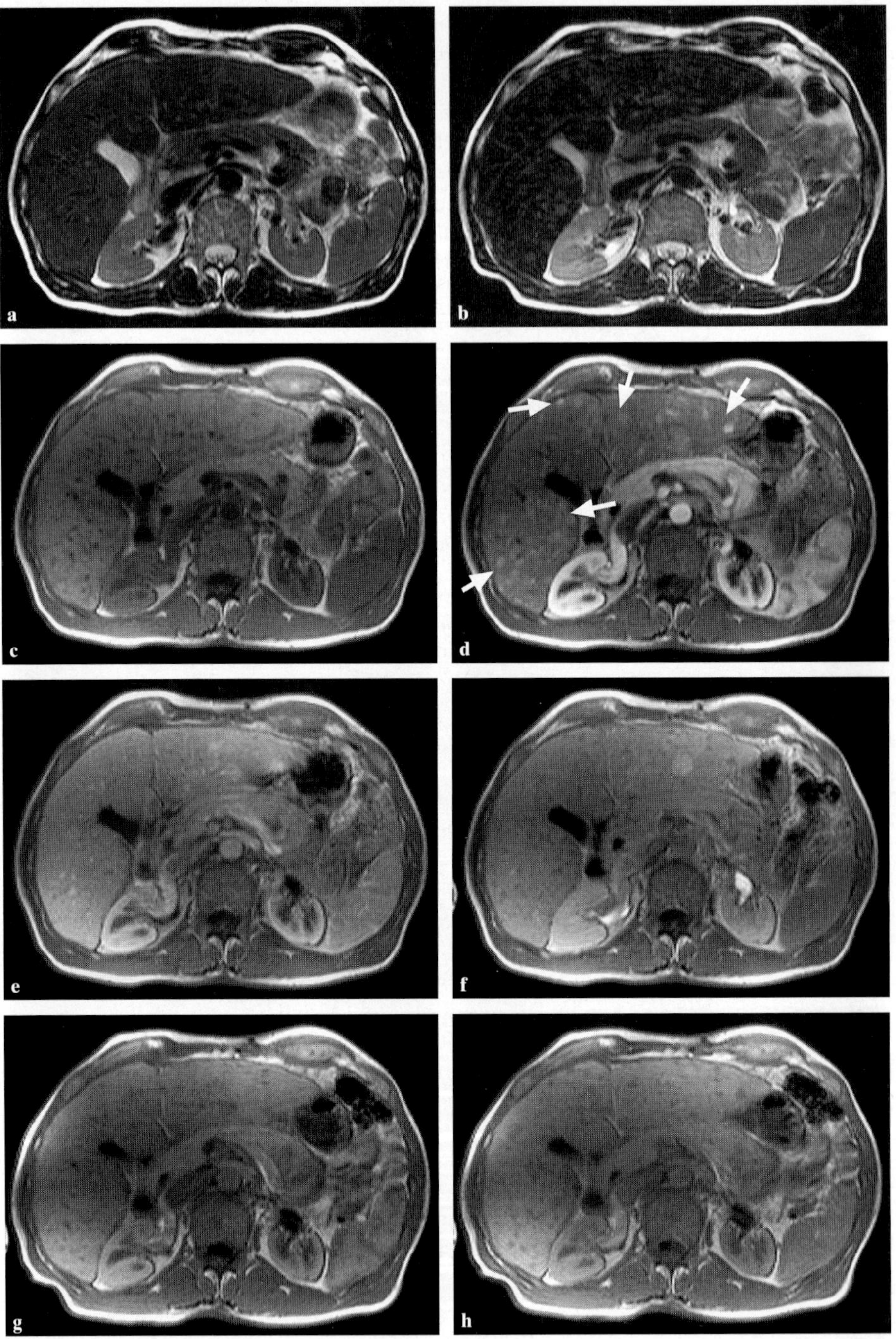

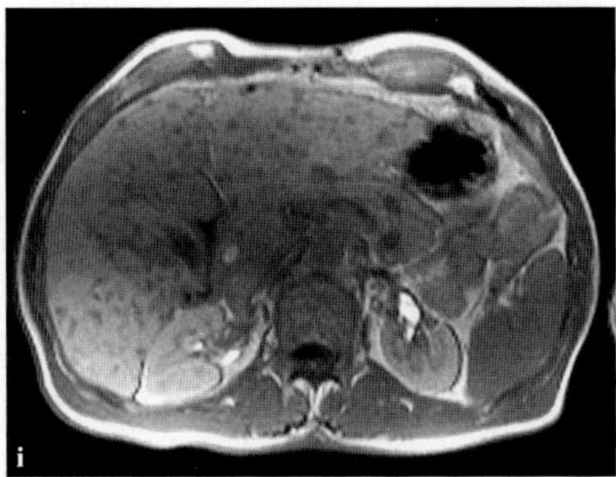

Fig. 13a-i. Diffuse hepatocellular carcinoma. Diffuse lesions in the liver parenchyma can be noted on T2-weighted images before (**a**), as well as after (**b**), the injection of iron oxide particles (SHU 555A). However, the nature of the lesions remains unclear since no signs of cirrhosis are present. On unenhanced T1-weighted images the lesions appear hypointense (**c**). Arterial phase images acquired after the injection of Gd-BOPTA (**d**) clearly reveal numerous hypervascular lesions (*arrows*). These lesions demonstrate rapid washout in the portal-venous phase (**e**) and hypointensity in the equilibrium phase (**f**). In contrast, the hypervascular nature of the lesions is not clearly depicted on dynamic imaging after the bolus injection of SHU 555A (**g**, **h**), hence the differential diagnosis is still unclear. An increase of contrast between the hypointense liver lesions and surrounding normal liver tissue can be observed on hepatobiliary phase T1-weighted images after the injection of Gd-BOPTA (**i**), indicating the malignant nature of the lesions. This case shows the importance of dynamic imaging for differential diagnosis, since the only hint to the diagnosis in a patient without obvious signs of liver cirrhosis is the hypervascular nature of the lesions

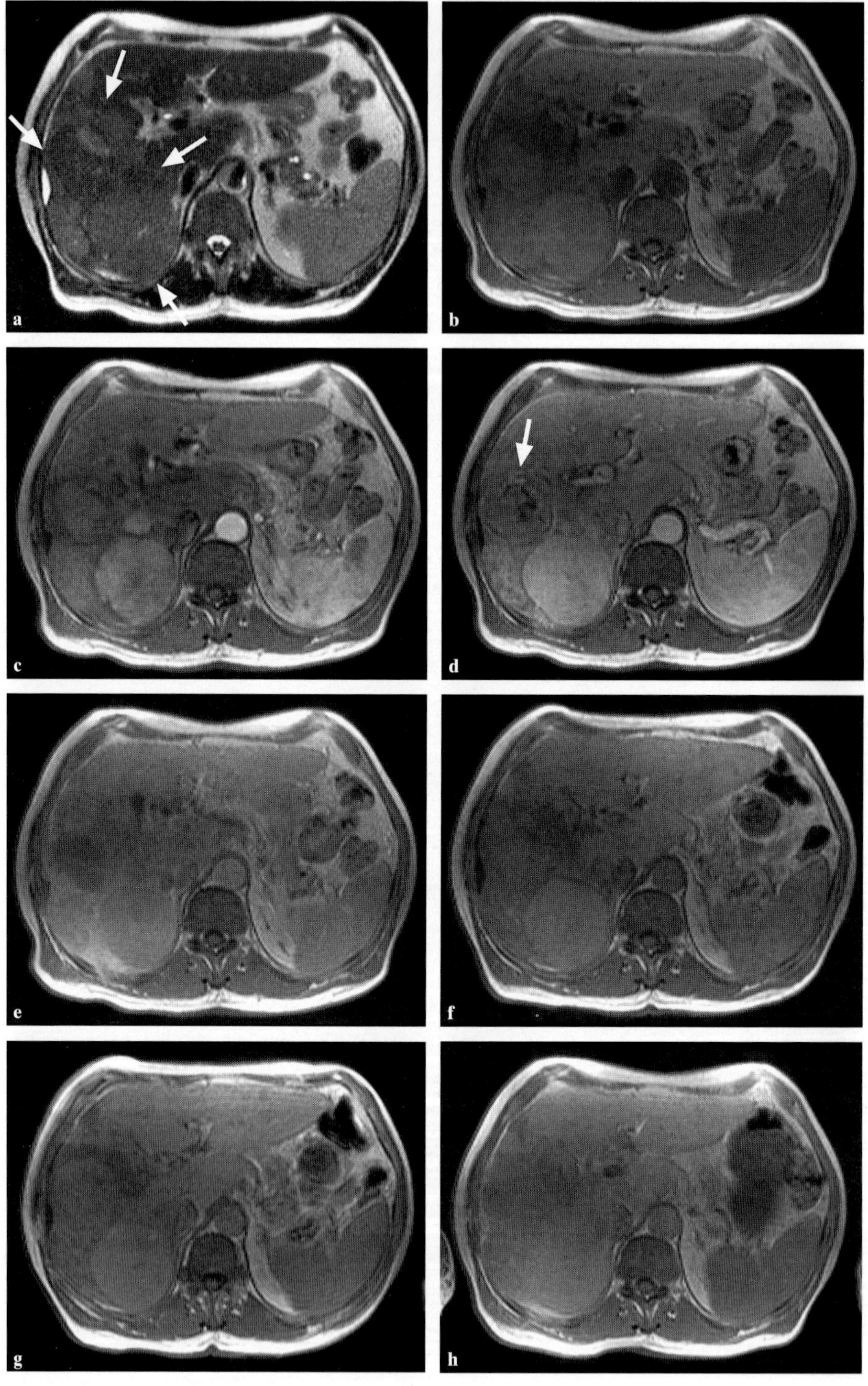

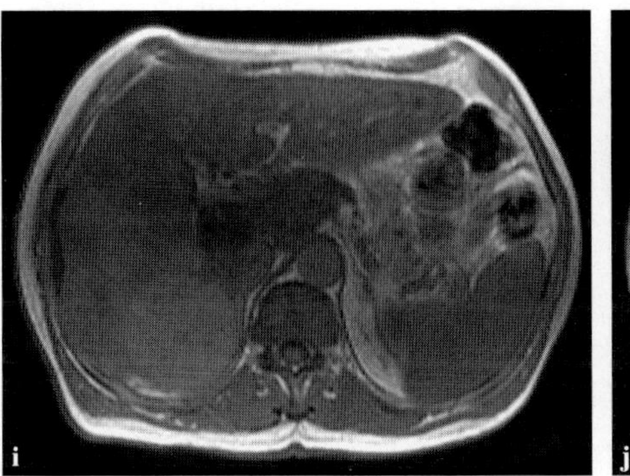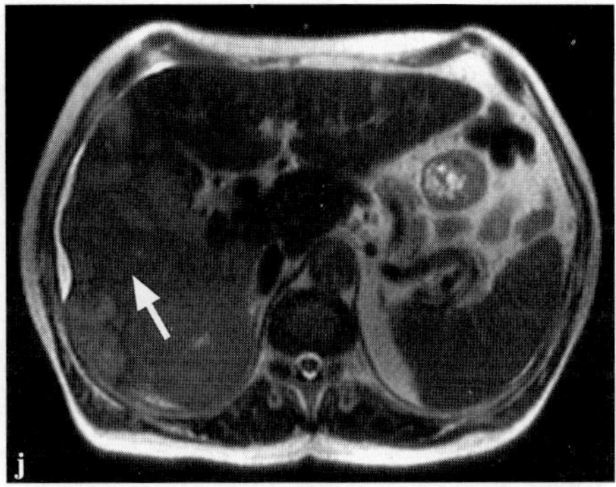

Fig. 14a-j. Hepatocellular carcinoma with different stages of differentiation. On unenhanced T2-weighted images (**a**) a large inhomogeneously hyperintense lesion can be noted in the right liver lobe (*arrows*). On the corresponding T1-weighted image (**b**), the lesion again shows inhomogeneous signal intensity with regions of hypo-, hyper- and isointensity. The hypervascularity of the lesion and the presence of numerous nodules is clearly depicted on arterial phase images after the bolus injection of Gd-BOPTA (**c**). In the portal-venous phase image (**d**), the more anterior aspect of the lesion demonstrates contrast agent washout (*arrow*), while the more posterior parts show contrast agent pooling. In the equilibrium phase (**e**) most of the lesion shows washout compared to the normal liver tissue, thereby indicating a hepatocellular carcinoma. On arterial (**f**) and portal-venous (**g**) phase images after the injection of iron oxide particles (SHU 555A), the hypervascular nature of the lesion cannot be appreciated to the same extent as after the application of a Gd-agent. In the hepatobiliary phase after the injection of Gd-BOPTA (**h**) parts of the lesion appear hypointense and parts isointense to the surrounding liver tissue. This is indicative of both well-differentiated and undifferentiated areas of the HCC. The same holds true for iron oxide enhanced T1-weighted (**i**) and T2-weighted (**j**) images in which parts of the lesion lose signal (*arrow*), due to uptake of contrast agent by Kupffer cells while other parts show higher signal intensity compared to normal liver tissue due to the lack of uptake

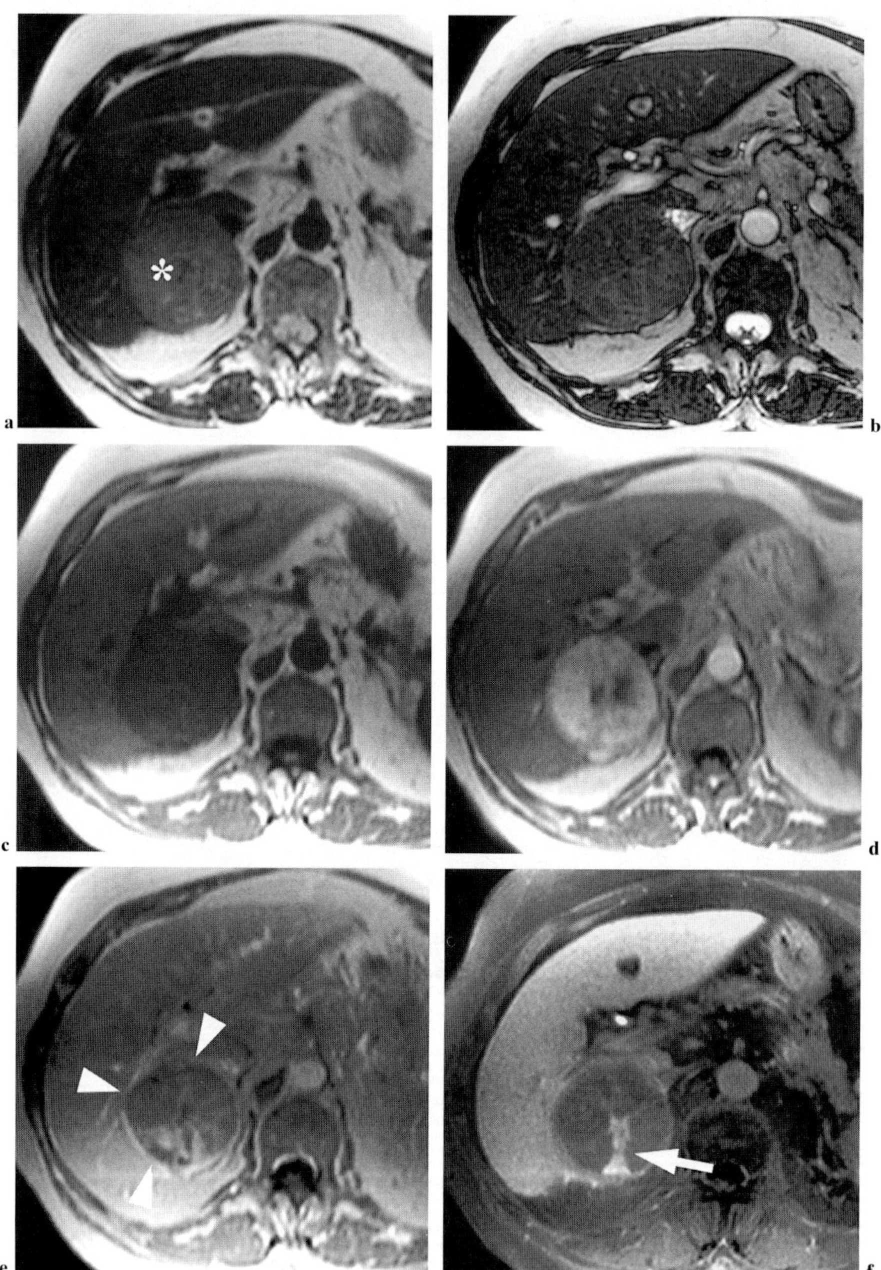

Fig. 15a-f. Large hepatocellular carcinoma. On T2-weighted HASTE (**a**) and TrueFISP (**b**) images, the HCC (*asterisk in* **a**) appears as a heterogeneous, slightly hyperintense mass. Conversely, on the unenhanced GE T1-weighted image (**c**), the lesion is seen as markedly hypointense. In the arterial phase after the administration of Gd-BOPTA (**d**), the mass appears as heterogeneously hyperintense while in the portal-venous phase (**e**) it is heterogeneously hypointense with a well-defined peripheral hyperintense pseudocapsule (*arrowheads*). In the delayed hepatobiliary phase (**f**) the lesion is again hypointense due to the lack of contrast medium uptake by the malignant hepatocytes. A rim of intermediate signal intensity surrounds the lesion while central areas of necrosis show unspecific contrast medium retention (*arrow*)

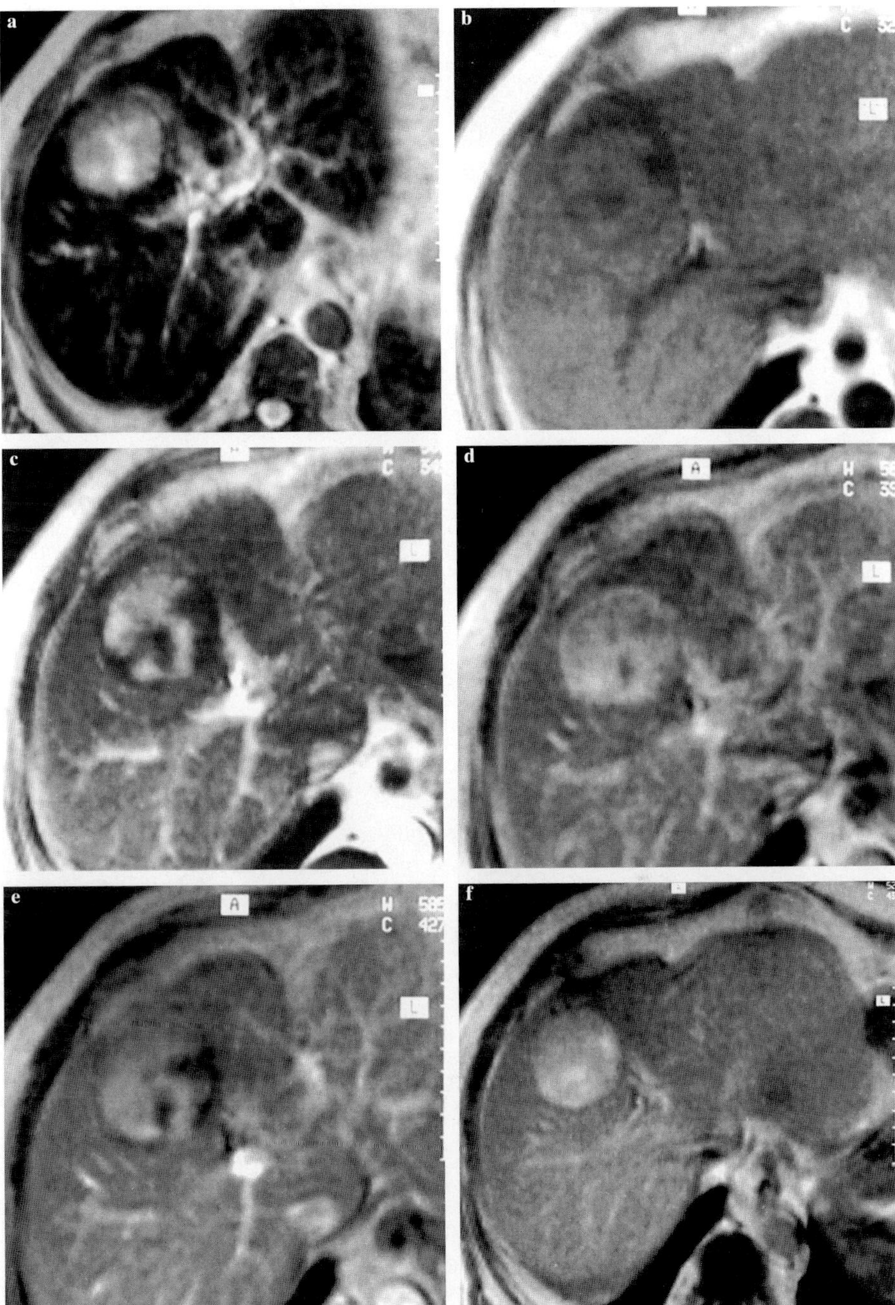

Fig. 16a-f. Well-differentiated hepatocellular carcinoma. The unenhanced Turbo SE T2-weighted (**a**) and GE T1-weighted (**b**) images reveal the lesion to be heterogeneously hyperintense and heterogeneously isointense to the normal liver, respectively. On dynamic imaging after the bolus administration of Gd-BOP-TA (**c-e**), the lesion enhances progressively, while on the delayed hepatobiliary phase image (**f**) it is seen as markedly hyperintense to the surrounding parenchyma. In this case, the malignant cells in the well-differentiated HCC retain the ability to take up the contrast agent and to produce bile

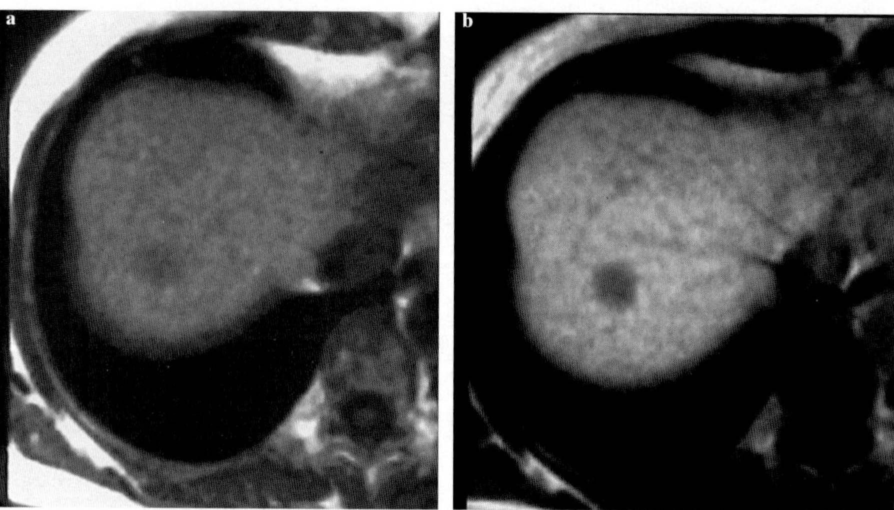

Fig. 17a,b. Poorly-differentiated hepatocellular carcinoma. On the unenhanced GE T1-weighted image (**a**) and on the image acquired during the delayed hepatobiliary phase after Gd-BOPTA administration (**b**) the nodule is seen as hypointense to the liver

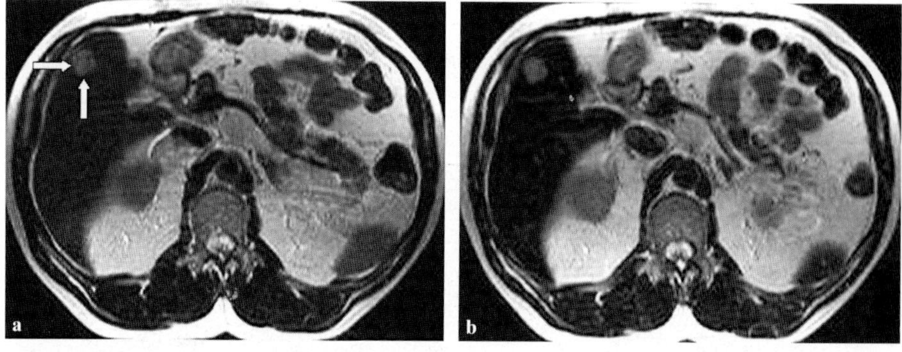

Fig. 18a,b. Hepatocellular carcinoma. On the unenhanced Turbo SE T2-weighted image (**a**) the nodule is well-defined and slightly hyperintense (*arrows*). On the image acquired during the delayed liver-specific phase after SPIO administration (**b**) the contrast-to-noise ratio is improved. The lesion does not show uptake of SPIO and remains hyperintense

HCCs generally do not show significant uptake of mangafodipir and thus appear as hypointense masses against enhanced normal parenchyma on mangafodipir-enhanced T1-weighted images. However, some well-differentiated HCCs do show uptake of mangafodipir (Fig. 19) and thus differentiation of HCC from benign lesions such as hepatic adenoma or focal nodular hyperplasia (FNH) may be problematic. Although mangafodipir is often employed to differentiate benign hepatocellular from non-hepatocellular tumors [93], a dynamic imaging capability is usually invaluable to obtain important additional information for the characterization of focal liver lesions. Thus, dual MR contrast agents such as Gd-BOPTA or Gd-EOB-DTPA, that allow both dynamic and hepatocyte-specific imaging may be of greater use (Fig. 20).

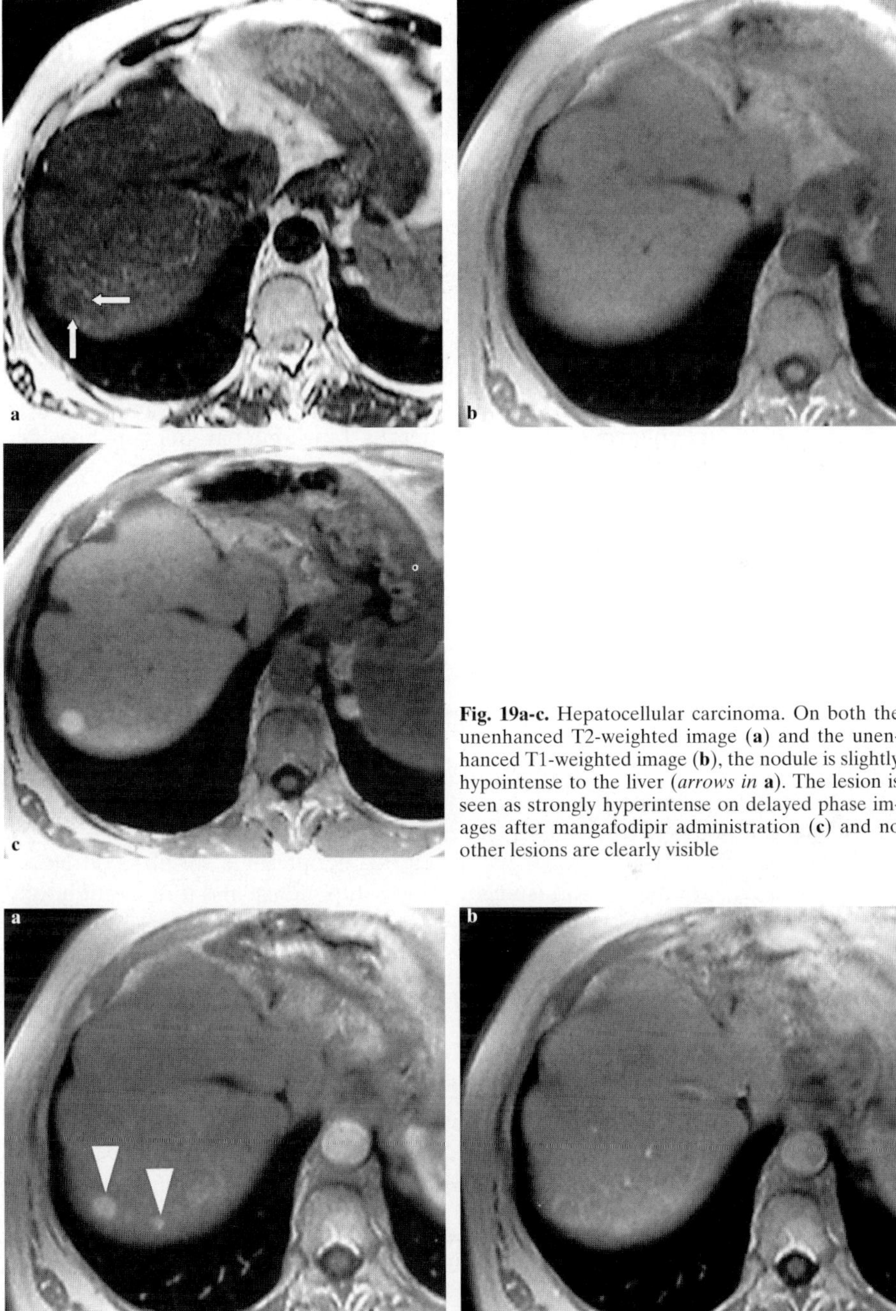

Fig. 19a-c. Hepatocellular carcinoma. On both the unenhanced T2-weighted image (**a**) and the unenhanced T1-weighted image (**b**), the nodule is slightly hypointense to the liver (*arrows in* **a**). The lesion is seen as strongly hyperintense on delayed phase images after mangafodipir administration (**c**) and no other lesions are clearly visible

Fig. 20a-b. Hepatocellular carcinoma. The same case as presented in Fig. 19. During dynamic imaging in the arterial phase after the bolus administration of Gd-BOPTA (**a**), the lesion shows intense enhancement. Another small satellite nodule can be seen only in this phase of contrast enhancement (*arrowheads*). In the portal-venous phase (**b**) the larger lesion is seen as mildly hypointense with a slightly hyperintense rim while the smaller lesion cannot be seen

5.1.2 Fibrolamellar Carcinoma

Fibrolamellar carcinoma (FLC) is an uncommon tumor with clinical and pathological features that are different from those of HCC. This neoplasm occurs predominantly in young adult patients who have no history of cirrhosis or chronic liver disease [28]. Macroscopically, the size of the tumors varies from 5–20 cm. The usual appearance of FLC is similar to that of FNH, with a central scar and multiple fibrous septa. Although hemorrhage is rare in FLC, necrosis and coarse calcifications have been reported in 20–60% of cases, especially in the central scar [28, 35, 53]. Commonly, FLC is present as a solitary mass, although sometimes FLC may appear as a bilobed mass or as a mass with small peripheral satellite lesions. Only rarely is FLC present as a diffuse multifocal mass. FLC lesions are usually intrahepatic, although sometimes pedunculated neoplasms may be found [133].

Histologically, FLCs are composed of sheets of large polygonal tumor cells separated by abundant collagen bundles which are arranged in parallel lamellae. The tumor cells have a cytoplasm that is deeply eosinophilic and granular due to the presence of mitochondria. Sometimes FLCs contain bile [6, 97, 103].

The clinical presentation is variable, although patients commonly have abdominal pain, hepatomegaly, a palpable right upper quadrant abdominal mass, and cachexia [28]. Less frequently, the disease is accompanied by pain and fever which simulates a liver abscess, gynecomastia in men, venous thrombosis, or jaundice. The gynecomastia is a result of the conversion of circulating androgens into estrogens by the enzyme aromatase, which is produced by the malignant hepatocytes. Venous thrombosis can occur due to invasion of the hepatic venous system or the inferior vena cava. Alternatively, it may form part of a paraneoplastic syndrome (Trousseau syndrome). Jaundice is a very rare condition, and can be caused either by invasion of the biliary vessels, by compression of the biliary vessels by the tumor or by enlarged nodes [1, 35].

On ultrasound scans, the echostructure of this neoplasm is variable. Often the tumor contains both hyper- and iso-echogenic components, and thus is not homogeneous. The central scar, when present, is frequently seen as a central area of hyperechogenicity (Fig. 21) [10, 88].

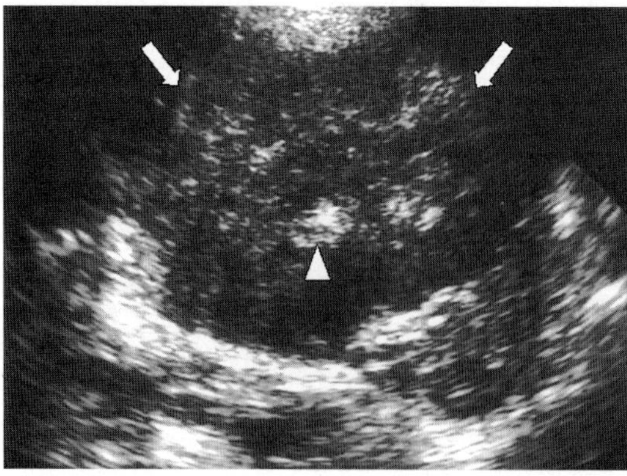

Fig. 21. Fibrolamellar carcinoma. Ultrasound reveals a non homogeneous hyper to isoechoic lesion (*arrows*) with a hyperechoic central area (*arrowhead*) that corresponds to the central scar

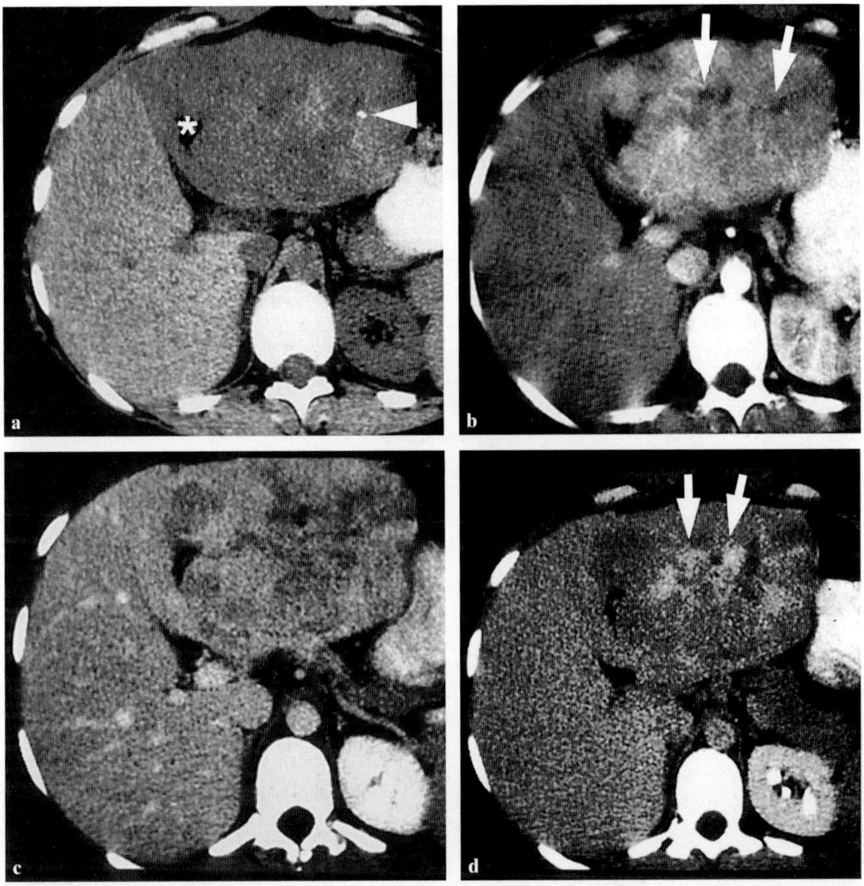

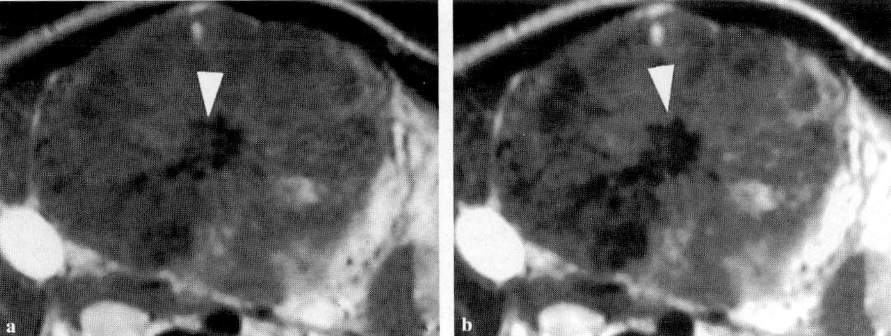

Fig. 22a-d. Fibrolamellar carcinoma. On unenhanced CT scans (**a**), the neoplasm appears as a hypodense mass compared to the liver, with coarse calcification (*arrowhead*) and a small area of necrosis (*asterisk*). On arterial and portal-venous phase images after the administration of contrast material (**b** and **c**, respectively), the nodule is seen as heterogeneously hyperattenuating with a hypodense central scar (*arrows in* **b**). In the delayed phase (**d**), the neoplasm is hypodense and the central scar hyperdense (*arrows*)

Fig. 23a,b. Fibrolamellar carcinoma. Unenhanced T1-weighted (**a**) and T2-weighted (**b**) images reveal a neoplasm that is hypointense and hyperintense to the normal parenchyma, respectively. On both images a hypointense central scar (*arrowhead*) is evident

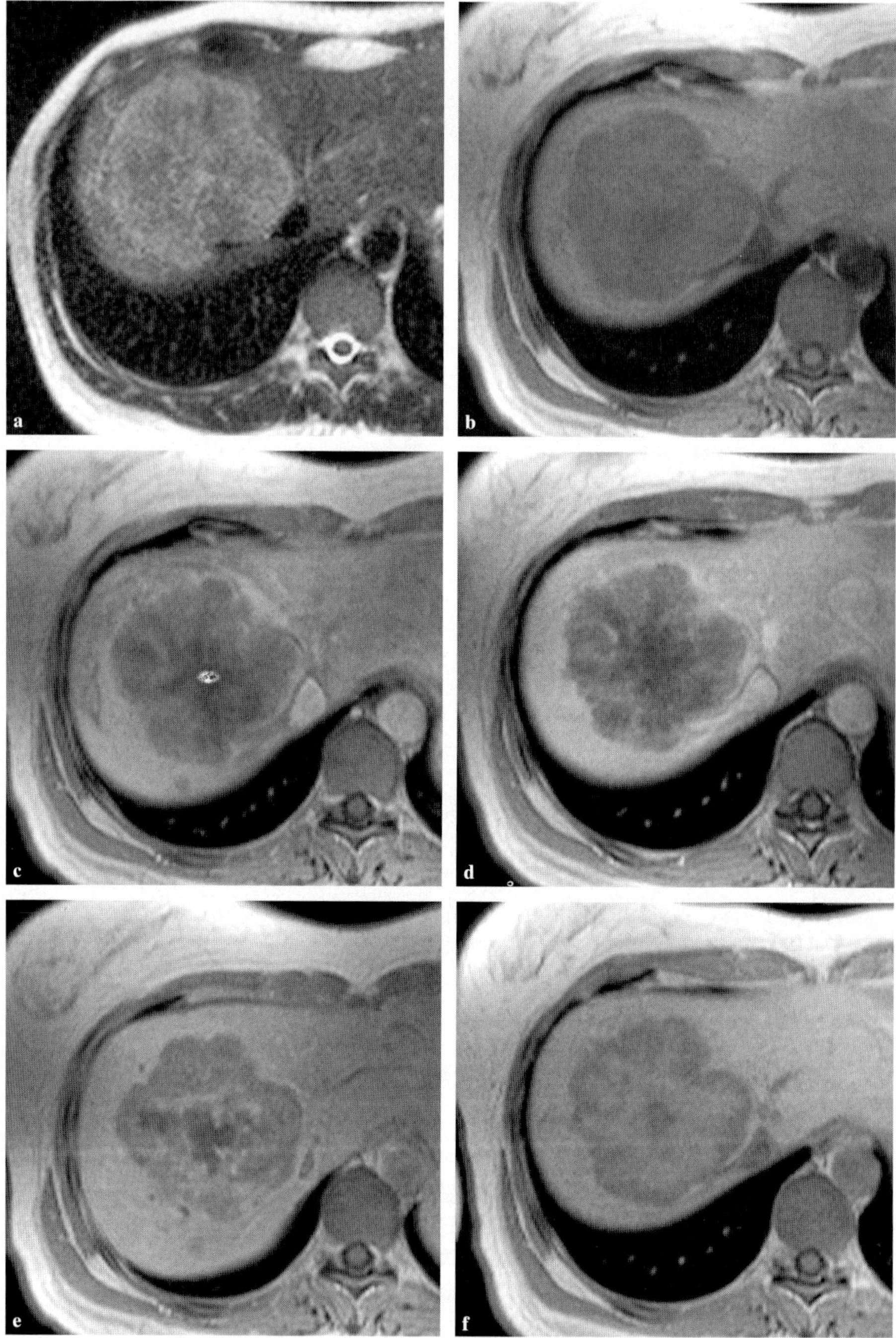

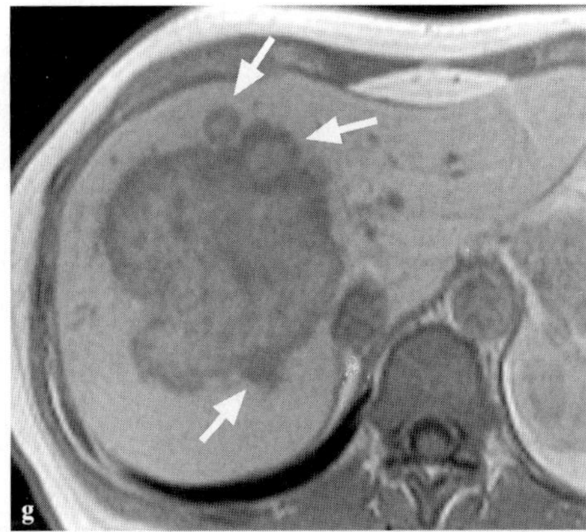

Fig. 24a-g. Fibrolamellar carcinoma. On the unenhanced T2-weighted image (**a**) a large hyperintense lesion can be noted in the dome of the liver. On the corresponding unenhanced T1-weighted image (**b**) this lesion appears as inhomogeneously hypointense. Dynamic imaging after the bolus injection of Gd-BOPTA reveals hypervascularization of the periphery of the lesion during the initial arterial phase (**c**), followed by filling-in in the subsequent portal-venous phase (**d**). During the equilibrium phase (**e**) a hypointense appearance is evident even of peripheral areas. In contrast to FNH, the central scar of this lesion shows no enhancement in the equilibrium phase. On T1-weighted images acquired during the hepatobiliary phase at 1 h after the injection of Gd-BOPTA (**f, g**), the lesion shows peripheral wash-out and a hypointense central scar. Non-specific enhancement due to diffusion of the contrast medium into different parts of the lesion can be noted. Additionally, peripheral satellite nodules (*arrows in* **g**) can be depicted on images acquired more caudally. In contrast to FNH, the lesion shows a higher signal intensity on unenhanced T2-weighted images and more pronounced hypointensity on unenhanced T1-weighted images. In the equilibrium phase no enhancement of the central scar can be noted and no uptake of Gd-BOPTA by the lesion is apparent on hepatobiliary phase images. This behavior is consistent with the presence of non-functioning hepatocytes and hence malignancy

On unenhanced CT images, FLC is usually seen as hypoattenuating compared with the liver and as well-defined with lobulated margins. Areas of low-density within the tumor correspond to the central scar or to necrosis and hemorrhage, while calcification may be seen in 15–30% of all central scars [53]. During the arterial and portal-venous phases after administration of contrast material, FLC is predominantly, but heterogeneously, hyperattenuating [53, 88]. On delayed phase images, sometimes parts of the non-necrotic portions of the tumor increase in attenuation relative to the liver (Fig. 22) [53]. The central scar usually shows minimal enhancement on arterial and portal-venous phase images and is best seen during the delayed phase. The appearance of the lesion in the arterial and portal-venous phases reflects the enhancement of the cellular and vascular components of the tumor and the presence of fibrous and necrotic components. The relative homogeneity of the tumor observed on delayed images may indicate washout of contrast material from the more vascular areas, together with delayed enhancement of the fibrous lamellae [53, 88, 131].

FLC is usually either hypointense or isointense to the liver on T1-weighted MR images. On T2-weighted images, 90% of the lesions are hyperintense and the remaining 10% are isointense. Because of its purely fibrous nature, the scar is hypointense on both T1- and T2-weighted images (Fig. 23) [53, 88].

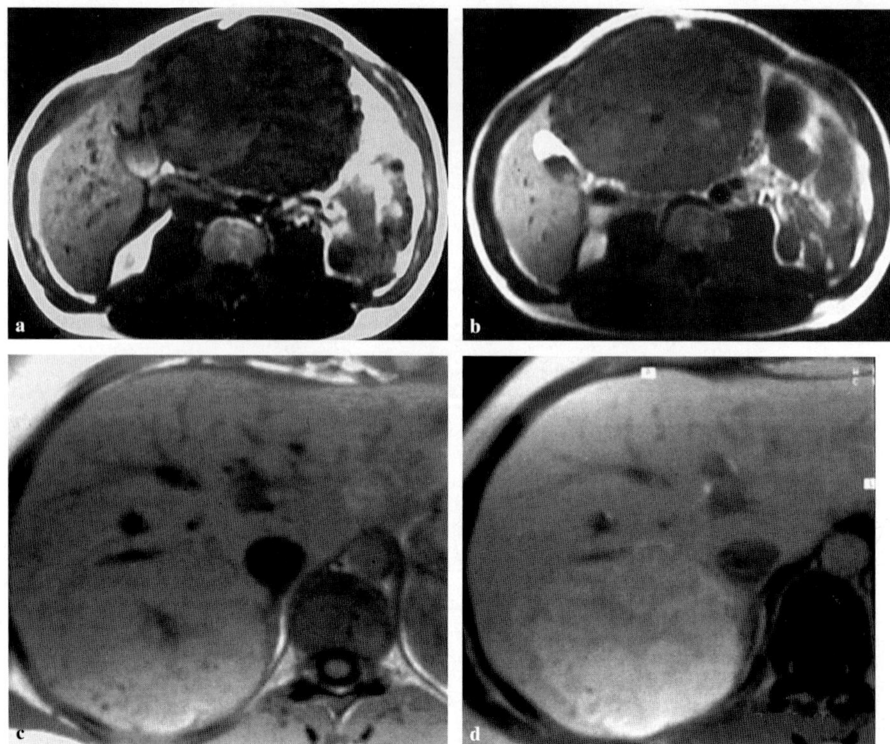

Fig. 25a-d. Fibrolamellar carcinoma. Fibrolamellar carcinoma does not show significant enhancement on delayed hepatobiliary phase images after the bolus administration of Gd-BOPTA (**a** and **b**, respectively). Conversely, FNH generally appears hyperintense on delayed phase images after Gd-BOPTA due to the accumulation of contrast agent within the nodule and impaired biliary elimination (**c** and **d**, respectively)

FLCs become heterogeneously hyperintense during the arterial phase after administration of gadolinium, but may appear as isointense or slightly hypointense during the portal-venous and equilibrium phases (Fig. 24) [26, 88]. As on CT scans, the central scar shows minimal or no enhancement on hepatic arterial and portal-venous phase images, but may show persistent enhancement on equilibrium phase images.

On images acquired during the delayed phase after Gd-BOPTA or mangafodipir administration, FLC usually appears as heterogeneously isointense or hypointense with areas of low signal intensity due to necrosis or, less frequently, hemorrhage. Irregular hyperintense areas, if present, may be related to the presence of fibrotic components. The lack of enhancement on delayed phase images is helpful in distinguishing fibrolamellar carcinoma from FNH (Fig. 25).

Similarly, FLC does not enhance significantly on SPIO-enhanced images. This absence of enhancement is helpful in distinguishing FLC from FNH in larger lesions, but may be less helpful in smaller lesions [88].

5.1.3 Cholangiocellular Carcinoma

Cholangiocarcinomas (CCC) are malignant tumors of the biliary system and comprise 15–25% of all liver and biliary tract cancers. They can be differentiated into proximal, perihilar, and distal biliary tumors. Proximally located hilar tumors of the bifurcation are often referred to as "Klatskin tumors" [68]. Primary sclerosing cholangitis, choledochal cyst, familial polyposis, congenital hepatic fibrosis, infection with the Chinese liver fluke *Clonorchis sinensis*, and a history of exposure to Thorotrast are risk factors for CCC [24, 78]. CCC occurs most frequently in patients in the sixth decade, although patients with these risk factors may develop this neoplasm at a much younger age. CCC occurs slightly more often in men than in women.

The histologic variants of CCC include: adenocarcinoma, mixed CCC-HCC, squamous-, mucoepidermoid-, cystadano- and granular cell carcinoma. Adenocarcinoma comprises 95% of the cases, and can range from well-differentiated mucin-producing to poorly differentiated [87]. Distinguishing morphological features allow further sub-classification of bile duct adenocarcinomas into papillary, sclerosing, and nodular variants. The sclerosing type is most common, followed by papillary and nodular cholangiocarcinoma [16].

Nearly 70% of bile duct cancers are located proximal to the junction of the cystic and hepatic duct. Peripheral or lobular cholangiocarcinoma arises from small biliary intrahepatic radicals and usually presents as a large hepatic mass [151]. Intrahepatic cholangiocarcinoma can be exophytic with intrahepatic masses, or may be polypoid or focally stenotic. Klatskin's tumor is usually scirrhous [68, 138].

The clinical signs and symptoms are related to the site of origin of the tumor. In intrahepatic CCC, the symptoms are usually vague until the tumor is in an advanced phase, when patients frequently present with anorexia, weight loss, abdominal pain, and a palpable mass in the upper abdomen. Jaundice is rarely a presenting symptom in intrahepatic CCC, although it is common with hilar or ductal CCC [68]. There are no specific tumor markers for cholangiocarcinoma, although elevations of serum carcinoembryonic antigen (CEA) and CA 19-9 are often found [149].

On ultrasound scans, CCCs may have mixed echogenicity or may be predominantly hypoechoic or hyperechoic. The sonographic features of Klatskin's tumors include duct dilatation, isolation of the right and left bile duct segments, mass or bile duct wall thickening at the hilus, and lobar atrophy with crowded, dilated bile ducts. Ultrasound is accurate for revealing the level of bile duct obstruction, but shows tumor mass in only 20–70% of patients. When a mass is seen, it is usually poorly defined and echogenic, reflecting the sub-mucosal, scirrhous nature of this fibrotic neoplasm (Fig. 26) [14, 39]. Focally stenotic or papillary CCCs often cause segmental bile duct dilatation and may induce lobar atrophy if the location of the tumor is central.

Peripheral CCC may appear as an ill-defined mass with mixed echogenecity (Fig. 27) with or without segmental bile duct dilatation. Satellite nodules, which contribute to the bad prognosis of CCC, are frequently seen.

CCCs are usually hypodense or isodense relative to the normal liver parenchyma on unenhanced CT scans. After administration of contrast material, most CCCs remain hypodense during the portal-venous phase but thereafter show enhancement on delayed phase images. This pattern of enhancement reflects the hypovas-

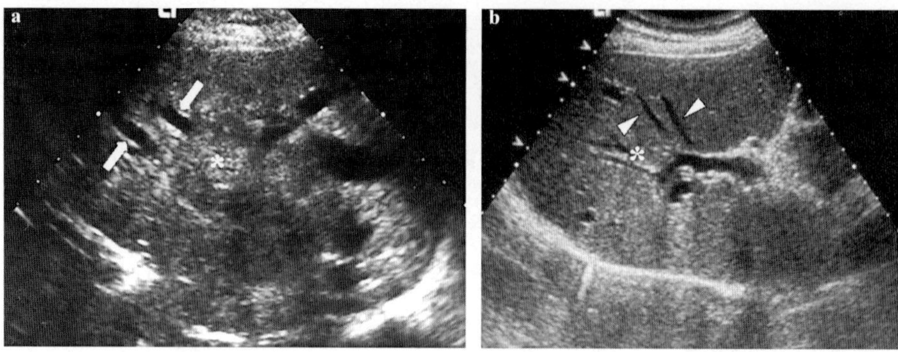

Fig. 26a-b. Hilar cholangiocellular carcinoma. Ultrasound reveals an ill-defined heterogeneous mass (*asterisk*) (**a**) with dilated bile ducts (*arrows*). An ill-defined infiltrative mass (*asterisk*) from the hilus through the hepatic parenchyma can also be depicted (**b**). Some bile ducts around the mass appear dilated (*arrowheads*)

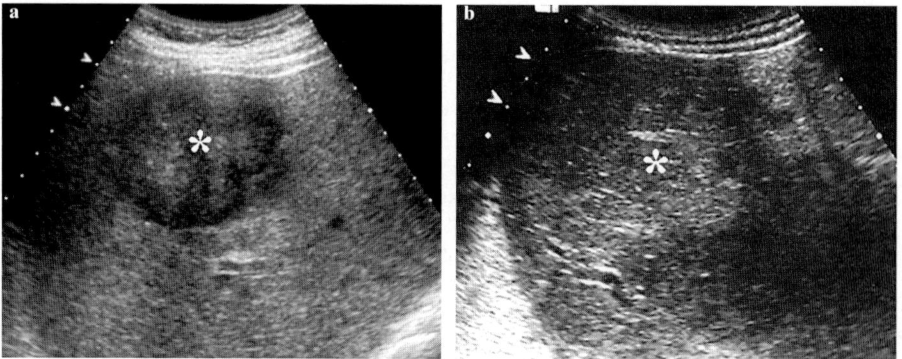

Fig. 27a,b. Peripheral cholangiocellular carcinoma. On ultrasound, the neoplasm (*asterisk*) appears as a well-defined heterogeneous nodule (**a**) or as an ill-defined mass (*asterisk*) (**b**) compared to the surrounding parenchyma

cular, desmoplastic composition of most CCCs; therefore, most lesions are better appreciated at 15–20 minutes after contrast medium administration. Small necrotic regions are common in larger lesions [14]. Segmental or diffuse bile dilatation is a common finding in hilar CCC (Fig. 28). The peripheral type of CCC may simulate other hepatic neoplasms, such as metastases or HCC. Its most common pattern consists of a hypodense ill-defined lesion on unenhanced CT scans, poor enhancement during the arterial and portal-venous phases, and iso- or hyperdensity on delayed phase images (Fig. 29).

CCCs are either isointense or hypointense relative to the normal liver on T1-weighted MR images, but may range from markedly to mildly hyperintense on T2-weighted images [148]. On dynamic T1-weighted MR images acquired after the intravenous administration of gadolinium, minimal or moderate incomplete enhancement is seen at the tumor periphery on early images, whereas progressive

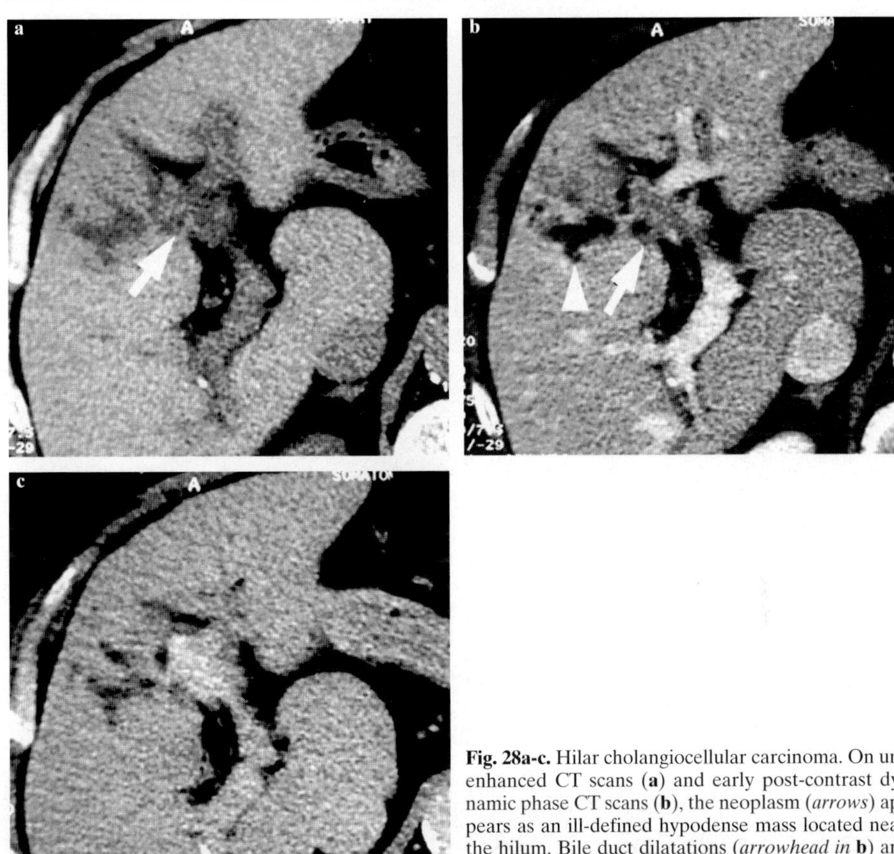

Fig. 28a-c. Hilar cholangiocellular carcinoma. On unenhanced CT scans (**a**) and early post-contrast dynamic phase CT scans (**b**), the neoplasm (*arrows*) appears as an ill-defined hypodense mass located near the hilum. Bile duct dilatations (*arrowhead in* **b**) are also evident. On delayed phase images after contrast medium administration (**c**), the lesion is seen as hyperattenuating

central contrast enhancement is seen on later images (Fig. 30). The degree of enhancement varies with the type of tumor. A greater peripheral enhancement is noted in the early phases in large CCCs, whereas greater enhancement is noted in the fibrous core of scirrhous CCCs on delayed phase images (Fig. 31). Small, incidentally discovered intrahepatic CCCs, as well as mixed CCC/HCC tumors, can show intense, homogeneous enhancement during the arterial phase with prolonged enhancement on delayed phases due to marked hypervascularity [148, 153].

Generally, lesions show peripheral hypointensity and central iso- or hyperintensity on delayed phase images after the administration of contrast agents with liver specific properties (see Fig. 30; Fig. 31). However, the central area may also show incomplete enhancement. Satellite nodules are also seen in about 10–20% of CCC cases and it is this that is chiefly responsible for the poor prognosis of this lesion (Fig. 32).

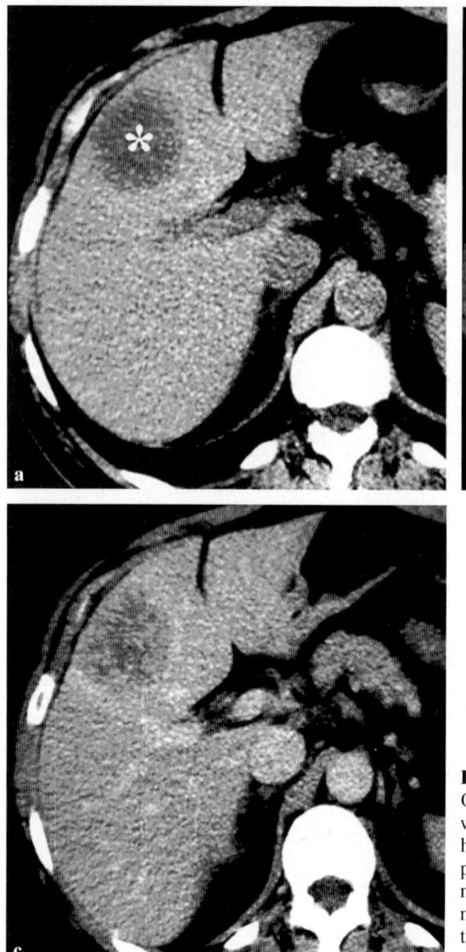

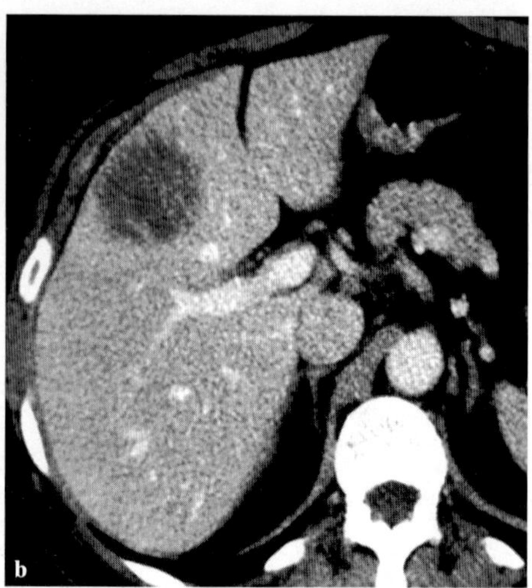

Fig. 29a-c. Peripheral cholangiocellular carcinoma. On unenhanced CT scans (**a**) the lesion appears as a well-defined hypodense mass (*asterisk*). Minimal enhancement is seen on images acquired during the portal-venous phase after administration of contrast material (**b**), while in the equilibrium phase (**c**) the neoplasm is seen as inhomogeneously hyperdense to the liver due to abundant fibrotic desmoplastic reaction

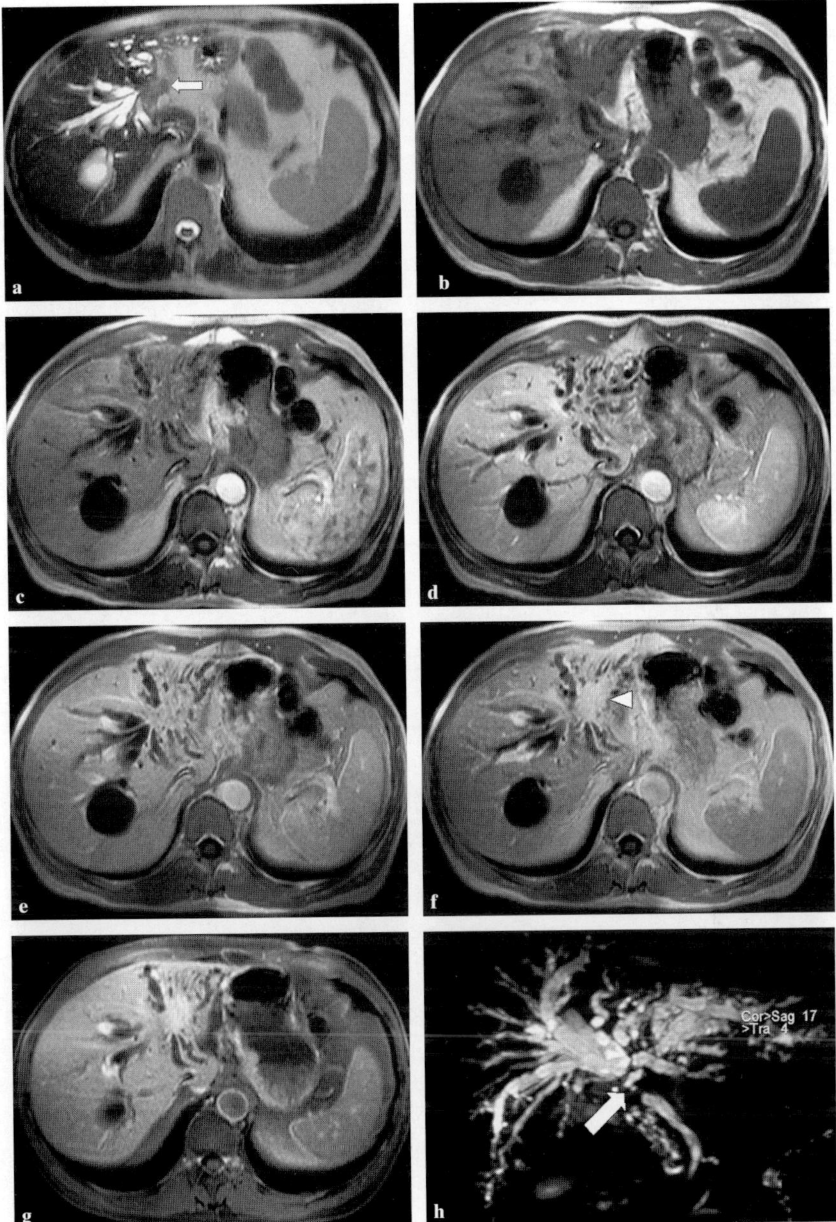

Fig. 30a-h. Hilar cholangiocellular carcinoma. On the unenhanced Turbo SE T2-weighted image (**a**) the neoplasm (*arrow*) appears slightly heterogeneously hyperintense to the normal liver and involvement of the bile duct system can be seen. On the unenhanced GE T1-weighted image (**b**), the lesion appears as a slightly hypointense ill-defined mass. Poor enhancement is seen during the arterial phase after the bolus administration of Gd-BOPTA (**c**). However, desmoplastic reaction determines a progressive increase of contrast enhancement in subsequent acquisitions during the portal-venous and equilibrium phases (**d** and **e**, respectively). After 20 min the lesion (*arrowhead*) appears hyperintense (**f**). Due to the large amount of fibrotic tissue which causes non-specific contrast agent retention, the lesion retains this hyperintense appearance on images acquired at 1 h after Gd-BOPTA administration (**g**). Nevertheless, the presence of a hypointense peripheral rim indicates the malignant nature of the lesion. The involvement of hilar bile ducts (*arrow*) is clearly demonstrated with MRCP (**h**)

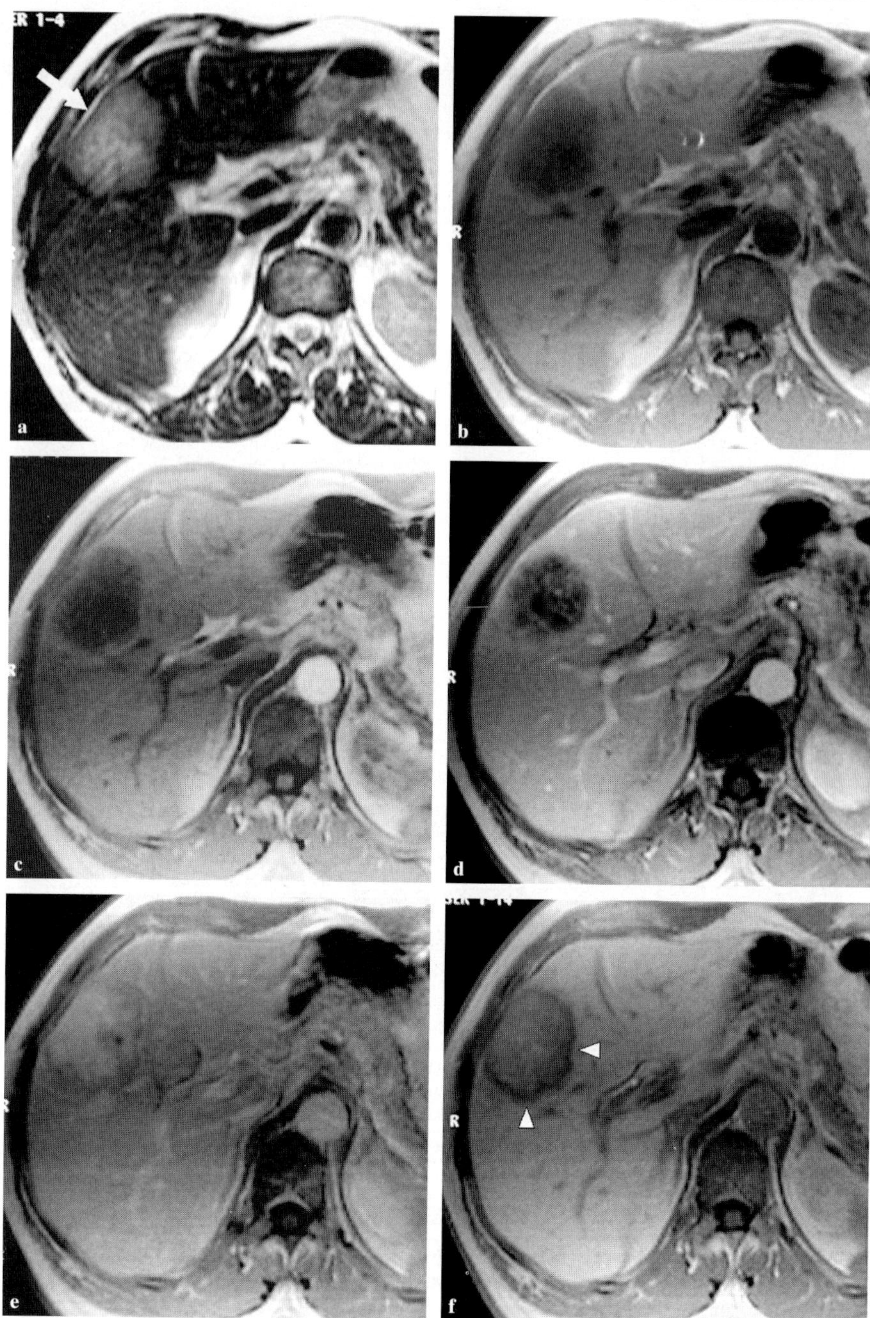

Fig. 31a-f. Peripheral cholangiocellular carcinoma. The neoplasm (*arrow*) appears heterogeneously hyperintense on unenhanced T2-weighted images (**a**) and hypointense on unenhanced T1-weighted images (**b**). Moderate peripheral enhancement is seen on images acquired during the arterial (**c**) and portal-venous (**d**) phases after the administration of Gd-BOPTA. On the equilibrium phase image (**e**) the enhancement appears progressive and complete due to desmoplastic reaction. A peripheral hypointense rim (*arrowheads*) can be seen on the delayed phase image (**f**) and the lesion appears hypointense compared to the surrounding parenchyma, indicating malignancy

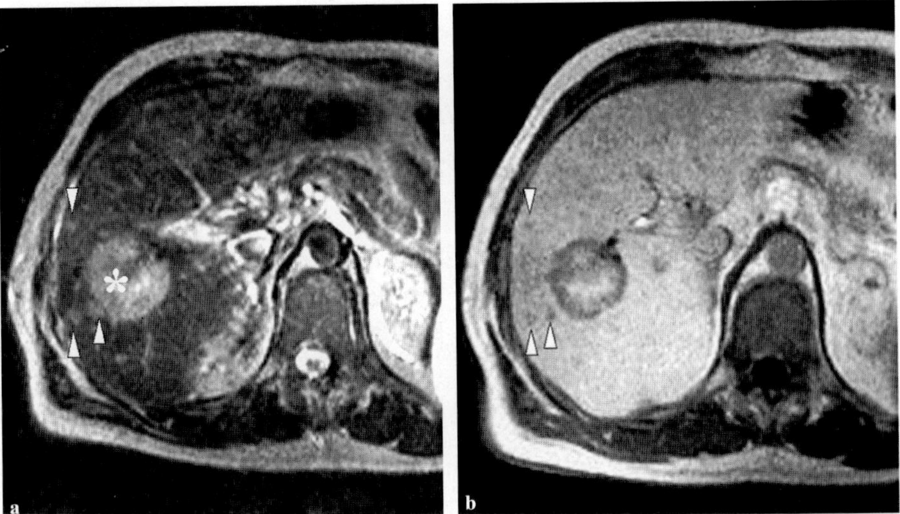

Fig. 32a,b. Cholangiocellular carcinoma. On the unenhanced T2-weighted image (**a**) a large heterogeneous hyperintense mass (*asterisk*) and numerous satellite nodules (*arrowheads*) can be seen. On the image acquired during the hepatobiliary phase after injection of Gd-BOPTA (**b**), the biggest nodule shows central enhancement and peripheral washout while the smaller satellite nodules (*arrowheads*) remain hypointense

5.1.4 Gallbladder Carcinoma

Gallbladder carcinoma is the fifth most common malignancy of the gastrointestinal tract (bile duct carcinoma occurs less frequently) [76]. The risk of gallbladder carcinoma is increased in patients with gallstones. Similarly, porcelain gallbladder is also a predisposing factor, an estimated 22% of patients with porcelain gallbladder develop carcinoma [5, 111].

Nearly 85% of primary carcinomas of the gallbladder are adenocarcinomas, the remainder are anaplastic or squamous cell carcinomas. Gallbladder carcinomas have three major patterns of presentation: 1) focal or diffuse thickening of the gallbladder wall; 2) polypoid mass originating in the gallbladder wall and projecting into the lumen; 3) mass obscuring or replacing the gallbladder, often invading adjacent liver [44, 130, 132].

Most patients with carcinoma of the gallbladder present with either acute cholecystitis or symptoms of malignancy, including constant right upper quadrant pain, malaise, weight loss, and jaundice. Patients sometimes have a long history of episodic cholecystitis. Gallbladder carcinoma is occasionally an incidental finding on abdominal imaging studies [80].

Mild to marked mural thickening in a focal or diffuse pattern with irregular and mixed echogenicity may be indicative of gallbladder carcinoma on ultrasound scans. Carcinomas confined to the gallbladder mucosa may appear as flat or slightly raised lesions with mucosal irregularity that are difficult to appreciate sonographically. On the other hand, polypoid carcinomas may be hyperechoic, hypoechoic, or isoechoic relative to the liver. These lesions are fixed to the gallbladder wall, and do not cause an acoustic shadow. Gallstones are usually present. A large mass obscuring or replacing the gallbladder is the most common presentation of this neoplasm (Fig. 33). The echotexture of this manifestation is often complex with regions of necrosis and small amounts of pericholecystic fluid often present [132, 145].

Focal malignant wall thickening and polypoid cancer are both usually enhanced on CT images acquired after the administration of intravenous contrast material. However, infiltrating carcinoma that replaces the gallbladder often shows irregular contrast enhancement with scattered regions of internal necrosis (Fig. 34) [132].

The MR findings for gallbladder carcinoma are similar to those reported for CT. The tumor usually has increased signal intensity relative to the liver on T2-weighted images and poorly delineated contours. These lesions are either isointense or hypointense relative to the liver on T1-weighted images. The tumor generally shows poor and heterogeneous enhancement on dynamic phase imaging and often appears hyperintense on fat suppressed T1-weighted images in the equilibrium phase. On delayed hepatobiliary phase images after the administration of Gd-BOPTA, the tumor appears as a heterogeneous hypointense mass (Fig. 35) [120].

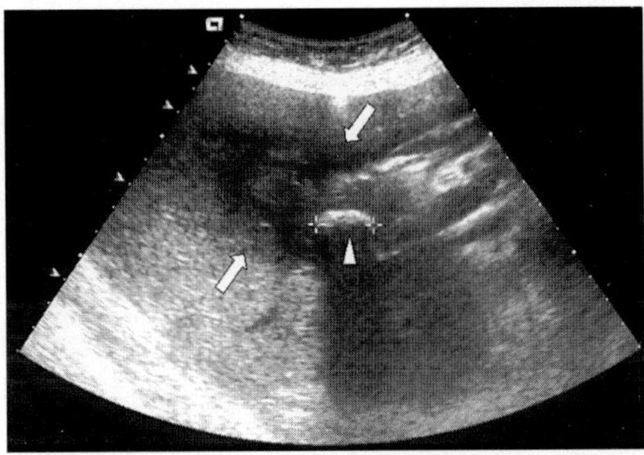

Fig. 33. Gallbladder carcinoma. Ultrasound reveals an inhomogeneous, hypo- and hyperechoic mass (*arrows*) that replaces the gallbladder. A coarse stone with acoustic shadow can be seen within the mass (*arrowhead*)

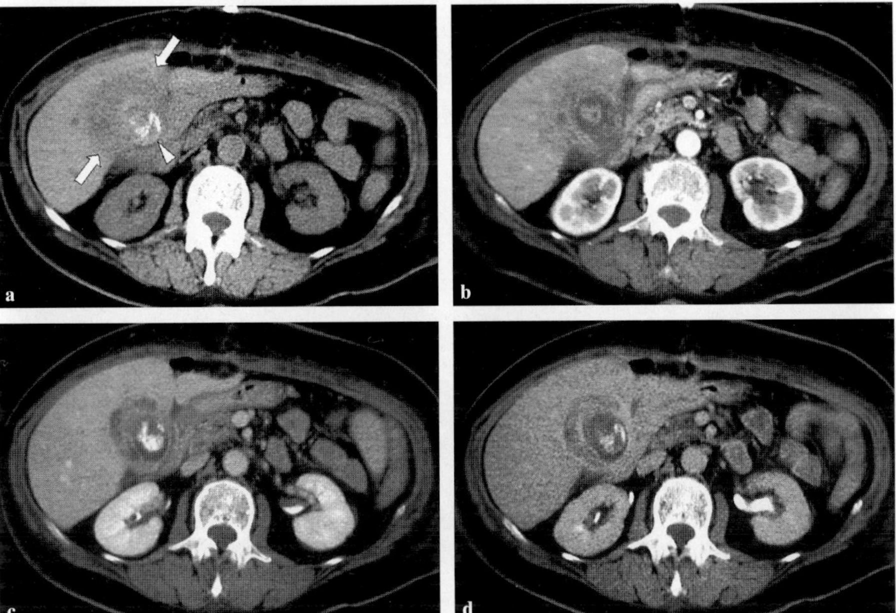

Fig. 34a-d. Gallbladder carcinoma. Unenhanced CT scan (**a**) reveals an ill-defined slightly hypodense mass (*arrows*) surrounding a coarse irregular and inhomogeneous stone (*arrowhead*). In the arterial phase after contrast material administration (**b**), the neoplasm remains poorly delineated and poorly enhanced. In the portal-venous phase (**c**) the lesion appears heterogeneously isodense, but better defined against the normal liver. In the equilibrium phase (**d**) the neoplasm is more homogeneous and a thin hyperdense peripheral rim can be seen

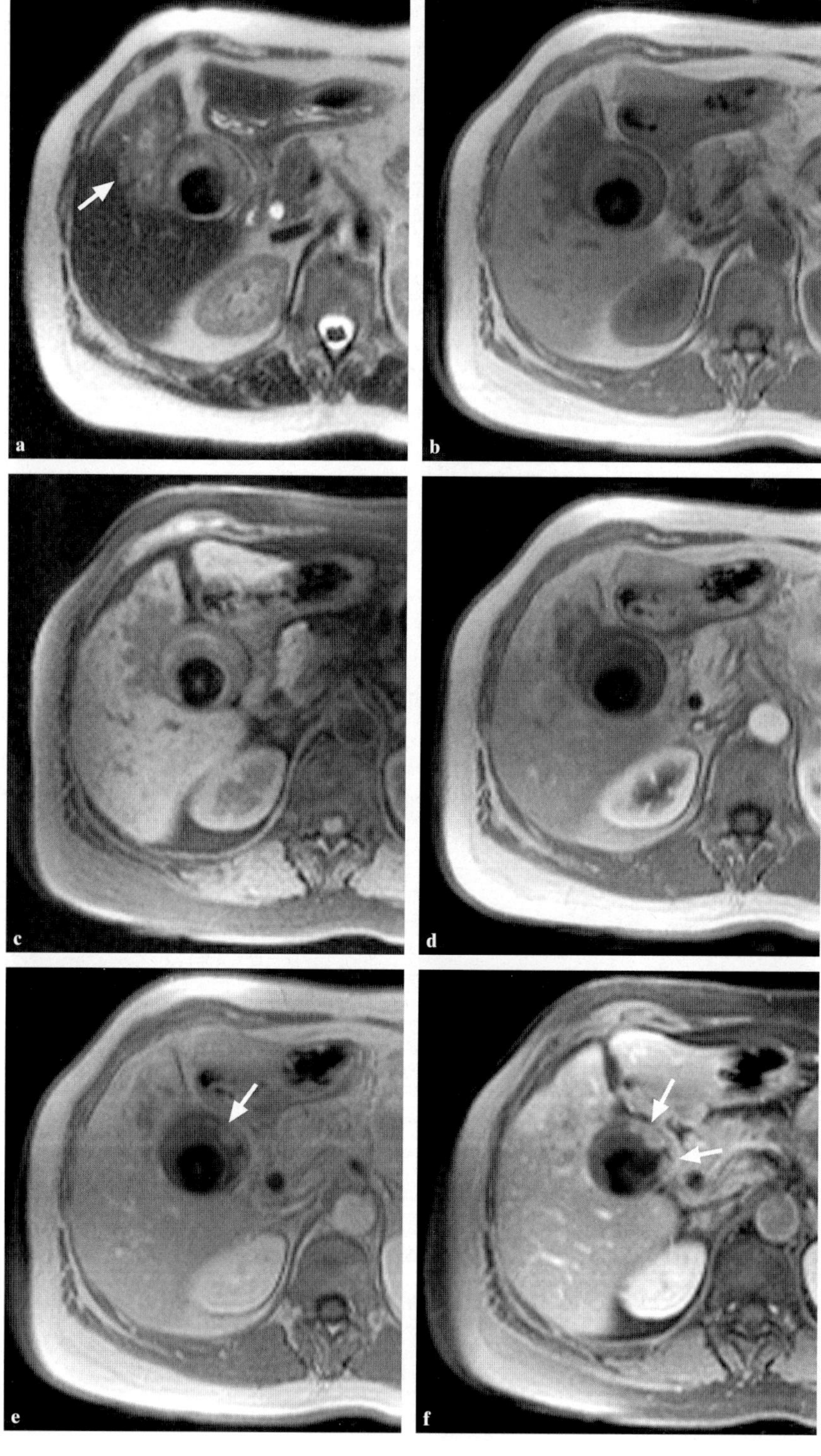

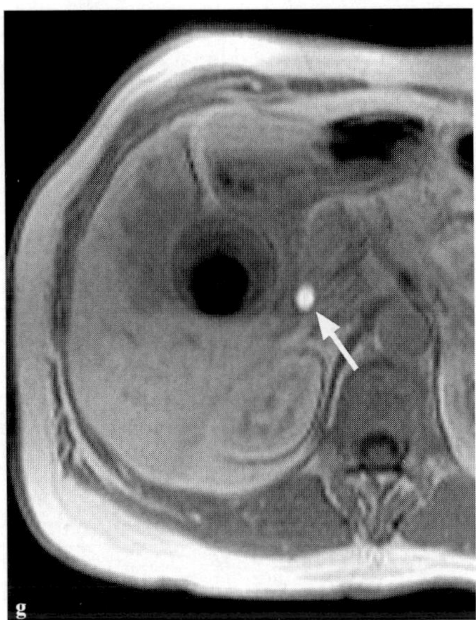

Fig. 35a-g. Gallbladder carcinoma. On T2-weighted images (**a**), a gallbladder stone together with some solid material in the gallbladder can be seen infiltrating the surrounding liver tissue of the right liver lobe (*arrow*). On the corresponding T1-weighted image the infiltrating tissue appears hypointense (**b**). On T1-weighted fs images (**c**) some hyperintense areas indicative of hemorrhage can be noted inside the solid components. On arterial phase T1-weighted images after the bolus administration of Gd-BOPTA, an irregular enhancement of the periphery of the infiltrated right liver lobe can be noted (**d**). Enhancement of papillary solid areas in the gallbladder can also be detected on the portal-venous phase image (**e**) (*arrow*). This is even more obvious on T1-weighted fs images in the equilibrium phase (**f**), in which tumor growth in the gallbladder is clearly visualized (*arrows*). Additionally, homogeneous enhancement of the infiltration of the right liver lobe can be noted, which is typical for cholangiocellular carcinoma. In the hepatobiliary phase (**g**) the infiltrated areas of the right liver lobe are once again hypointense, indicating the malignant nature of the lesion. Note the excretion of the contrast medium in the bile duct (*arrow*) and the enhancement of the surrounding liver tissue compared with unenhanced T1-weighted images

5.1.5 Hepatoblastoma

Hepatoblastoma (HB) is the most common primary hepatic malignancy in children and represents approximately 45% of liver neoplasms in this age group. It can be considered the infantile form of hepatocellular carcinoma and is generally detected in children younger than 5 years old. Approximately two thirds of all patients are younger than 2 years old [29]. A correlation has been observed with pre-maturity, with a gestational age of < 37 weeks, as well as with a birth weight of < 1000 g. Other risk factors are trisomy 18, hemi-hypertrophy, Beckwith-Wiedemann syndrome, familial adenomatous polyposis, fetal alcoholic syndrome, maternal use of gonadotropin, and maternal exposure to metals or petroleum products. Liver cirrhosis is not considered a risk factor [67, 114].

Histological classification divides HB into two main types: a pure epithelial form and a mixed epithelial-mesenchymal form. The pure epithelial form includes fetal, embryonal, macrotrabecular and undifferentiated small cell variants. The mixed epithelial-mesenchymal form contains an epithelial component identical to that of epithelial hepatoblastoma plus a mesenchymal component with osteoid, chondroid and rhabdomyoblastic elements. It is often associated with areas of calcification, hemorrhage and necrosis [15, 127].

This type of histological classification carries prognostic implications: the survival rate for patients with the pure fetal variant is 90%, as opposed to 54% for the mixed form and 33% for the embryonal variant. The anaplastic variant has a survival rate of 0% [15].

HB frequently presents as a single, large, bulky mass, most often in the right lobe of the liver. Macroscopically, its appearance varies according to the histological type. Epithelial hepatoblastoma tends to be homogeneous, while the mixed form is more heterogeneous due to calcifications, fibrotic bands and osteoid and cartilaginous material [114]. Although nodules may sometimes be multiple and affect both lobes, diffuse involvement of the entire liver is less common. Generally, multifocal nodules, diffuse involvement and vascular invasion is encountered in approximately 50% of cases and is associated with a worse prognosis and unresectability. In 30% of cases, remote metastases are detected. The organs most often involved are the lung, kidney, brain and abdominal lymph nodes.

On the basis of the above considerations, two categories of risk have been established for HB: (1) *standard risk hepatoblastoma,* for patients with single or apparently multifocal neoplasms involving no more than three hepatic segments in the absence of metastases and extrahepatic abdominal involvement; (2) *high risk hepatoblastoma,* with neoplastic disease extending to four liver segments and evidence of extrahepatic spread.

HB can also be seen, albeit infrequently, in older children, in which case it tends to have clinical and anatomo-pathological characteristics in common with HCC. Approximately 50% of children with HB are symptom-free. In such cases, the diagnosis is frequently made during a medical check-up due to the incidental finding of a palpable mass or an increase in abdominal circumference. Abdominal pain, fever, loss of appetite and weight loss are reported in 25% of patients, although jaundice occurs in fewer than 10% of cases [127].

Serum α-fetoprotein elevation in pediatric HB and HCC is much higher than in adult HCC, with high values being detected in more than 90% of cases. The values of this tumor marker are indicative of a worse prognosis when they are higher than 1, 000, 000 ng ml^{-1} or lower than 100 ng ml^{-1}. The reason for such low values in the latter case, which corresponds to the undifferentiated form of HB, is that the tumor cells are too immature and undifferentiated to produce the protein [139]. High values of human chorionic gonadotropin (HCG) are sometimes observed and in these cases the HB is associated with signs of early puberty. Thrombocytosis is present in more than 90% of cases [49].

Ultrasound findings vary according to the histological type. The mass is normally well-defined, multilobulated and septate. The epithelial variant is usually homogeneously slightly hypo- or hyperechogenic, while the mixed form is generally a heterogeneous mass with hyper- and hypoechogenic areas reflecting calcification and tumor necrosis, respectively. Color Doppler ultrasound is very sensitive in demonstrating the rich vascularization of the tumor (Fig. 36) and high-velocity vascular shunts [4, 114].

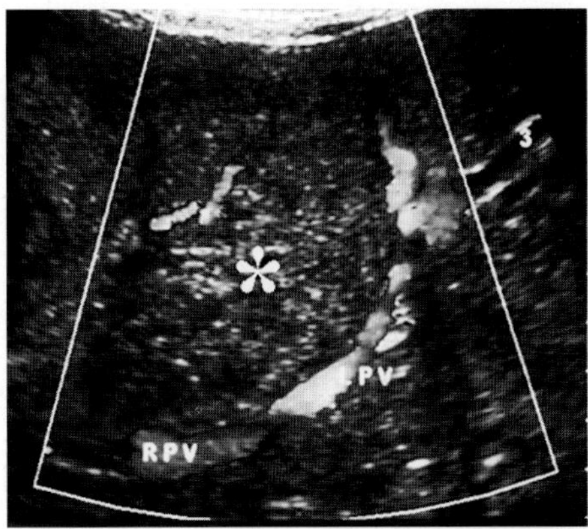

Fig. 36. Hepatoblastoma. Color Doppler Ultrasound reveals a slightly hyperechoic and hypervascular mass (*asterisk*). An impression on the portal vein (*PV*) and on the right branch of the portal vein (*RPV*) can be seen

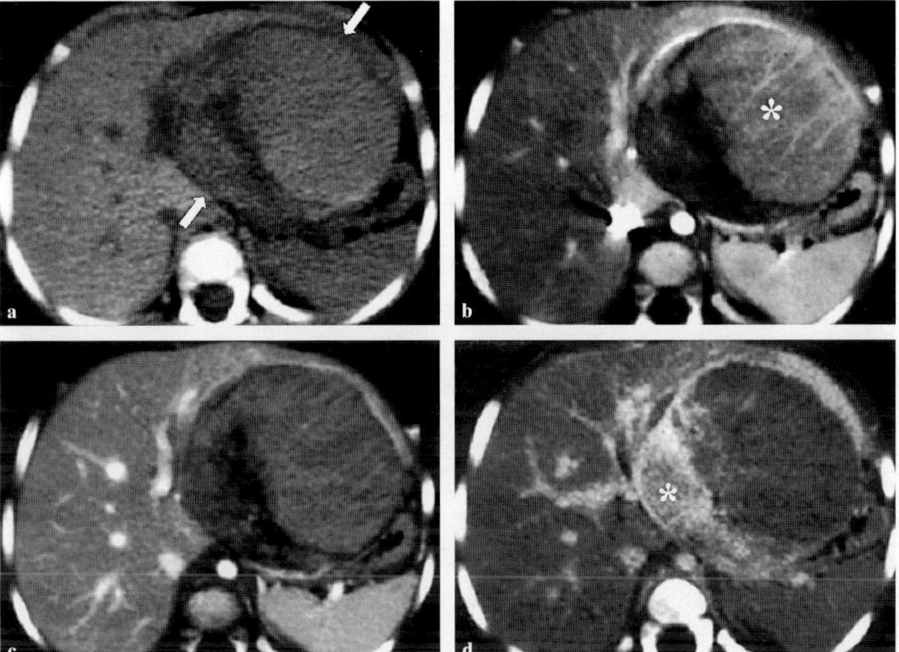

Fig. 37a-d. Mixed hepatoblastoma. On an unenhanced CT scan (**a**) the neoplasm (*arrows*) is heterogeneously iso- and hypoechoic. The cellular component of the lesion (*asterisk*) enhances during the arterial phase after contrast material administration (**b**), but becomes hypodense in the portal-venous (**c**) and delayed (**d**) phases. Conversely, the stromal component (*asterisk*) enhances markedly in the delayed phase

On unenhanced CT scans the epithelial form of HB is generally homogeneously hypodense with small and punctiform calcifications, whereas the mixed form is more heterogeneous with large and coarse calcifications. On enhanced CT images after the injection of contrast material, most HBs demonstrate enhancement during the arterial phase that subsequently fades in the portal-venous phase. The enhancement is frequently heterogeneous and inferior to that of healthy parenchyma. A peripheral rim and/or hyperdense septa may be seen in the late phase, due to the stromal component (Fig. 37) [49, 114, 128].

With MR, the signal intensity of the tumor varies in relation to the histological type. Whereas epithelial HB is usually seen as homogeneously hypointense on T1-weighted images and hyperintense on T2-weighted images, the mixed form is much more heterogeneous due to the presence of necrosis, hemorrhage and fibrosis (Fig. 38) [49, 110]. On dynamic phase images after the administration of extracellularly distributed Gd-agents HBs demonstrate early enhancement and rapid washout (Fig. 39) [46, 136]. During the arterial phase after the administration of Gd-BOPTA, the lesion is seen as heterogeneously hyperintense with internal hypointense areas corresponding to fibrotic and necrotic areas. In the portal-venous and equilibrium phases, the neoplasm is normally seen as isointense and then hypointense with hyperintense areas corresponding to the stromal component. On delayed, hepatobiliary phase images, the tumor is usually heterogeneously hypo- or isointense.

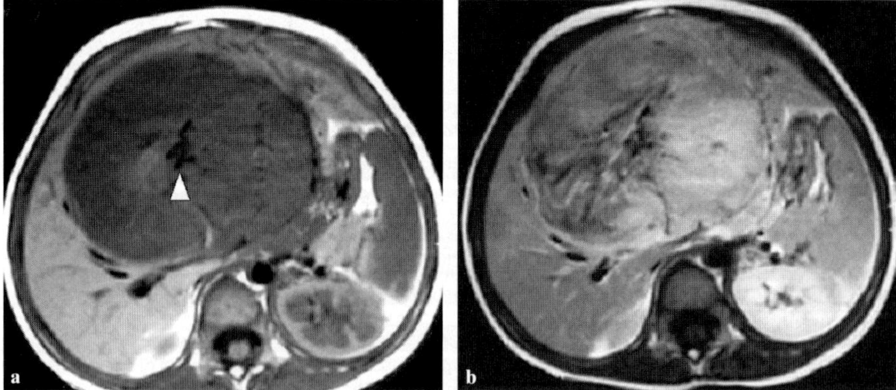

Fig. 38a,b. Hepatoblastoma. The unenhanced T1-weighted image (**a**) reveals a large, well-defined, lobulated hypointense mass with a small central area of lower signal intensity (*arrowhead*), that corresponds to calcification. After contrast medium administration (**b**), the neoplasm demonstrates early, inhomogeneous enhancement

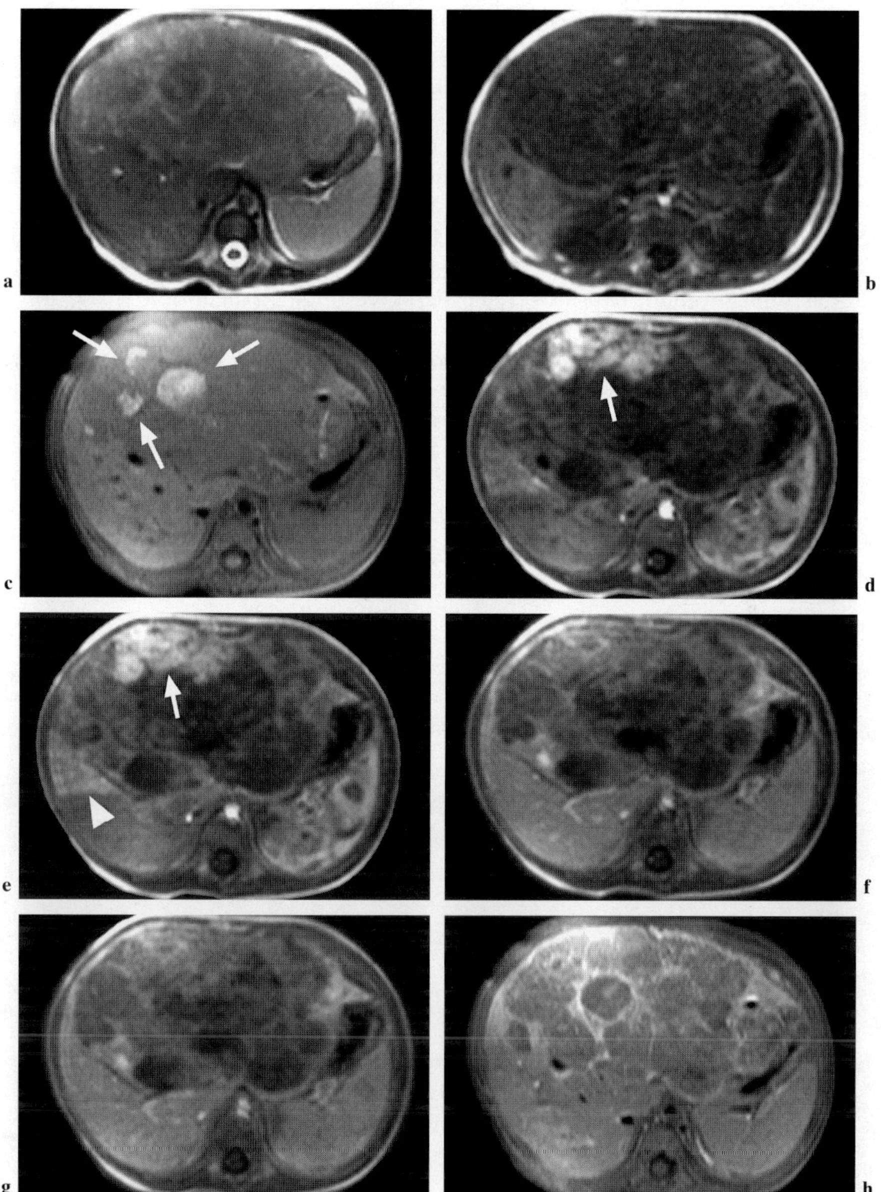

Fig. 39a-h. Hepatoblastoma. A slightly hyperintense lesion compared with the surrounding liver tissue can be seen on the unenhanced T2-weighted image (**a**). On the unenhanced T1-weighted image (**b**) the lesion can be seen as a giant inhomogeneous hypointense mass with small areas of hyperintensity indicative of hemorrhage. The unenhanced T1-weighted fs image (**c**) more clearly reveals the areas of high signal intensity indicative of hemorrhage and regressive changes (*arrows*). The lesion appears slightly hypointense in comparison to the normal liver parenchyma. On dynamic imaging after the bolus administration of Gd-BOPTA (**d-g**) the more ventrally located parts of the lesion show hypervascularity (*arrow in* **d** *and* **e**) whereas most of the remaining parts show only slightly inhomogeneous contrast agent uptake. Due to the mass effect of the lesion, inhomogeneous perfusion of the remaining liver tissue can also be noted (*arrowhead*). T1-weighted fs images acquired during the delayed hepatobiliary phase (**h**) reveal inhomogeneous uptake of Gd-BOPTA. The lesions have a multinodular appearance with hypointense areas indicative of regressive changes

5.1.6   Epithelioid Hemangioendothelioma

Epithelioid hemangioendothelioma (EHE) is a rare malignant hepatic neoplasm of vascular origin that develops in adults. It is more common in women than in men. No risk factors or specific causes have been identified [143].

Two different types of EHE have been described [37]. The nodular type represents an early manifestation of the disease. In the majority of cases there are multiple nodular lesions ranging in size from 1–3 cm. Frequently, the nodules are found in both lobes of the liver and in 50–65% of cases are located at sub-capsular sites. Lesions adjacent to the capsule often produce capsular retraction [37]. The diffuse type of EHE develops in the later stages of the disease. It originates from the nodular type with the lesions increasing in size until they finally coalesce, forming extensive peripheral lesions [91]. The route of lesion spread follows the hepatic veins or the different branches of the portal vein [36].

Histologically, EHE is composed of fibrous myxoid stroma with a relatively hypocellular center and two cell types: epithelioid and dendritic. The epithelioid cells stain positive for factor VIII-related antigen, indicating the vascular nature of this neoplasm and distinguishing it from metastasis. Intratumoral necrosis and hemorrhage are common findings [91].

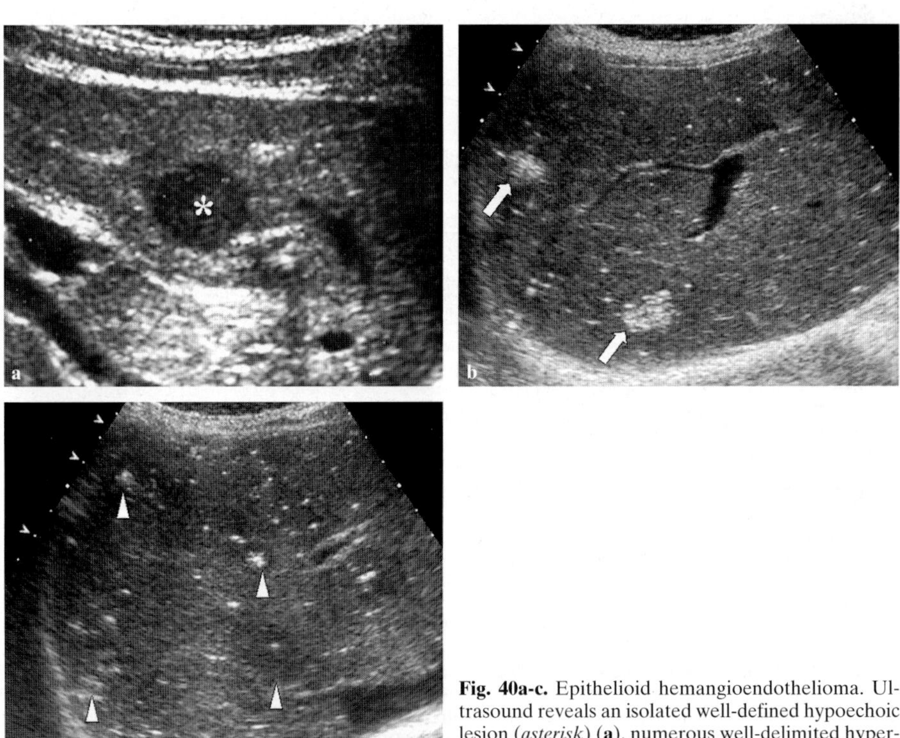

Fig. 40a-c. Epithelioid hemangioendothelioma. Ultrasound reveals an isolated well-defined hypoechoic lesion (*asterisk*) (**a**), numerous well-delimited hyperechoic nodules (*arrows*) (**b**), or hypoechoic and hyperechoic lesions (*arrowheads*) with peripheral hypoechoic rims (**c**)

The clinical manifestation is non-specific and variable, ranging from the complete absence of symptoms to hepatic failure. Generally, the symptoms are non-specific, such as right upper quadrant or epigastric discomfort or pain, weight loss, and weakness. Less common symptoms at initial presentation include jaundice, fever, and tiredness. Raised levels of serum alkaline phosphatase (AP) are found in approximately 70% of patients. Occasionally, rupture with hemoperitoneum may be present [57, 77]. Hepatomegaly and abdominal pain are present in 50–70% of cases.

On ultrasound, EHE is usually well-defined and hypoechoic, although hyperechoic examples are seen occasionally. Sometimes, it is possible to find hypoechoic, hyperechoic and hyperechoic lesions with a peripheral hypoechoic rim in the same patient (Fig. 40) [91]. Echo-color Doppler may demonstrate vascularization within the nodule.

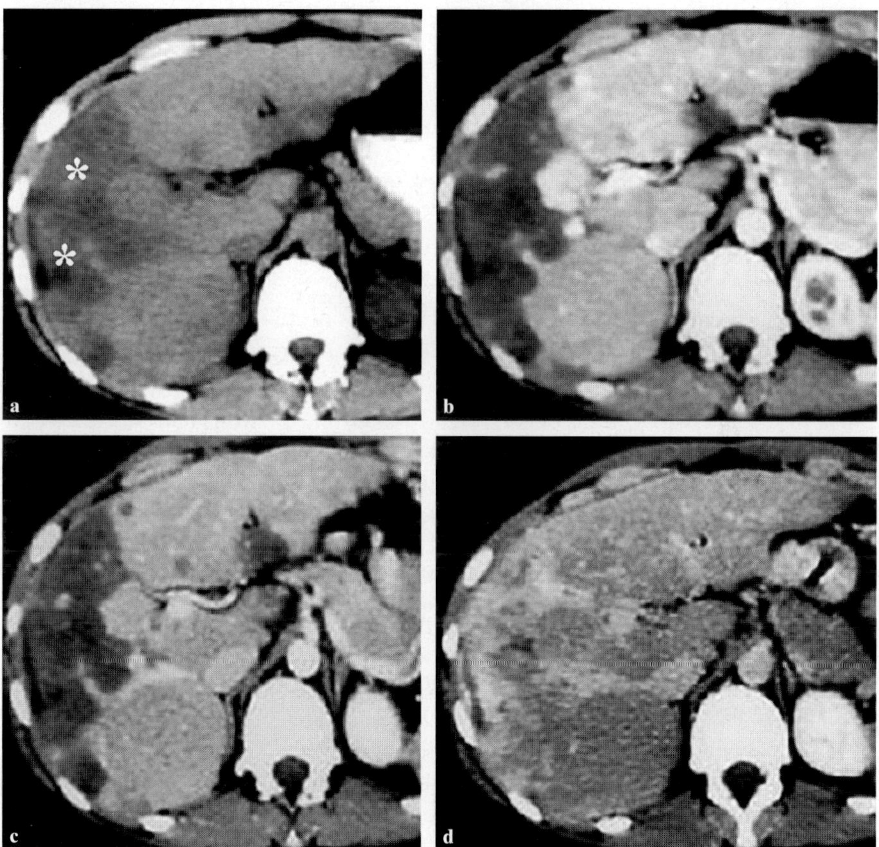

Fig. 41a-d. Epithelioid hemangioendothelioma. Unenhanced CT scans (**a**) reveal large hypodense, confluent diffuse nodules (*asterisks*). Arterial (**b**) and portal-venous (**c**) phase images acquired after the administration of contrast material reveal enhancement at the periphery of the nodules, but few contrast enhancing areas at the center of the lesions. In the equilibrium phase (**d**), the nodules become heterogeneously hyperdense to the normal liver, while compensatory hypertrophy and capsular retraction can be clearly seen

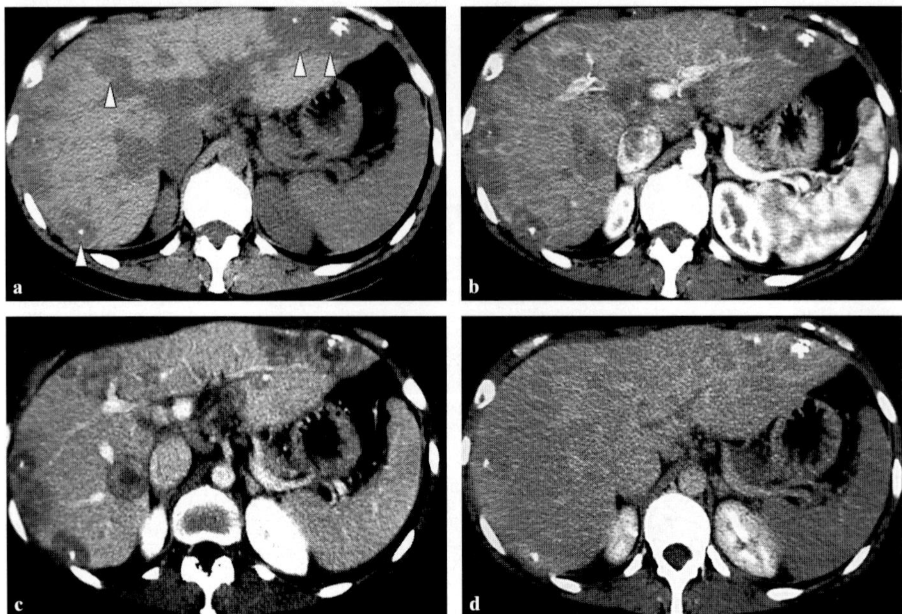

Fig. 42a-d. Epithelioid Hemangioendothelioma (diffuse type). On the unenhanced CT scan (**a**) several hypodense peripheral nodules (*arrowheads*) can be seen; several of these lesions show central calcification. Dynamic evaluation of these lesions after administration of contrast material reveals peripheral enhancement in the early post-contrast phases (**b** and **c**) but isodensity with the normal parenchyma on images acquired in the equilibrium phase (**d**)

On unenhanced CT images, the nodular type of EHE is of low attenuation, corresponding to myxoid stroma. After intravenous administration of contrast material, areas of high density can be observed in the periphery of the tumor, however, the center of the tumor shows very few or no contrast-enhancing areas [11, 91, 140]. Unenhanced CT scans of the diffuse type of EHE reveal large, hypodense, diffuse areas throughout the liver extending toward the periphery. The organ outline is irregularly shaped. Focal calcifications within the tumor are found in about 20% of cases. Compensatory hypertrophy of unaffected liver segments, as well as splenomegaly, are common findings. The liver capsule is not usually affected, although confluent nodules may produce capsular retraction (Fig. 41). After intravenous administration of contrast material, enhancement at the periphery of the tumor can be observed, corresponding to a proliferating zone of active growth. Hypervascular areas, indicative of the vasoformative structure of the tumor or of a more distinct representation of blood vessels due to an obstruction of the portal vein, can sometimes be detected within the tumor [91, 140]. The tumor itself takes up only a little contrast medium. During the delayed phase, the tumor becomes increasingly isodense, which makes it difficult to distinguish from normal liver tissue. Usually, slightly ill-defined areas can be seen in the delayed phase (Fig. 42). Therefore, the extension of the tumor is often better defined on unenhanced CT images [11].

The MR imaging features of EHE are similar to the CT findings: either peripheral nodules or larger confluent lesions are seen. The tumors are hypointense on

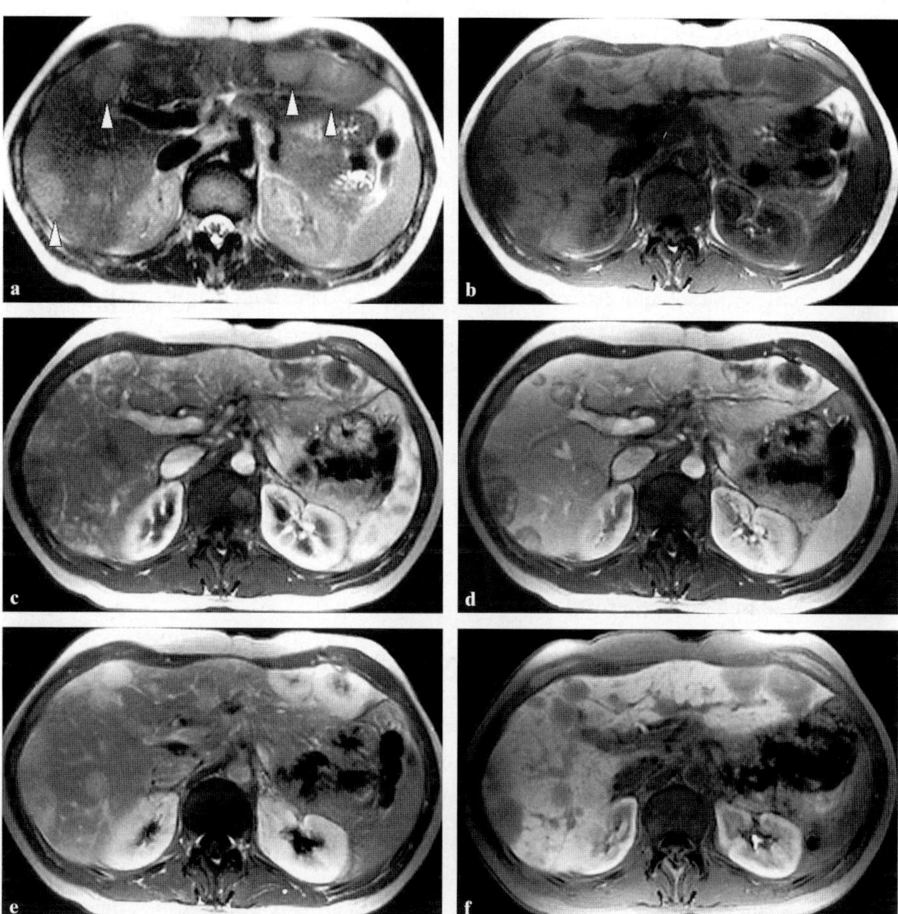

Fig. 43a-f. Epithelioid hemangioendhotelioma. Same case as shown in Fig. 42. The lesions (*arrowheads*) are seen as hyperintense and hypointense on unenhanced T2-weighted (**a**) and T1-weighted (**b**) images, respectively. Peripheral enhancement and progressive filling-in of the lesions are seen on arterial (**c**) and portal-venous (**d**) phase images after the bolus injection of Gd-BOPTA. In the equilibrium phase (**e**) these lesions are seen as either completely or incompletely hyperintense against the normal parenchyma. Images acquired during the delayed hepatobiliary phase (**f**) show the lesions to be homogeneously hypointense to the normal liver

T1-weighted images and hyperintense on T2-weighted images, although a hypointense center corresponding to calcification, necrosis, and hemorrhage may be seen on both sequences. After intravenous administration of extracellularly distributed contrast material, moderate peripheral enhancement, progressive filling-in and delayed central enhancement can usually be seen, particularly in larger lesions. Peripheral washout can also be seen, which is useful for characterization. Lesions are generally seen as hypointense on delayed hepatobiliary phase images, compared to the surrounding liver parenchyma and pre-contrast images after the administration of Gd-BOPTA (Fig. 43) [140].

5.1.7 Hepatic Sarcomas

5.1.7.1 Angiosarcoma

Hepatic angiosarcoma (HAS) is a very rare neoplasm that occurs more frequently in males than in females and most typically in the seventh decade of life. In the general population, angiosarcoma accounts for only 1.8 % of all primary hepatic neoplasms and is 30 times less common than HCC [55]. It is associated with previous exposure to toxins such as Thorotrast, vinyl chloride, arsenicals, steroids, radium and possibly copper [9, 137] and also with chronic idiopathic hemochromatosis [135] and von Recklinghausen disease [2]. Angiosarcoma represents approximately 25% of liver tumors in patients with proven thorium exposure. Although 40% of patients have hepatic fibrosis or cirrhosis at autopsy, the nature of the association between chronic liver disease and HAS is unknown. Further study is also required to delineate the cause of HAS in the remaining 60% of cases without definitive etiologic association.

Histologically, angiosarcoma is composed of malignant endothelial cells lining vascular channels of variable size, from cavernous to capillary, which attempt to form sinusoids. Thorotrast particles can be found within the malignant endothelial cells in cases of Thorotrast-induced angiosarcoma [59].

Macroscopically, the majority of angiosarcoma present as multiple nodules, often with areas of internal hemorrhage. When present as a single, large mass, it does not have a capsule and frequently contains large cystic areas filled with blood debris [11].

The clinical presentation is non-specific, with abdominal pain, weakness and weight loss as frequent complaints, and with hepatomegaly, ascites and jaundice as common findings. Liver function parameters are usually altered but no parameter or set of parameters is specific for the tumor. The occurrence of thrombocytopenia and disseminated intravascular coagulation is characteristic of angiosarcoma and may be related to the local derangement of clotting factors and blood cells. Massive intra-abdominal hemorrhage is a complication which occurs in 25% of all cases and is probably related to the high incidence of coagulation deficits and to the vascular nature of the neoplasm [56, 85].

On ultrasound scans, angiosarcomas are seen as single or multiple hyperechoic masses. The echo architecture is usually heterogeneous due to the presence of hemorrhage of various ages [114].

CT images reveal the reticular pattern of deposition of Thorotrast extremely well in both the liver and the spleen. Circumferential displacement of Thorotrast in the periphery of a nodule is a characteristic finding of angiosarcoma. When there is no evidence of Thorotrast deposition, angiosarcomas present with unenhanced CT as single or multiple hypodense masses containing hyperdense areas of fresh hemorrhage. Many angiosarcomas are hypoattenuating to the liver on both arterial and portal-venous phase images after the administration of contrast material. However, a few lesions are hyperattenuating on arterial phase images, becoming isoattenuating on portal-venous phase images [108]. Centripetal contrast enhancement simulating the pattern of enhancement in hemangioma may occur. The earlier CT reports of angiosarcoma mimicking hemangioma can likely be attributed to imaging in a single temporal phase, often during the delayed phase of contrast enhance-

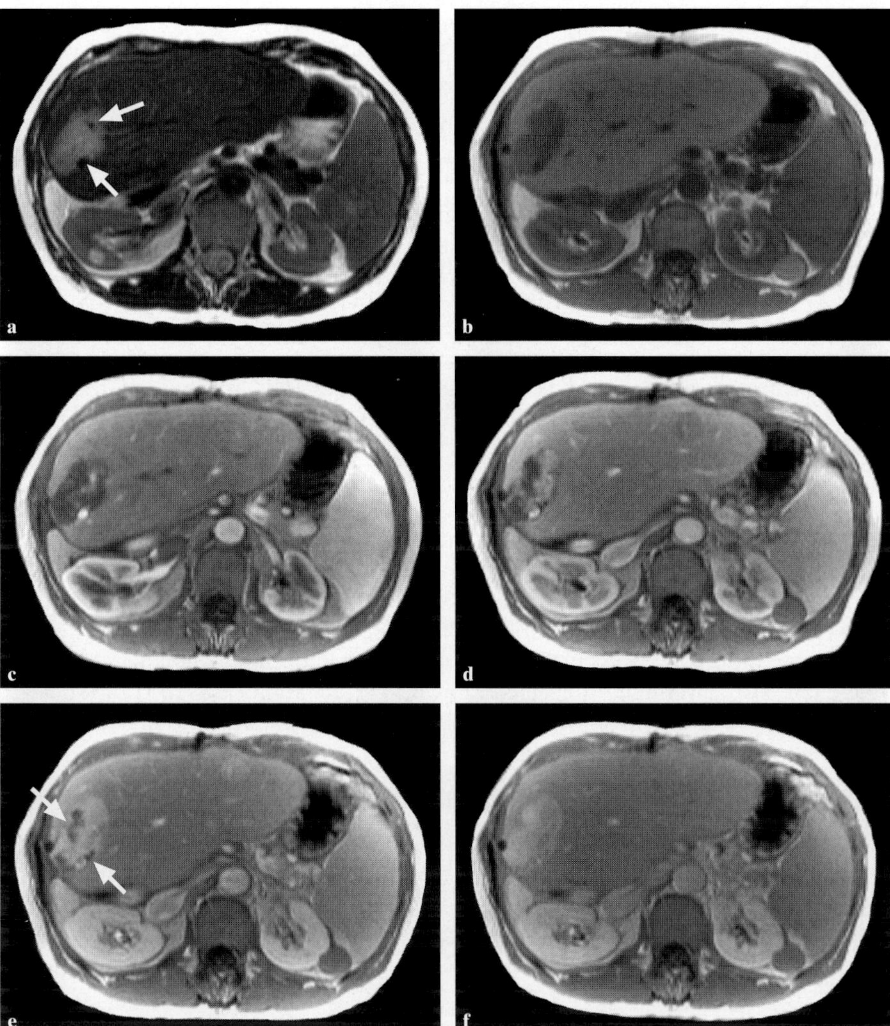

Fig. 44a-f. Angiosarcoma. The unenhanced T2-weighted image (**a**) reveals a high signal intensity mass with hypointense areas that represent large vessels with flow void (*arrows*). The signal intensity of the lesion is comparable to that seen with hemangioma. On the corresponding unenhanced T1-weighted gradient echo image (**b**), the mass again is sharply demarcated and shows homogeneous signal intensity. In contrast to hemangioma, enhancement is seen in central areas of the lesion on arterial phase images (**c**) with subsequent centrifugal filling-in of the lesion in the portal-venous phase (**d**). The peripheral areas of the lesion still do not show enhancement on T1-weighted images acquired 5 min after contrast agent injection (**e**) (*arrows*). However, 10 min after contrast agent administration (**f**), homogeneous enhancement of the lesion can be observed, comparable to a hemangioma. The hint to the diagnosis in this case is the centrifugal enhancement in the lesion rather than the nodular peripheral enhancement typically observed in hemangioma ment, and to the evaluation of lesion enhancement relative to liver parenchyma rather than the aorta or hepatic artery. Temporal assessment by means of multiphasic helical CT of the various patterns of angiosarcoma enhancement in comparison with the pattern of normal vascular enhancement allows confident exclusion of the diagnosis of hemangioma [108].

On T1-weighted MR images, angiosarcomas are usually seen as hypointense with central areas of hyperintensity corresponding to hemorrhage. Conversely, on T2-weighted images the signal intensity is predominantly high, with central areas of low signal [147]. On dynamic contrast-enhanced MR images, the enhancement pattern of angiosarcoma is usually different to that of cavernous hemangioma and is not dissimilar to that observed with spiral CT [108]. Generally, diffuse or central enhancement is seen, although in some cases peripheral enhancement and centripetal filling-in of the lesion is observed. In these cases, irregular borders may contribute to the diagnosis. On equilibrium phase images, the lesion appears as a well-defined hyperintense mass (Fig. 44).

5.1.7.2 Undifferentiated Embryonal Sarcoma

Undifferentiated embryonal sarcoma (UES) is the fourth most common hepatic neoplasm in children after hepatoblastoma, hemangioendothelioma and hepatocellular carcinoma. UES occurs predominantly in children between 6 and 10 years of age [30, 110], although it has been known to affect adults as well [12]. UES was first recognized as a clinical pathological entity in 1978 [134]. The incidence is almost the same in males and females.

Microscopically, UES is composed of primitive, undifferentiated spindle cells, with frequent mitoses and myxoid stroma, that resemble primitive (embryonal) cells [52].

Macroscopically, it is a large, spherical well-defined mass. It is usually solitary and located more frequently in the right lobe of the liver. In some cases a pseudocapsule is present. It can reach 20 cm in diameter and may contain cystic, hemorrhagic and/or necrotic areas. Cystic variants are more frequent than solid forms and this is related to the rapid growth of the neoplasm [115].

UES presents as an abdominal mass with or without pain, fever, jaundice, and weight loss. Sometimes, the tumor may rupture leading to acute abdominal crisis (115). There are no reliable changes in laboratory data, although mild leukocytosis and anemia may be seen in 50% of cases and elevated liver enzymes in 30% of cases. Typically, serum α-fetoprotein levels are normal [27, 141].

In cases of UES, the prognosis depends on the possibility of achieving complete resection of the neoplasm. This is often difficult, but resection combined with adjuvant chemotherapy offers the best chance of cure [141].

On ultrasound images, the appearance of UES ranges from a multiseptate cystic mass to a non inhomogeneous, predominantly echogenic, solid mass. This diversity of echostructure depends on the greater or lesser prevalence of myxoid, solid and hemorrhagic or necrotic components [12, 62, 92].

On CT scans, UES appears as a large intrahepatic mass that has lower attenuation than the surrounding liver. The abundant myxoid matrix of the tumor may be the cause of the hypodense appearance on CT. A dense, peripheral enhancing thin

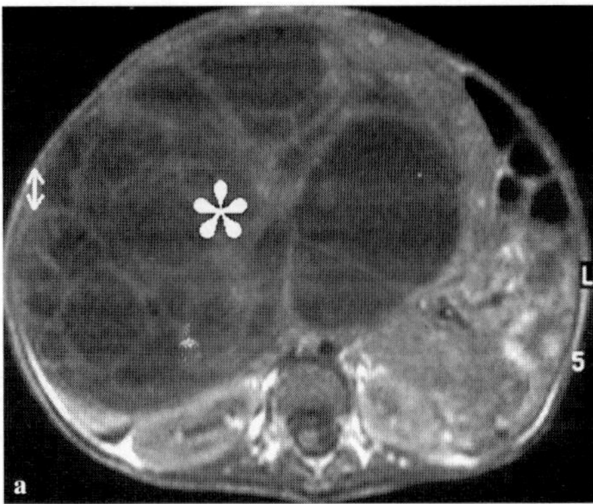
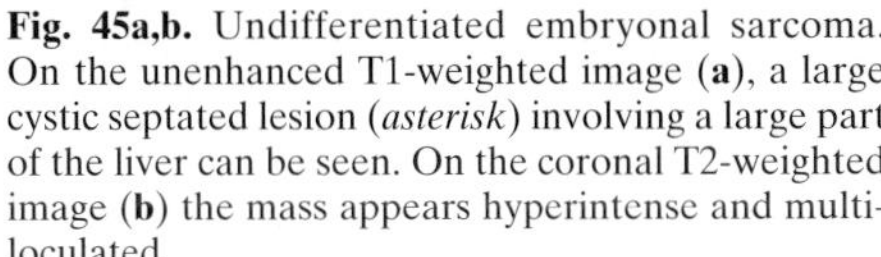
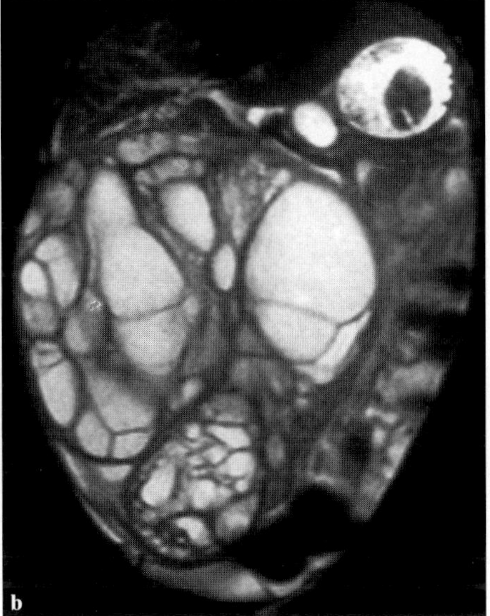

Fig. 45a,b. Undifferentiated embryonal sarcoma. On the unenhanced T1-weighted image (**a**), a large cystic septated lesion (*asterisk*) involving a large part of the liver can be seen. On the coronal T2-weighted image (**b**) the mass appears hyperintense and multi-loculated

rim corresponding to the fibrous pseudocapsule, can sometimes be depicted on CT images, as can the hyperdense septations [92, 115].

On MR, UES is usually seen as heterogeneously hypointense on T1-weighted images and hyperintense on T2-weighted images, correlating with the predominately cystic nature of the lesion. Hemorrhage, if present, is seen as an area of high signal intensity on T1-weighted images, while the pseudocapsule and septations are of low signal on both T1- and T2-weighted images (Fig. 45) [115, 152].

5.1.7.3 Hepatobiliary Rhabdomyosarcoma

Although hepatobiliary rhabdomyosarcoma (RMS) is the most common neoplasm of the biliary tree in children, it is a rare disease, accounting for approximately 1% of all RMS in pediatric patients. RMS usually occurs in children of about 3 years of age and is rarely seen after the first decade of life. There may be a slight predominance among males [118].

Although the early histological classification of RMS was different in the United States [51] and Europe [13], a universal classification now exists [98]. Hepatobiliary RMS in childhood can be of the embryonal or botryoid types [118]. It may arise in the liver or intrahepatic bile ducts [84], in intrahepatic cysts [123], the gallbladder [89], the cystic duct [74], the extrahepatic bile duct [74], the ampulla [17] or in choledocal cysts [105].

Microscopically, RMS contains spindle cell tumors in a myxoid stroma. A few cells have eosinophilic cytoplasmic tails resembling rhabdomyoblasts with or without cross striations [52]. Macroscopically, RMS tends to be well-demarcated from the surrounding tissue with a "pushing" margin. The mean diameter at diagnosis is usually about 8 cm [52, 118].

The most common clinical features are jaundice and abdominal distension. Pain, nausea, vomiting and fever are less frequent. The α-fetoprotein values are normal [118, 123].

Ultrasound typically reveals biliary dilatation and an intraductal mass [34, 40]. Although the portal vein may be displaced by a large tumor, portal vein thrombosis has not yet been described. Larger masses may have fluid, cystic areas within them, possibly reflecting tumor necrosis [90]. When the tumor arises in the liver, there may be no distinguishing ultrasound features. Color Doppler ultrasound may reveal numerous abnormal tumor arteries with low resistive index [112].

CT also reveals an intraductal mass with or without biliary dilatation. Hypodense and heterogeneous attenuation patterns have been described [40] and areas of low attenuation within the tumor may be present [17, 84, 90, 105]. Enhancement patterns after the administration of contrast material have been described as strong heterogeneous, incomplete globular, mild and none [112] indicating that enhancement may be variable.

RMS is generally hypointense on unenhanced T1-weighted MR images and moderately or markedly hyperintense on T2-weighted images. Following the administration of a gadolinium contrast agent, intense but inhomogeneous contrast enhancement is usually seen [112].

5.2 Secondary Malignant Liver Lesions

5.2.1 Non-Hodgkin's Lymphoma and Hodgkin's Disease

Hepatic lymphoma can be either primary or secondary and can occur in patients with Hodgkin's disease (HD) and in patients with non-Hodgkin's lymphoma. Most lymphomas of the liver are secondary. Primary lymphoma is rare because the amount of lymphatic tissue in the liver is very small, present only in the periportal spaces. Normally, primary hepatic lymphomas are non-Hodgkin's lymphomas of B-cell origin [119]. However, secondary lymphoma of the liver is found in more than 50% of patients with HD or non-Hodgkin's lymphoma [101]. Primary hepatic lymphoma occurs most commonly in middle-aged white men [126]. Organ transplant recipients and patients with AIDS are at high risk for developing hepatic lymphoma.

Whereas in well-differentiated non-Hodgkin's lymphoma, numerous miliary small nodules may be present in the liver, in less well-differentiated non-Hodgkin's lymphomas, the lesions are often larger and more infiltrative. In Burkitt's lymphoma subcapsular infiltration may also be found as a consequence of peritoneal spread [60].

In Hodgkin's lymphoma, the hepatic involvement may range from multiple small nodes to large infiltrations. This involvement occurs more frequently with lymphocyte depletion and mixed cellular sub-types than with the lymphocyte-rich sub-type of HD. Concomitant peliosis hepatis may also be present [125].

Clinically, patients with primary non-Hodgkin's lymphoma most often present with pain in the right upper quadrant or hepatomegaly. Secondary lymphomas as well as Hodgkin's lymphoma may induce jaundice, fever and hepatomegaly, but these signs are non-specific and often result from chemotherapy [7].

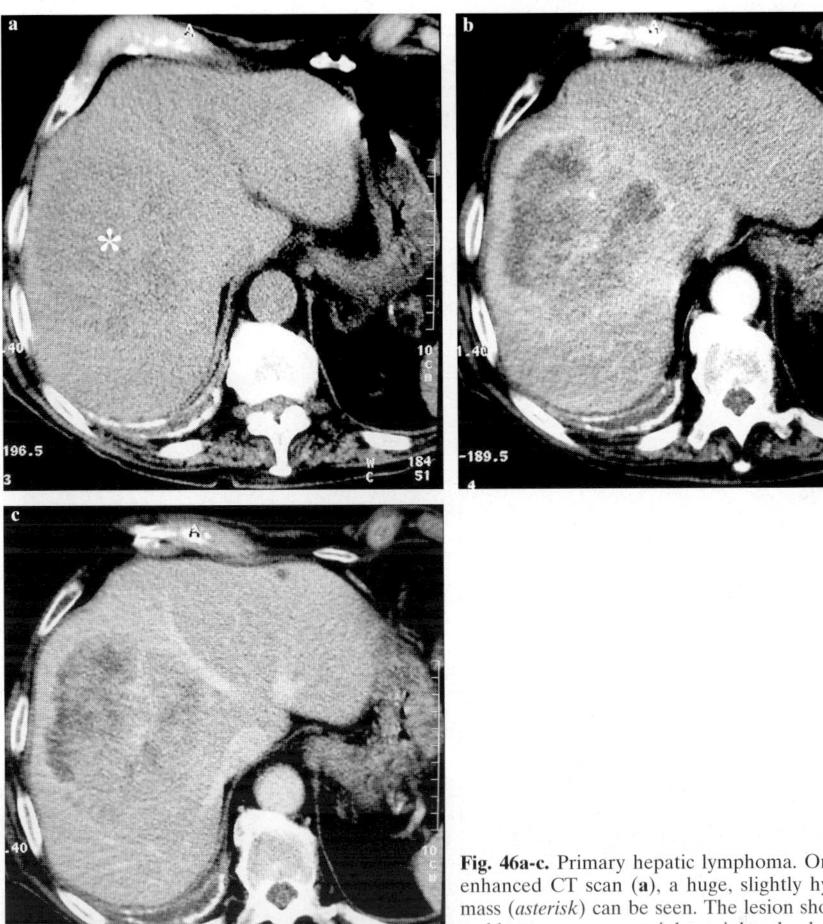

Fig. 46a-c. Primary hepatic lymphoma. On the unenhanced CT scan (**a**), a huge, slightly hypodense mass (*asterisk*) can be seen. The lesion shows weak and heterogeneous, mainly peripheral enhancement during the arterial phase (**b**), and remains heterogeneously hypodense in the portal-venous phase (**c**)

On ultrasound, both Hodgkin's and non-Hodgkin's lymphoma commonly appear as single or multiple hypoechoic masses, often with indistinct margins. Multiple hypoechoic lesions may mimic the appearance of a diffuse infectious process such as candidiasis. In the diffuse lymphomatous form, the echogenicity of the hepatic parenchyma may be normal or heterogeneous and the overall architecture of the liver may be altered. Occasionally, patients with non-Hodgkin lymphoma have echogenic or target-like lesions [144]. If there is bleeding within the tumor, the ultrasonographic characteristics of a cyst may be seen [126].

On CT, these tumors appear as large discrete masses, with decreased attenuation relative to the surrounding liver parenchyma on both unenhanced and portal-venous phase enhanced images (Fig. 46) [122].

On MR images, focal hepatic lymphoma is seen as homogeneously hypointense on unenhanced T1-weighted images and hyperintense on T2-weighted images, compared to the normal parenchyma. Dynamic imaging after the administration of a gadolinium contrast agent typically reveals a hypointense appearance on arterial phase images, followed by homogeneous, delayed enhancement on portal-venous phase images and isointensity on equilibrium phase images (Fig. 47). Susceptibility artifacts may be caused by hemorrhage in pre-treated focal infiltrations and may be more clearly delineated on fat-suppressed T1-weighted images [63]. Although lymphoma is readily distinguishable from normal liver, the difference in relaxation times from either metastases or HCC is not significant.

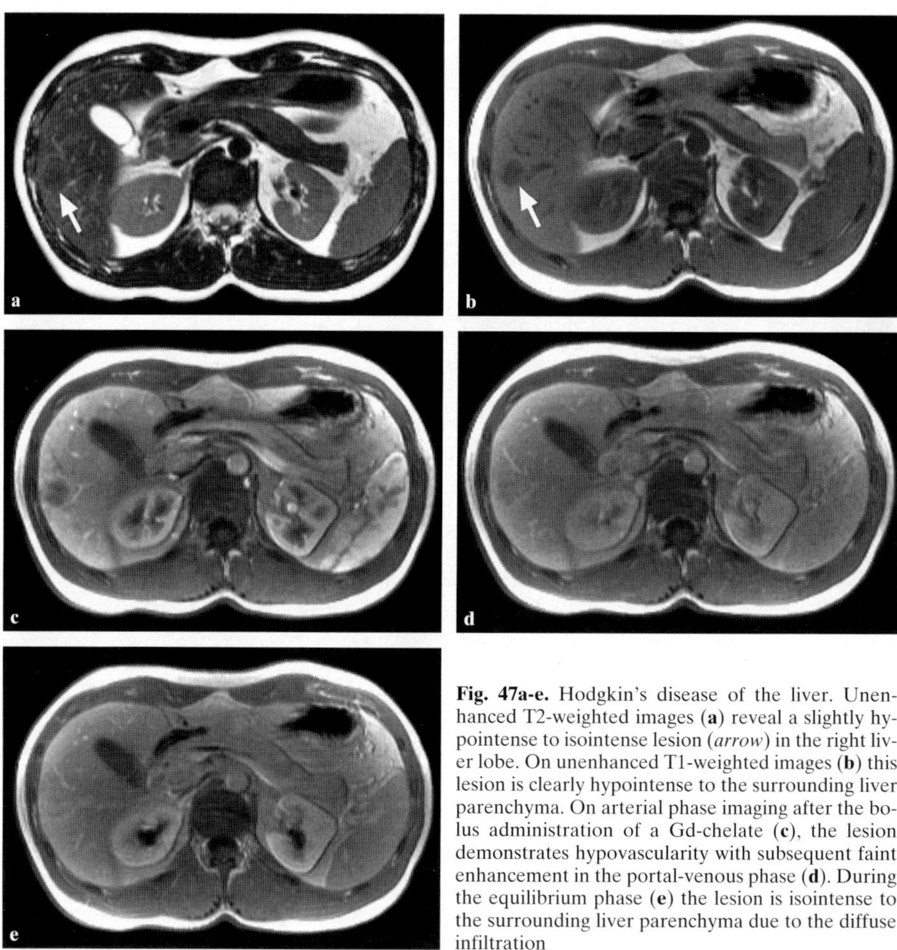

Fig. 47a-e. Hodgkin's disease of the liver. Unenhanced T2-weighted images (**a**) reveal a slightly hypointense to isointense lesion (*arrow*) in the right liver lobe. On unenhanced T1-weighted images (**b**) this lesion is clearly hypointense to the surrounding liver parenchyma. On arterial phase imaging after the bolus administration of a Gd-chelate (**c**), the lesion demonstrates hypovascularity with subsequent faint enhancement in the portal-venous phase (**d**). During the equilibrium phase (**e**) the lesion is isointense to the surrounding liver parenchyma due to the diffuse infiltration

5.2.2 Metastases

Metastases are the most common malignant focal liver lesions in the non-cirrhotic liver. However, metastases are relatively uncommon in the cirrhotic liver where HCC is more frequent. The liver is second only to regional lymph nodes as a site of metastatic disease; autopsy series of patients with primary tumors indicate that at the time of death, approximately 50% of patients have metastatic disease of the liver [104]. Although metastases can develop in the liver via hematogenous spread from most solid tumors, certain primary neoplasms are particularly virulent in causing liver-dominant disease and often isolated liver metastases. These include colorectal cancer and neuroendocrine tumors, gastrointestinal sarcomas, uveal melanomas and other neoplasms [41].

The gross features of liver metastases vary. Lesions may be expansive, infiltrative, surface spreading, or miliary, depending on the primary tumor of origin. Within each of these categories, metastatic lesions may be massive, nodular, or diffuse and may range in size from less than 1 mm to many centimeters in diameter. Metastases from colon carcinoma usually appear as a few large nodules with central umbilication. Nodules from breast or lung carcinoma have a early central umbilication. Metastatic lesions of the miliary type are seen more frequently in breast, prostate or stomach cancers.

Microscopically, metastases resemble the primary tumors. Fibrous reaction to the metastatic tumor is common for breast and pancreatic carcinomas, while a "fish flesh" texture is common for cellular and undifferentiated tumors such as small cell cancer, adenocarcinoma of the lung, some sarcomas, and melanoma [41, 73].

Clinically, hepatomegaly is the most common finding, followed by ascites, jaundice, and varices [31].

On ultrasound images, metastases to the liver usually take on one of the following appearances: hypoechoic, mixed echogenicity, target pattern, hyperechoic, cystic, heterogeneous or coarse echo texture without focal mass [3]. Most metastatic lesions exhibit a hypoechoic halo. This hypoechoic halo is composed of compressed normal liver parenchyma, proliferating tumor edema, and a rim of hypervascularity in the periphery of the lesion (Fig. 48). In addition to a halo, metastases may take on a target or bull's-eye appearance due to alternating layers of hyper- and hypoechoic tissue (Fig. 49). These patterns are highly suggestive for malignancy [106].

Hypoechoic metastases tend to be hypovascular, and can be secondary to lymphoma, melanoma, breast and lung carcinoma. Hyperechoic metastases in many cases correspond to hypervascular lesions, and frequently arise from colon, renal, breast, and islet cell carcinomas (Fig. 50). Cystic metastases are rare, and include those from sarcomas, ovarian cancer (Fig. 51) colon cancer and squamous cell carcinoma. Calcified metastases derive frequently from mucinous adenocarcinomas of the colon (Fig. 52), pancreas or ovary [106]. Color and power Doppler can frequently differentiate metastases from HCC, since the former are often avascular.

Since the majority of liver metastases are supplied by the hepatic artery and do not have a significant vascular supply from the portal system, most metastases are hypovascular relative to the normal liver parenchyma [106]. These metastases nearly always demonstrate decreased attenuation compared with normal liver parenchyma on unenhanced CT scans, and are best seen during the portal-venous phase of contrast enhancement following the administration of contrast material when the

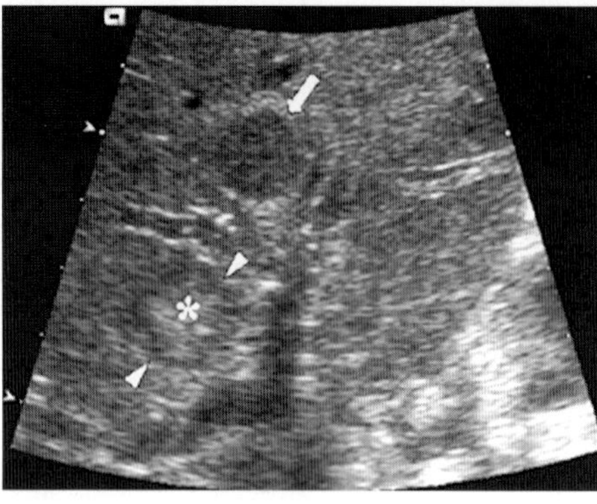

Fig. 48. Metastases with halo pattern. Ultrasound reveals a hyperechoic lesion (*asterisk*) surrounded by a regular hypoechoic rim (*arrowheads*). Another metastatic homogeneous hypoechoic nodule (*arrow*) coexists in the same patient

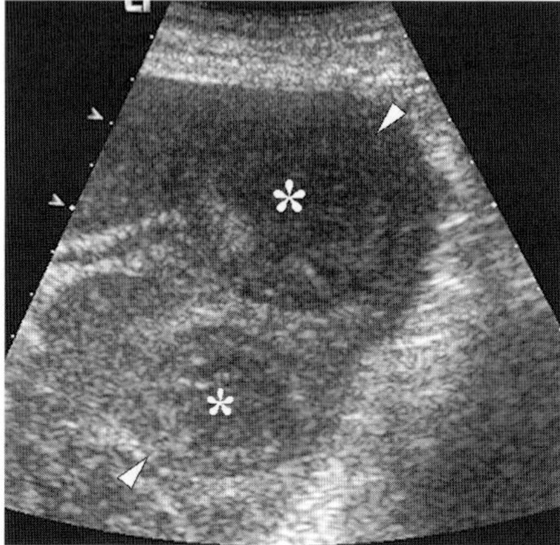

Fig. 49. Metastases with bull's eye pattern. Ultrasound reveals two large nodular lesions (*asterisks*) with hyper- and hypoechoic peripheral layers (*arrowheads*)

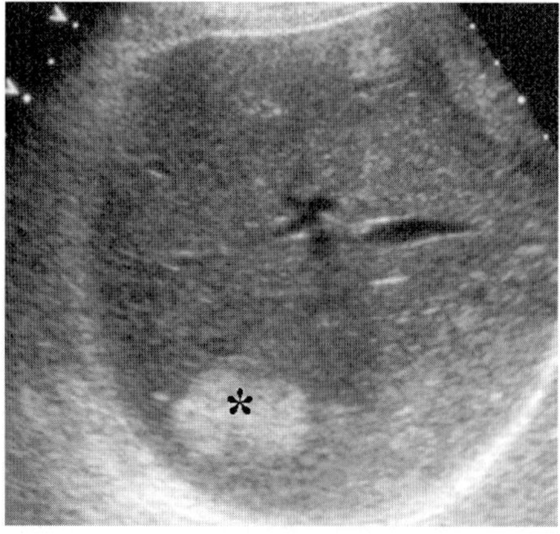

Fig. 50. Hyperechoic metastases from renal cancer. A large lobulated, homogeneous, hyperechoic nodule simulating an hemangioma can be seen in liver segment VII (*asterisk*)

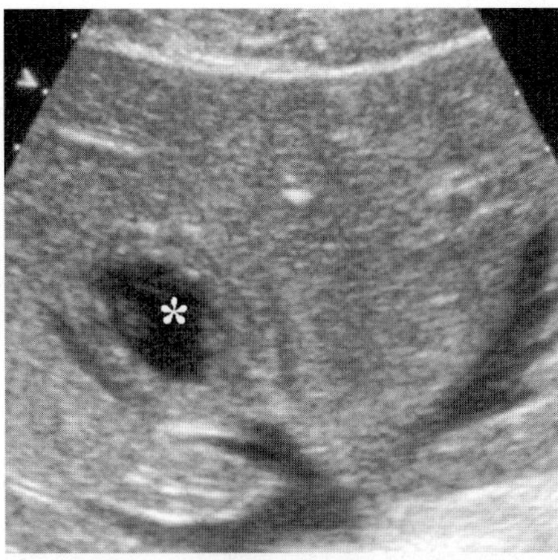

Fig. 51. Cystic metastases from ovarian cancer. An anechoic nodule with slighty irregular margins (*asterisk*) is surrounded by a thick hyperechoic and a thin hypoechoic rim

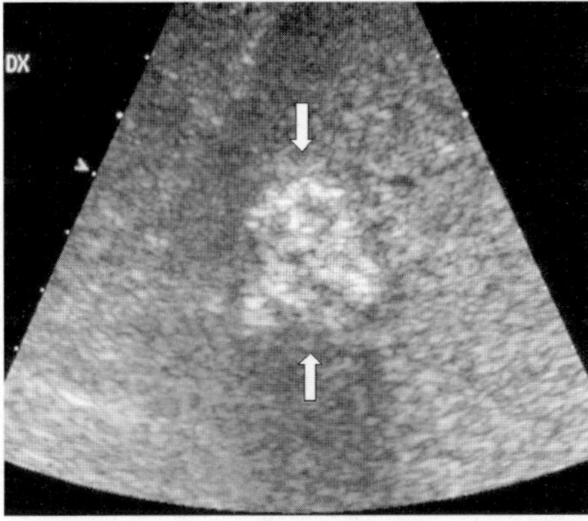

Fig. 52. Calcified metastases from colon cancer. Ultrasound reveals a nodular lesion with irregular margins (*arrows*) and numerous small calcifications with acoustic shadow

normal liver parenchyma is maximally enhanced (Fig. 53) [72]. They most commonly arise from colon, stomach, pancreas, lung, breast, and cervix neoplasms.

On the other hand, hypervascular metastases tend to be more vascular than normal liver parenchyma and are best seen during the arterial phase of contrast enhancement when they are maximally enhanced. During the portal-venous phase these lesions are often isodense with the normal liver and difficult to detect (Fig. 54). Metastases of this type include those deriving from renal cell carcinoma, breast carcinoma, islet cells tumors, melanoma and sarcomas, pheochromocytoma, carcinoid and thyroideal carcinoma [8].

Regardless of the hypo- or hypervascular nature of the lesion, arterial phase imaging is generally considered essential for the visualization of metastases smaller than 1 cm in size. This is due to the fact that the predominant blood supply derives from the hepatic artery in small lesions, with the result that they appear isointense in the portal-venous phase [50]. Since small tumors do not usually outgrow their blood supply, they generally do not have necrotic, and thus hypovascular, central areas.

Visualization of the hyperdense rim of typical hypovascular lesions, such as colon carcinoma metastases, is frequently best achieved during the arterial phase

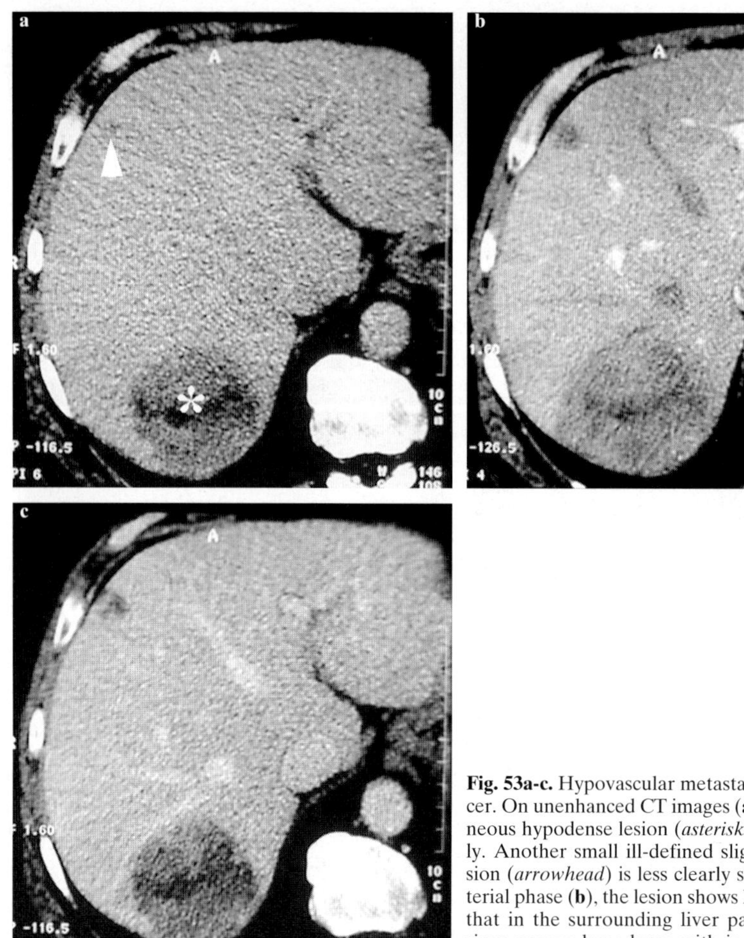

Fig. 53a-c. Hypovascular metastases from colon cancer. On unenhanced CT images (**a**), a large heterogeneous hypodense lesion (*asterisk*) can be seen clearly. Another small ill-defined slightly hypodense lesion (*arrowhead*) is less clearly seen. During the arterial phase (**b**), the lesion shows less vascularity than that in the surrounding liver parenchyma. The lesions appear hypodense with increased conspicuity in the portal-venous phase (**c**)

[19]. The equilibrium phase, however, enables an evaluation of enhancement pattern and contrast washout and is thus important for lesion characterization. In this phase some metastases show central pooling and peripheral washout due to desmoplastic reaction and peripheral edema (Fig. 55).

With MR, the signal intensity of metastases varies considerably, depending on the degree of vascularity, necrosis, and hemorrhage. Generally, on unenhanced T1-weighted images metastases are of low signal intensity relative to the surrounding parenchyma, but may demonstrate increased signal intensity whenever intralesional hemorrhage is present. On T2-weighted images, metastases are usually of high signal intensity relative to surrounding liver parenchyma, although the signal intensity is generally lower than that typically observed for hemangiomas or cysts. The presence of coagulative necrosis, fibrous tissue or calcifications decreases the signal intensity on T2-weighted images, while colliquative necrosis or edema leads to an increase of signal intensity (Fig. 56). For metastases from adenocarcinomas, a

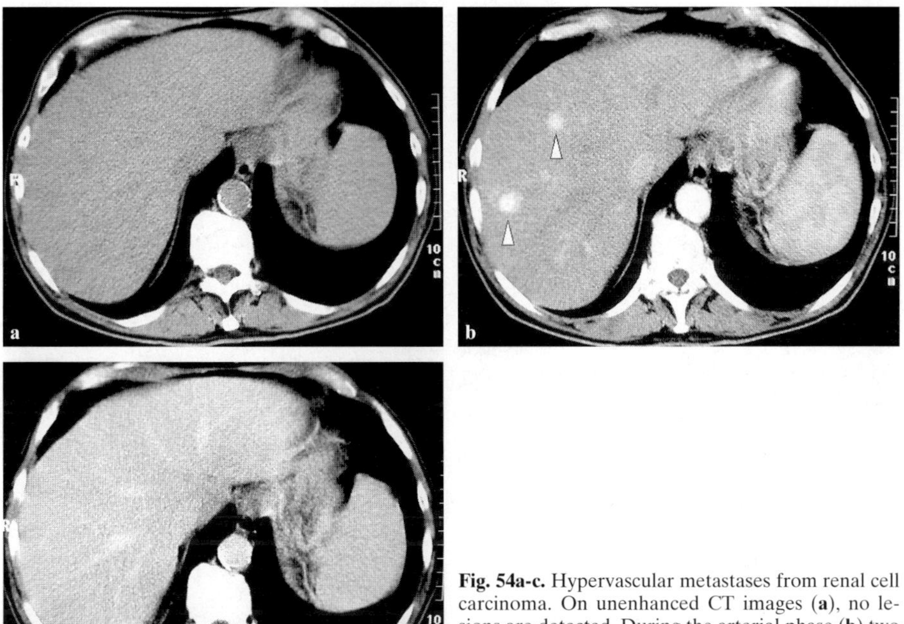

Fig. 54a-c. Hypervascular metastases from renal cell carcinoma. On unenhanced CT images (**a**), no lesions are detected. During the arterial phase (**b**) two homogeneous hypervascular nodules (*arrowheads*) are seen. The nodules are seen as isodense on the portal-venous phase image (**c**)

Fig. 55a,b. Metastases with central pooling from colon cancer. The unenhanced CT scan (**a**) shows numerous ill-defined hypodense nodules (*arrows*). In the equilibrium phase (**b**) the nodules demonstrate central contrast agent pooling and peripheral washout (*arrowheads*)

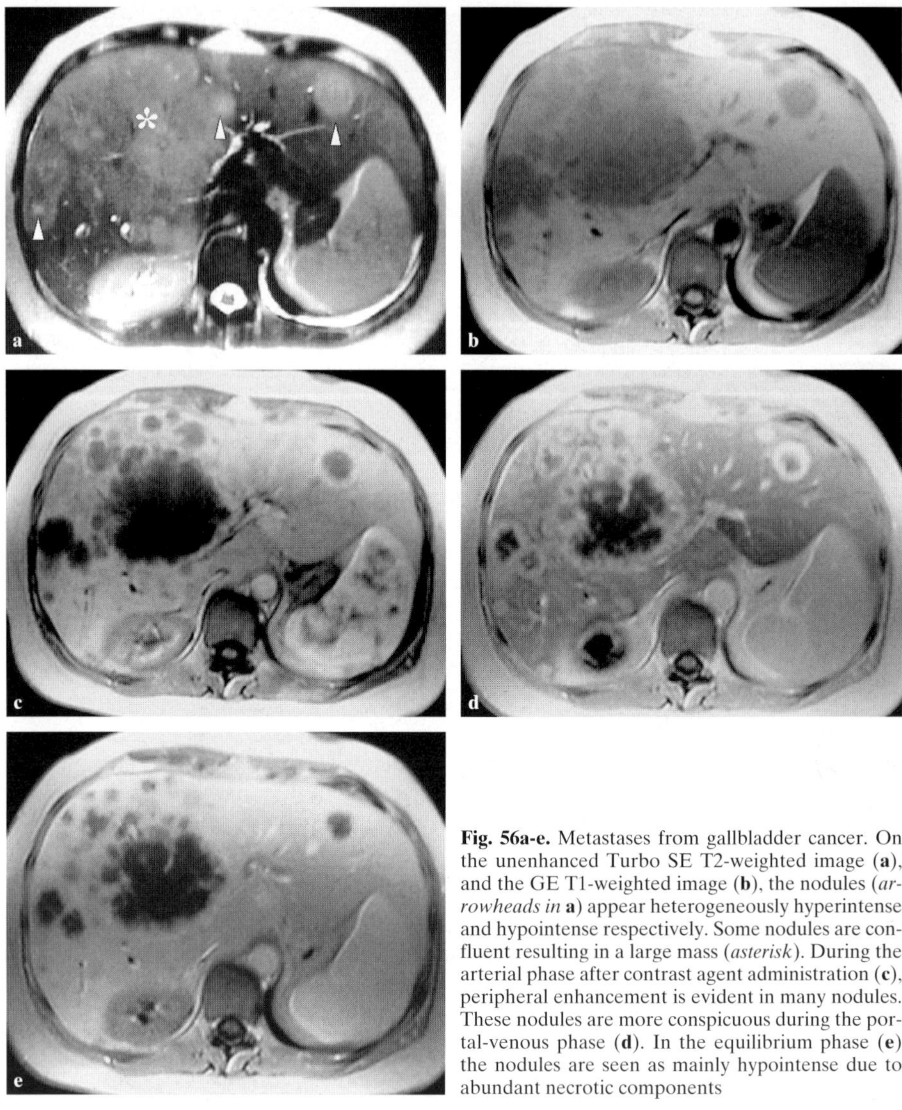

Fig. 56a-e. Metastases from gallbladder cancer. On the unenhanced Turbo SE T2-weighted image (**a**), and the GE T1-weighted image (**b**), the nodules (*arrowheads in* **a**) appear heterogeneously hyperintense and hypointense respectively. Some nodules are confluent resulting in a large mass (*asterisk*). During the arterial phase after contrast agent administration (**c**), peripheral enhancement is evident in many nodules. These nodules are more conspicuous during the portal-venous phase (**d**). In the equilibrium phase (**e**) the nodules are seen as mainly hypointense due to abundant necrotic components

characteristic "doughnut" or "target" sign is often seen on T2-weighted images, in which a central hypointense area corresponding to necrosis is surrounded by a less hypointense area corresponding to the growth margins of the tumor.

During the arterial phase after the administration of an extracellularly-distributed contrast agent, weak peripheral heterogeneous enhancement can usually be seen, while nodular or globular enhancement aspects are rarely present. A hypointense rim caused by edema may delineate the lesion in the portal-venous and equilibrium phases. Often, larger metastases demonstrate heterogeneous enhancement due to the presence of non-enhancing central necrotic areas.

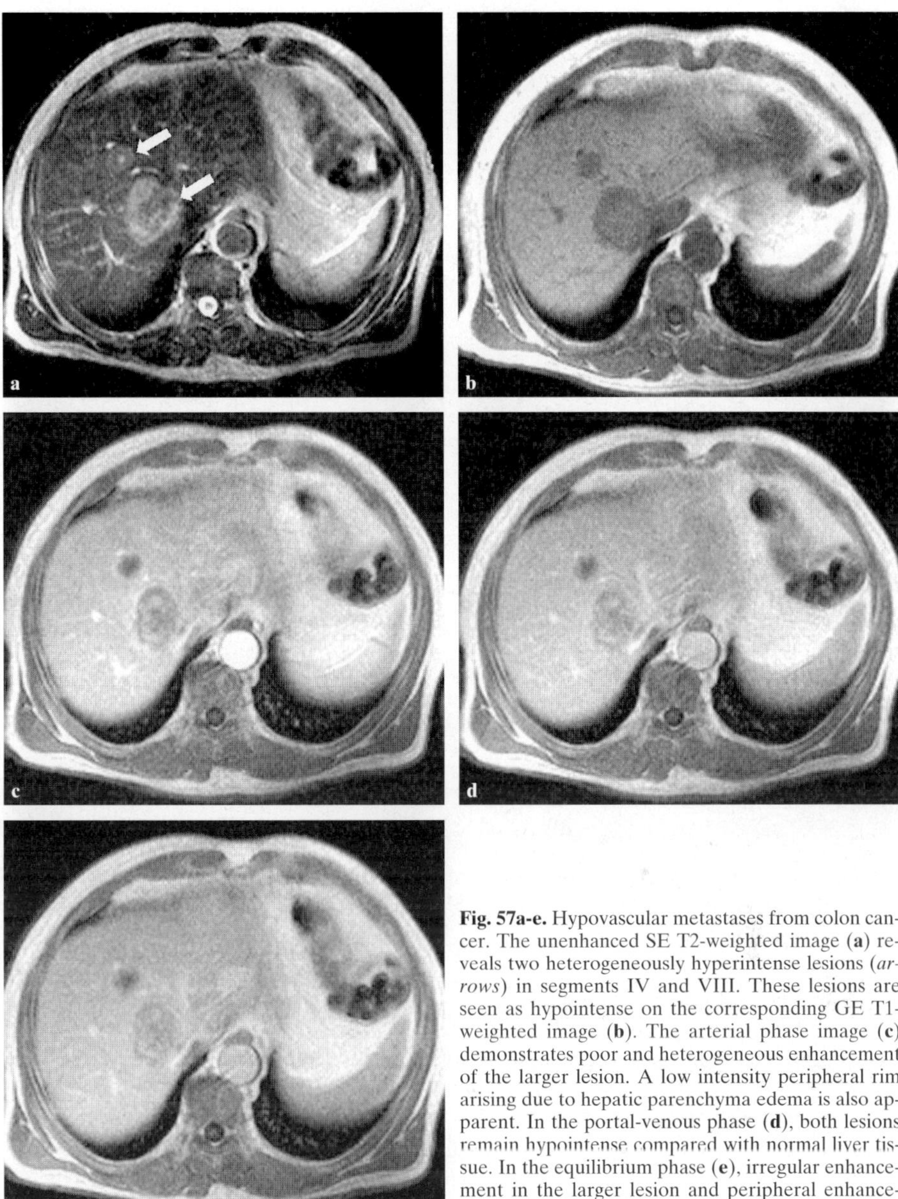

Fig. 57a-e. Hypovascular metastases from colon cancer. The unenhanced SE T2-weighted image (**a**) reveals two heterogeneously hyperintense lesions (*arrows*) in segments IV and VIII. These lesions are seen as hypointense on the corresponding GE T1-weighted image (**b**). The arterial phase image (**c**) demonstrates poor and heterogeneous enhancement of the larger lesion. A low intensity peripheral rim arising due to hepatic parenchyma edema is also apparent. In the portal-venous phase (**d**), both lesions remain hypointense compared with normal liver tissue. In the equilibrium phase (**e**), irregular enhancement in the larger lesion and peripheral enhancement of the smaller one can be noted

On late phase images, lesions are typically heterogeneously hypointense, often with characteristic "target", "halo", "peripheral washout" or "doughnut" aspects (Fig. 57). Hypervascular metastases are usually hypo- to isointense on unenhanced T1-weighted images and reveal strong transient enhancement in the arterial phase followed by isointensity in the portal-venous and equilibrium phases (Fig. 58) [81].

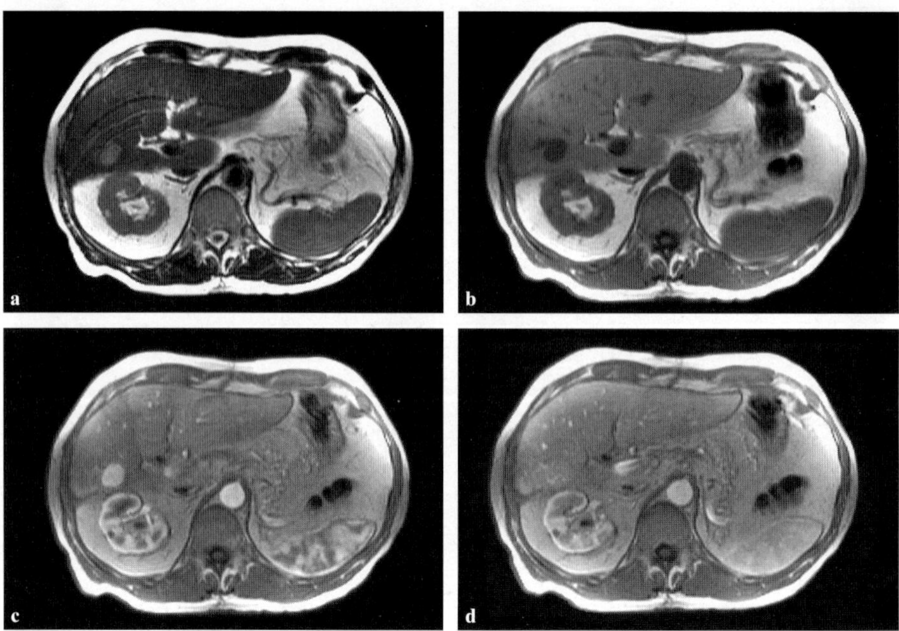

Fig. 58a-d. Hypervascular metastases from gastrinoma. On the unenhanced Turbo SE T2-weighted image (**a**) the nodule is seen as homogeneously hyperintense with distinct borders. The GE T1-weighted image (**b**) reveals a sharply demarcated, hypointense lesion with homogeneous signal intensity. During the dynamic study after the administration of gadolinium contrast agent, the lesion demonstrates initial strong homogeneous hypervascularization during the arterial phase (**c**) followed by isointensity in the portal-venous phase (**d**) due to rapid wash-out

The use of contrast agents with liver-specific properties is generally considered appropriate for both the detection and diagnosis of metastases. Both positive and negative contrast agents improve significantly the detection capability compared with spiral CT [18, 45, 113, 124].

Dual contrast agents such as Gd-BOPTA, which have both extracellular and hepatobiliary properties, enable improved characterization which can be particularly important in cases in which benign and malignant lesions coexist in the same patient (Fig. 59). On dynamic phase images the pattern of enhancement seen after Gd-BOPTA or after bolus injection of another Gd-chelate may provide useful information on the extent of tumor vascularization, and thus aid in tumor characterization (Fig. 60). Lesion detectability can also be improved on MR by the acquisition of liver-specific delayed scans after Gd-BOPTA (Fig. 61). The greatest increase has been observed for metastases smaller than 1 cm in diameter [117].

With mangafodipir, metastases usually appear as hypointense against a strongly enhanced normal liver (Fig. 62) [142]. In some cases, it is possible to observe a rim of peripheral enhancement surrounding the metastasis, which can be useful for discriminating metastases from other liver lesions such as cysts and hemangiomas [113]. Unfortunately, metastases from neuroendocrine tumors may show enhancement after mangafodipir. Moreover, some hemangiomas may be confused with

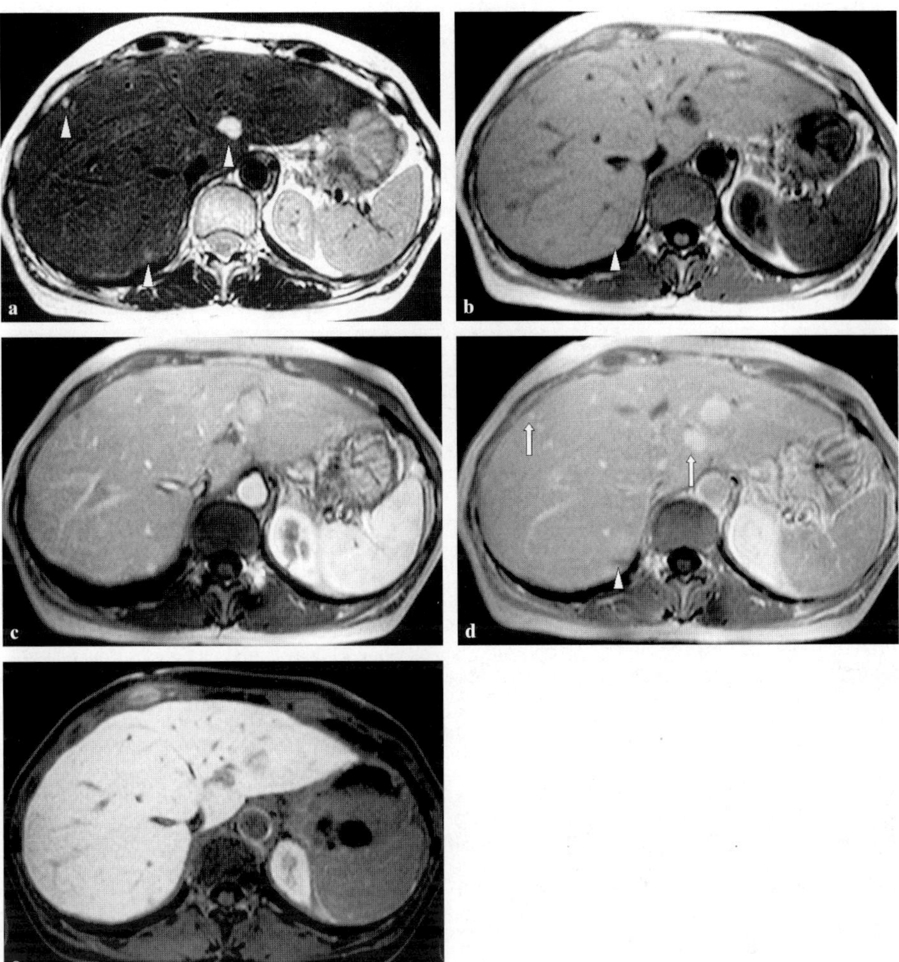

Fig. 59a-e. Detection and characterization of liver metastases from melanoma with Gd-BOPTA. On unenhanced Turbo SE T2-weighted images (**a**) three nodules (*arrowheads*) demonstrating different degrees of hyperintensity can be seen. On the GE T1 weighted image (**b**) two of these lesions are seen as hypointense while the third small nodule (*arrowhead*) appears slightly hyperintense. Dynamic evaluation (**c, d**) after Gd-BOPTA administration characterizes two lesions as hemangiomas (*arrows in* **d**), due to the presence of peripheral nodular enhancement, centripetal filling-in and complete filling-in. The metastatic lesion (*arrowhead in* **d**) shows homogeneous enhancement in the arterial phase (**c**) and washout in the equilibrium phase (**d**). While the metastasic lesion appears as an ill defined hypointense nodule in the equilibrium phase, the hemangiomas are both hyperintense. Each of the lesions is seen as hypointense on the hepatobiliary phase image (**e**)

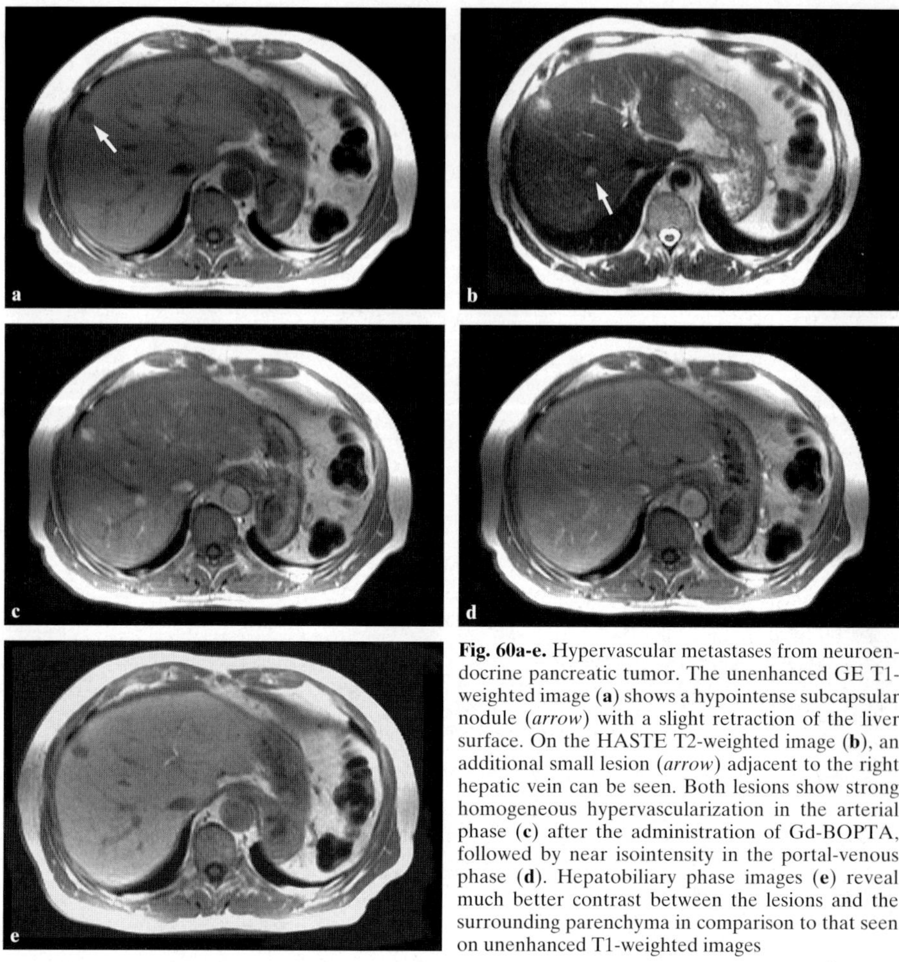

Fig. 60a-e. Hypervascular metastases from neuroendocrine pancreatic tumor. The unenhanced GE T1-weighted image (**a**) shows a hypointense subcapsular nodule (*arrow*) with a slight retraction of the liver surface. On the HASTE T2-weighted image (**b**), an additional small lesion (*arrow*) adjacent to the right hepatic vein can be seen. Both lesions show strong homogeneous hypervascularization in the arterial phase (**c**) after the administration of Gd-BOPTA, followed by near isointensity in the portal-venous phase (**d**). Hepatobiliary phase images (**e**) reveal much better contrast between the lesions and the surrounding parenchyma in comparison to that seen on unenhanced T1-weighted images

metastases, due to the low signal intensity on T2-weighted images and hypointensity on delayed hepatobiliary phase T1-weighted images (Fig. 63).

SPIO contrast agents are particularly helpful for lesion detection. Due to the absence of Kupffer cells, metastases generally do not show significant signal drop after SPIO administration and thus appear as hyperintense nodules against a darkened normal liver (Fig. 64). However, the lack of a dynamic imaging capability means that SPIO agents often present the same problem as mangafodipir when the need is to differentiate between metastases and coexisting benign lesions. To a certain extent the problem inherent to SPIO agents may be overcome by USPIO agents for which both dynamic and late phase imaging is possible (Fig. 65) [45].

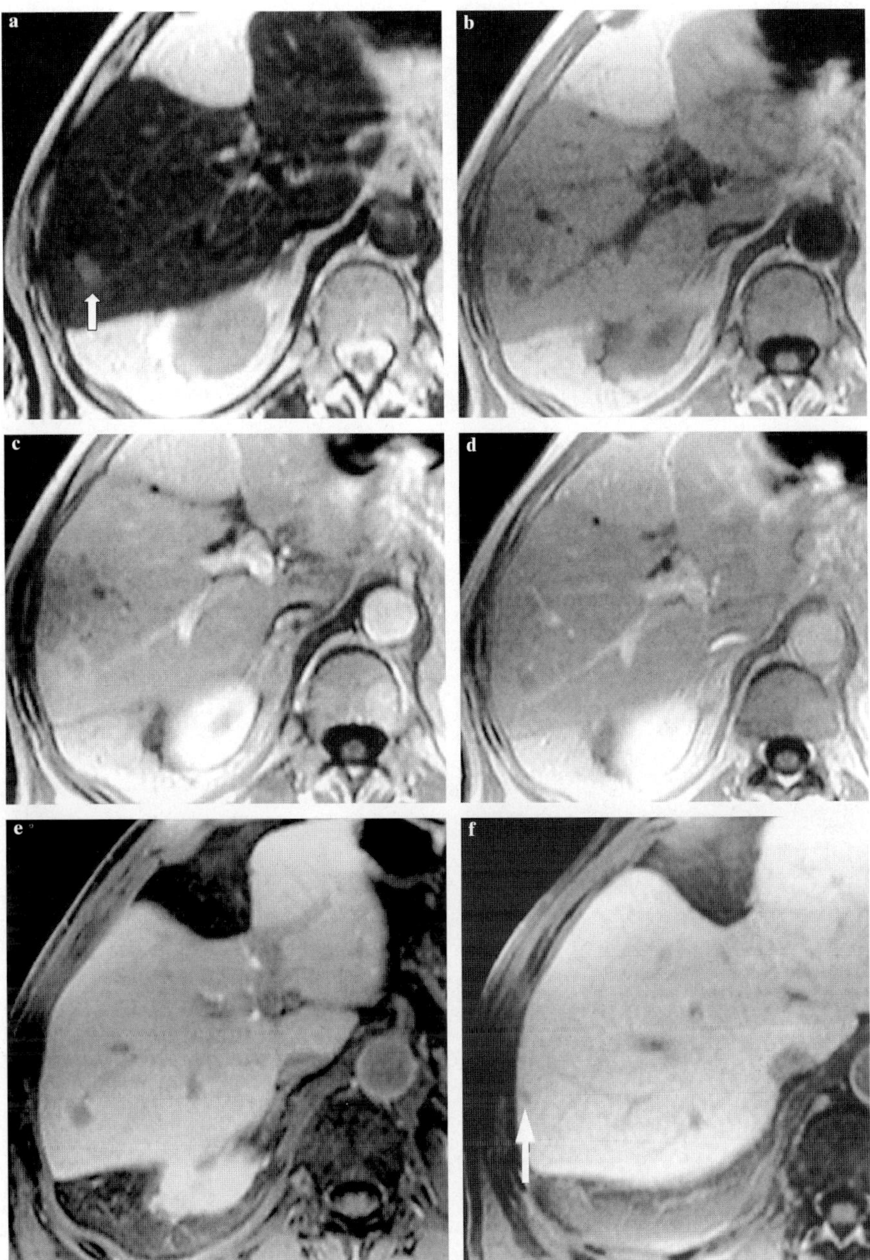

Fig. 61a-f. Metastases from endocrine tumor. A small, slightly hyperintense lesion (*arrow*) can be seen on the HASTE T2-weighted image (**a**). The lesion appears as hypointense on the unenhanced T1-weighted image (**b**). Dynamic imaging after the bolus administration of Gd-BOPTA reveals that the lesion demonstrates initial enhancement during the arterial phase (**c**) and wash-out in the portal-venous phase (**d**). On the hepatobiliary phase image (**e**) the nodule does not show any capacity to take up Gd-BOPTA and appears hypointense. Another very small nodule (*arrow*) can be seen only in the hepatobiliary phase (**f**)

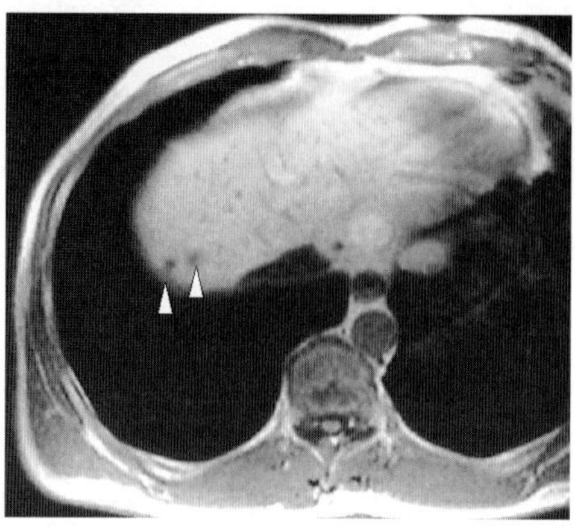

Fig. 62. Metastases from pancreatic cancer. After administration of mangafodipir, the liver metastases (*arrowheads*) appear as hypointense nodules against the surrounding enhanced normal liver parenchyma

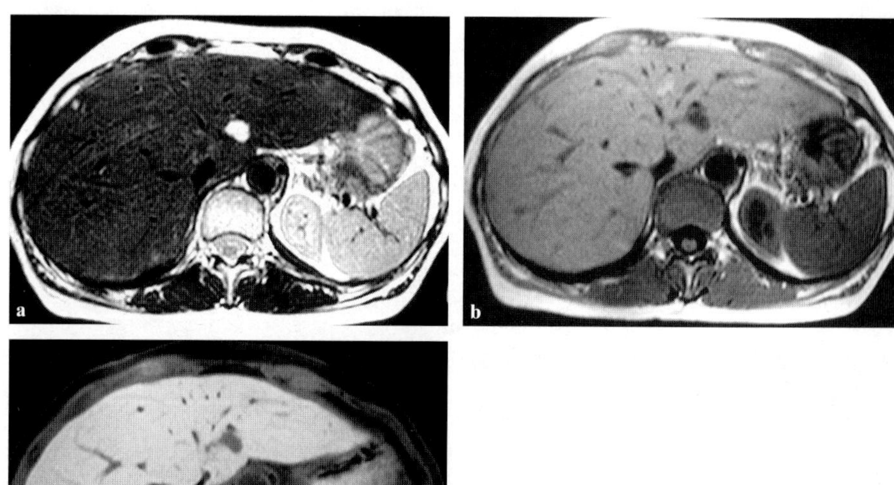

Fig. 63a-c. Metastases from melanoma. The same case as demonstrated in Fig. 59. All the lesions are hypointense on the hepatobiliary phase image after the administration of mangafodipir. On the basis of the signal intensity on unenhanced and hepatobiliary phase images, it is difficult to distinguish metastases from hemangioma

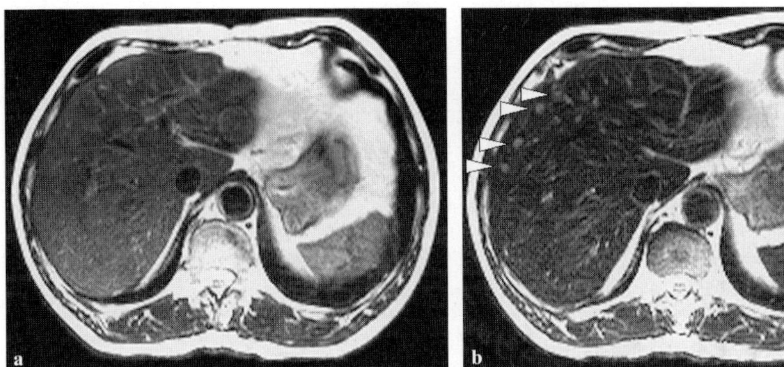

Fig. 64a,b. Metastases from colon cancer. Several small hyperintense nodules are demonstrated on the unenhanced Turbo SE T2-weighted image (**a**). After administration of ferumoxides (**b**), the lesions (*arrowheads*) do not show signal drop and are therefore better delineated. Additional nodules can also be seen

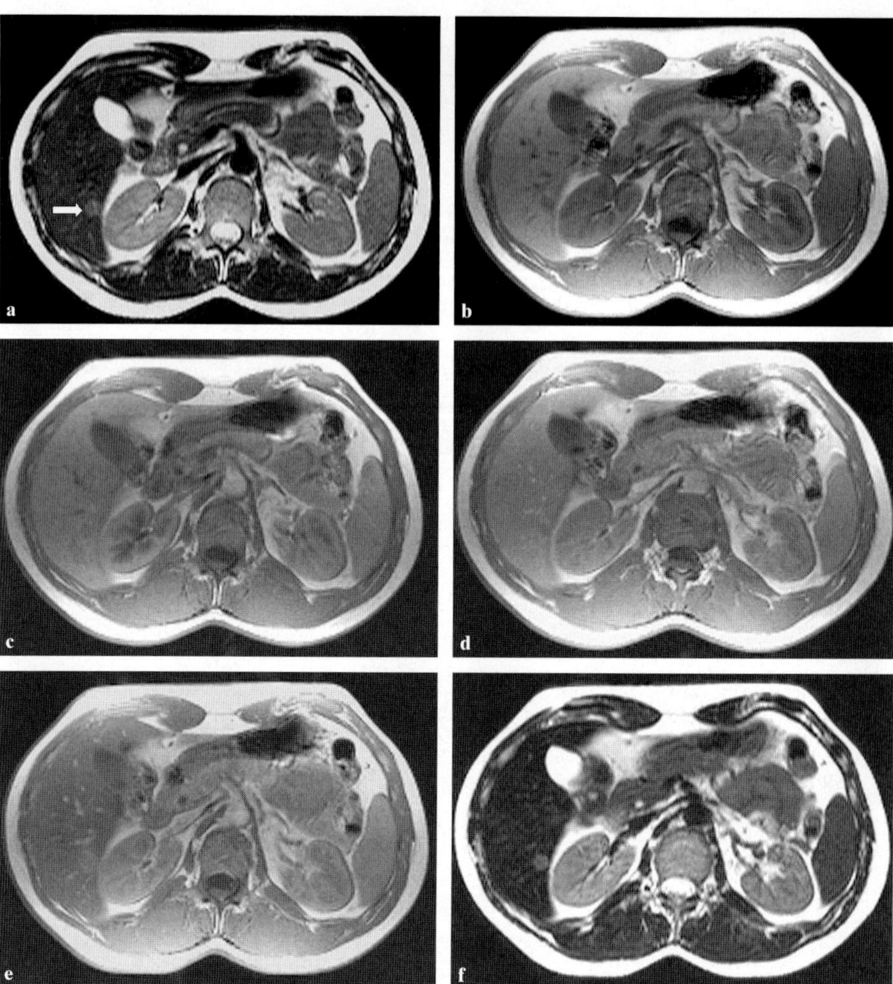

Fig. 65a-f. Metastases from melanoma. On the unenhanced Turbo SE T2-weighted image (**a**), a small hyperintense nodule (*arrow*) can be seen. On the GE T1-weighted image (**b**), the lesion is seen as hypointense and well-delineated. On dynamic phase images after the bolus injection of SHU 555 A, the nodule does not show significant enhancement (**c**, **d**). On GE T1-weighted images acquired 10 min after SHU 555 A administration (**e**), the signal of the parenchyma is decreased compared to that of the lesion, indicating the inability of the latter to take up the contrast agent. On the delayed phase Turbo SE T2-weighted image (**f**), the lesion appears brighter and better delineated as compared with unenhanced images

References

1. Agarwal VR, Takayama K, Van Wyk JJ, Sasano H, Simpson ER, Bulun SE. Molecular basis of severe gynecomastia associated with aromatase expression in fibrolamellar hepatocellular carcinoma. J Clin Endocrinol Metab 1998; 83:1797-1800.
2. Andreu V, Elizalde I, Mallafre C, Caballeria J, Salmeron JM, Sans M, Mas A, Bruguera M, Rods J. Plexiform neurofibromatosis and angiosarcoma of the liver in von Recklinghausen Disease. Am J Gastroenterol 1997; 92:1229-1230.
3. Baker ME, Paulson EK. Hepato metastatic disease. In Meyers M.A., ed. Neoplasms of the digestive tract: imaging, staging, and management. Philadelphia: Lippincott-Raven; 1998:361-395.
4. Bates SM, Keller MS, Ramos IM, Carter D, Taylor KJ. Hepatoblastoma: detection of tumor vascularity with Duplex Doppler US. Radiology 1990; 176:505-507.
5. Berk RN. Armbuster TG, Saltztein SL. Carcinoma in the porcelain gallbladder. Radiology 1973; 106:29-31.
6. Berman MM, Libbey NP, Foster JH. Hepatocellular carcinoma: polygonal cell type with fibrous stroma – an atypical variant with a favorable prognosis. Cancer 1980; 46:1448-1455.
7. Biemer JJ. Hepatic manifestation of lymphoma. Ann Clin Lab 1984; 14:252-260.
8. Bluemke DA, Soyer P, Fishman E. Helical (spiral) CT of the liver. Radiol Clin North Am 1995; 33:863-885.
9. Brady J, Liberatore F, Harper P, Greenwald P, Burnett W, Davies JN, Bishop M, Polan A, Vianna N. Angiosarcoma of the liver: an epidemiology survey. J Natl Cancer Inst 1977; 59:1383-1385.
10. Brandt DJ, Johnson CD, Stephens DH, Weiland LH. Imaging of fibrolamellar hepatocellular carcinoma. AJR 1988; 151:295-299.
11. Buetow PC, Buck JL, Ros PR, Goodman ZD. Malignant vascular tumors of the liver: radiologic-pathologic correlation. Radiographics 1994; 14:153-166.
12. Buetow PC, Buck JL, Pantongrag-Brown L, Marshall WH, Ros PR, Levine MS, Goodman ZD. Undifferentiated (embryonal) sarcoma of the liver: pathologic basis of imaging findings in 28 cases. Radiology 1997; 203:779-783.
13. Caillaud JM, Gerard-Marchant R, Marsden HB, van Unnik AJ, Rodary C, Rey A, Flamant F. Histopathological classification of childhood rhabdomyosarcoma: a report from the International Society of Pediatric Oncology pathology panel. Med Pediatr Oncol 1989; 17:391-400.
14. Campbell WL, Ferris JV, Holbert BL, Thaete FL, Baron RL. Biliary tract carcinoma complicating primary sclerosing cholangitis: evaluation with CT, cholangiography, US, and MR imaging. Radiology 1998; 207:41-50.
15. Carceller A, Blanchard H, Champagne J, St-Vil D, Bensoussan AL. Surgical resection and chemotherapy improve survival rate for patients with hepatoblastoma. J Ped Surg, 2001; 36:755-759.
16. Cariaga MT, Henson DE. Liver, gallbladder, extrahepatic bile ducts, and pancreas. Cancer 1995; 75:171-190.
17. Caty MG, Oldham KT, Prochownik EV. Embryonal rhabdomyosarcoma of the ampulla of Vater with long-term survival following pancreaticoduodenectomy. J Pediatr Surg 1990; 25:1256-1258.
18. Caudana R, Morana G, Pirovano GP, Nicoli N, Portuese A, Spinazzi A, Di Rito R, Pistolesi GF. Focal malignant hepatic lesions: MR imaging enhanced with Gadolinium Benzyloxypropionictetra-acetate (BOPTA)-preliminary results of phase II clinical application. Radiology 1996; 199:513-520.
19. Ch'en IY, Katz DS, Jeffrey RB Jr, Daniel BL, Li KC, Beaulieu CF, Mindelzun RE, Yao D, Olcott EW. Do arterial phase helical CT images improve detection or characterization of colorectal liver metastases?. Comput Assist Tomogr 1997; 21(3):391-397.
20. Chiao R, Mo L, Hall A, et al.. B-mode blood flow imaging. AIUM Annual Convention, San Francisco, California, USA, April 2-5 2000.
21. Choi BI, Kim CW, Han MC, Kim CY, Lee HS, Kim ST, Kim YI. Sonographic characteristic of small hepatocellular carcinoma. Gastrointestinal Radiol. 1989; 14:25-261.
22. Choi BI, Takayasu K, Han MC. Small hepatocellular carcinomas and associated nodular lesions of the liver: pathology, pathogenesis, and imaging findings. AJR 1993; 160:1177-1187.
23. Choi BI, Han JK, Hong SH, Kim TK, Song CS, Kim KW, Kim MJ, Han MC. Dysplastic nodules of the liver: imaging findings. Abdom Imaging 1999; 24:250-257.
24. Coffey RJ, Wiesner RH, Beaver SJ, et al.. Bile duct carcinoma: a late complication of end-stage primary sclerosing cholangitis. Hepatology 1984; 14:1056-1059.
25. Collier JD, Carpenter M, Burt AD, Bassendine MF. Expression of mutant p53 protein in hepatocellular carcinoma. Gut 1991; 35:98-100.
26. Corrigan K, Semelka RC. Dynamic contrast-enhanced MR imaging of fibrolamellar hepatocellular carcinoma. Abdom Imaging 1995; 20:122-125.
27. Craig JR. Mesenchymal tumors of the liver. Diagnostic problems for the surgical pathologist. Pathology 1994; 3:141-160.
28. Craig JR, Peters RL, Edmondson HA, Omata M. Fibrolamellar carcinoma of the liver: a tumor of adolescents and young adults with distinctive clinicopathologic features. Cancer 1980; 46:372-379.

29. Dachman AH, Pakter RL, Ros PR, Fishman EK, Goodman ZD, Lichtenstein JE. Hepatoblastoma: radiologic-pathologic correlation in 50 cases. Radiology 1987; 164:15-19.

30. Davey MS, Cohen MD. Imaging of gastrointestinal malignancy in childhood. Radiol Clin North Am. 1996; 34:717-742.

31. Del Pilar F, Redvanley RD. Primary hepatic malignant neoplasms. Radiol Clin North Am 1998; 36:333-348.

32. Enwonwu CO. The role of dietary aflatoxin in the genesis of hepatocellular cancer in the developing countries. Lancet 1984; 2:956-958.

33. Freeny PC, Baron RL, Teefey SA. Hepatocellular carcinoma: reduced frequency of typical findings with dynamic contrast-enhanced CT in a non-Asian population. Radiology 1992; 182:143-148.

34. Friedburg H, Kauffmann GW, Bohm N, Fiedler L, Jobke A. Sonographic and computed tomographic features of embryonal rhabdomyosarcoma of the biliary tract. Pediatr Radiol 1984; 14:436-438.

35. Friedman AC, Lichtenstein JE, Goodman Z, Fishman EK, Siegelman SS, Dachman AH. Fibrolamellar hepatocellular carcinoma. Radiology 1985; 157:583-587.

36. Fukayama M, Nihei Z, Takizawa T, Kawaguchi K, Harada H, Koike M. Malignant epithelioid hemangioendothelioma of the liver, spreading through the hepatic veins. Virchiws Arch A Pathol Anat Histopathol 1984; 404:275-287.

37. Furui S, Itai Y, Ohtomo K, Yamauchi T, Takenaka E, Iio M, Ibukuro K, Shichijo Y, Inoue Y. Hepatic epithelioid hemangioendothelioma: report of five cases. Radiology 1989; 171:63-68.

38. Gabata T, Matsui O, Kadoya M, Yoshikawa J, Ueda K, Kawamori Y, Takashima T, Nonomura A. Delayed MR imaging of the liver: correlation of delayed enhancement of hepatic tumors and pathologic appearance. Abdom Imaging 1998; 9:167-182.

39. Garber SJ, Donald JJ, Lees WR. Cholangiocarcinoma: ultrasound features and correlation with survival. Abdom Imaging 1993; 18:66-69.

40. Geoffray A, Couanet D, Montagne JP, Leclere J, Flamant F. Ultrasonography and computed tomography for diagnosis and follow-up of biliary tract rhabdomyosarcomas in children. Pediatr Radiol 1987; 17:127-131.

41. Goodman ZD. Nonparenchymal and metastatic malignant tumors of the liver. In Haubrich W.S., Schaffner F, Berk J.E. (eds): Bockus Gastroenterology. Philadelphia: WB Saunders, 1995; pp 2488-2500.

42. Grazioli L, Olivetti L, Fugazzola C, Benetti A, Stanga C, Dettori E, Gallo C, Matricardi L, Giacobbe A, Chiesa A. The pseudocapsule in hepatocellular carcinoma: correlation between dynamic MR imaging and pathology. Eur Radiol 1999; 9:62-67.

43. Grazioli L, Morana G, Caudana R, Benetti A, Portolani N, Talamini G, Colombari R, Pirovano G, Kirchin MA, Spinazzi A..: Hepatocellular carcinoma. Correlation between gadobenate Dimeglumine-enhanced MRI and pathologic findings. Invest Radiol 2000; 35 (1):25-34.

44. Gupta S, Udupa KN, Gupta S. Primary carcinoma of the gallbladder: a review of 328 cases. J Surg Oncol 1980; 14:35-44.

45. Hagspiel KD, Neidl KF, Eichenberger AC, Weder W, Marincek B. Detection of liver metastases: comparison of superparamagnetic Iron Oxide-enhanced and unenhanced MR imaging at 1.5 T with dynamic CT, intraoperative US, and percutanous US. Radiology 1995; 196:471-478.

46. Haliloglu M, Hoffer FA, Gronemeyer SA, Furman WL, Shochat SJ. 3D Gadolinium-enhanced MRA: evaluation of hepatic vasculature in children with hepatoblastoma. J Magn Reson Imaging 2000; 11:65-68.

47. Hardell L, Bengtsson NO, Jonsson U, Eriksson S, Larsson LG. Aetiological aspects of primary liver cancer with special regard to alcohol, organic solvents and acute intermittent porphyria – an epidemiological investigation. Br J Cancer 1984; 50:389-397.

48. Hayashi M, Matsui O, Ueda K, Kawamori Y, Kadoya M, Yoshikawa J, Gabata T, Takashima T, Nonomura A, Nakanuma Y. Correlation between the blood supply and grade of malignancy of hepatocellular nodules associated with liver cirrhosis: evaluation by CT during intraarterial injection of contrast medium. AJR 1999; 172:969-976.

49. Helmberger TK, Ros PR, Mergo PJ, Tomczak R, Reiser MF. Pediatric liver neoplasms: a radiologic-pathologic correlation. Eur Radiol 1999; 9:1339-1347.

50. Hollett MD, Jeffrey RB Jr, Nino-Murcia M, Jorgensen MJ, Harris DP. Dual phase helical CT of the liver: value of arterial-phase scans in the detection of small (<1.5 cm) malignant hepatic neoplasms. AJR 1995; 164:879-884.

51. Horn RC, Enterline HT. Rhabdomyosarcoma: a clinicopathological study and classification of 39 cases. Cancer 1958; 11:181-199.

52. Horowitz ME, Etcubanas E, Webber BL, Kun LE, Rao BN, Vogel RJ, Pratt CB. Hepatic undifferentiated (embryonal) sarcoma and rhabdomyosarcoma in children. Cancer 1987; 59:396-402.

53. Ichikawa T, Federle MP, Grazioli L, Madariaga J, Nalesnik M, Marsh W. Fibrolamellar hepatocellular carcinoma: imaging and pathologic findings in 31 recent cases. Radiology 1999; 213:352-361.

54. Imai Y, Murakami T, Yoshida S, Nishikawa M, Ohsawa M, Tokunaga K, Murata M, Shibata K, Zushi S, Kurokawa M, Yonezawa T, Kawata S, Takamura M, Nagano H, Sakon M, Monden M, Wakasa K,

Nakamura H. Superparamagnetic iron oxide-enhanced magnetic resonance images of hepatocellular carcinoma: correlation with histological grading. Hepatology 2000; 32:205-212.

55. Ishak KG. Mesenchymal tumors of the liver. In Okuda K, Peter R.L. (eds): Hepatocellular Carcinoma. New York: John Wiley e Sons, 1976, pp 228-587.

56. Ishak KG. Pathogenesis of liver diseases. In Farber E, Philips M.J., Kaufman N (eds): International Academy of Phatology Monograph, No.28. Baltimore: Williams & Wilkins, 1987, pp 314-315.

57. Ishak KG, Sesterhenn IA, Goodman ZD, Rabin L, Stromeyer FW. Epithelioid hemangioendothelioma of the liver: a clinicopathologic and follow-up study of 32 cases. Hum pathol 1984; 15:839-852.

58. Itai Y, Matsui O. Blood flow and liver imaging. Radiology 1997; 202:306-314.

59. Ito Y, Loijiro M, Nakshima T, et al. Pathomorphologic characteristics of 102 cases of thorotrast-related hepatocellular carcinoma, cholangiocarcinoma, and hepatic angiosarcoma. Cancer 1988; 62:1153-1162.

60. Jaffe ES: Malignant lymphoma: pathology of hepatic involvement. Semin Liver Dis 1987; 7:257-268.

61. Jang HJ, Lim HK, Lee WJ, Kim SH, Kim KA, Kim EY. Ultrasonographic evaluation of focal hepatic lesions: comparison of pulse inversion harmonic, tissue harmonic, and conventional imaging techniques. J Ultrasound Med 2000; 19:293-299.

62. Joshi SW, Merchant NH, Jambhekar NA. Primary multilocular cystic undifferentiated (embryonal) sarcoma of the liver in childhood resembling hydatid cyst of the liver. Br J Radiol 1997; 70:314-316.

63. Kelekis NL, Semelka RC, Siegelman ES, Ascher SM, Outwater EK, Woosley JT, Reinhold C, Mitchell DG. Focal hepatic lymphoma: magnetic resonance demonstration using current techniques including gadolinium enhancement. Magn Reson Imaging 1997; 15:625-636.

64. Kew MC. Hepatic tumors and cysts. In Feldman M, Scharschmidt B.F., Sleisenger M.H. (eds): Sleisenger and Fordtran's Gastrointestinal and Liver Disease (6th ed). Philadelphia: WB Saunders, 1998, pp 1364-1387.

65. Kim AY, Choi BI, Kim TK, et al.: Hepatocellular carcinoma: power Doppler US with a contrast agent-preliminary results. Radiology 1998; 209:135-140.

66. Kim T, Murakami T, Takahashi S, Tsuda K, Tomoda K, Narumi Y, Oi H, Sakon M, Nakamura H. Optimal phases of dynamic CT for detecting hepatocellular carcinoma: evaluation of unenhanced and triple-phase images. Abdom Imaging 1999; 24:473-480.

67. Kirks DR, Griscom NT. Hepatobiliary tumors. In Practical Pediatric Imaging. Diagnostic Radiology of Infants and Children. Lippincott-Raven 1998:954-969.

68. Klatskin G. Adenocarcinoma of the hepatic duct at its bifurcation within the porta hepatis. Am J Med 1965; 38:241-256.

69. Kojiro M. Hepatocellular nodular lesions. In Kojiro M (ed) Pathology of early hepatocellular carcinoma and related lesions. Tokyo: Medical Publishers, 1996; 148-165.

70. Kojiro M, Nakashima T. Pathology of hepatocellular carcinoma. In: Okuda K, Ishak K.G., eds. Neoplasms of the Liver. New York: Springer-Verlag, 1987, pp 81-104.

71. Krinsky GA, Lee VS, Theise ND, Weinreb JC, Rofsky NM, Diflo T, Teperman LW. Hepatocellular carcinoma and dysplastic nodules in patients with cirrhosis: prospective diagnosis with MR imaging and explanation correlation. Radiology 2001; 219:445-454.

72. Kuszyk BS, Bluemke DA, Urban BA, Choti MA, Hruban RH, Sitzmann JV, Fishman EK. Portal-phase contrast enhanced helical CT for the detection of malignant hepatic tumors: sensitivity based on comparison with intraoperative and pathologic findings. AJR 1996; 166:91-95.

73. LaBrecque DR. Neoplasia of the liver. In Kaplowitz N (ed): Liver and biliary disese (2nd ed). Baltimore: Williams and Wilkins, 1996, pp 391-438.

74. Lack EE, Perez-Atayde AR, Schuster SR. Botryoid rhabdomyosarcoma of the biliary tract: report of five cases with ultrastructural observations and literature review. Am J Surg Pathol 1981; 5:643-652.

75. Lai CL, Gregory PB, Wu PC, Lok AS, Wong KP, Ng MM. Hepatocellular carcinoma in Chinese males and females: Possible causes for male predominance. Cancer 1987; 60:1107-1110.

76. Landis SH, Murray T, Bolden S, Wingo PA. Cancer statistics. Cancer 1999, 49.8-31.

77. Lauffer JM, Zimmermann A, Krahenbuhl L, Triller J, Baer HU. Epithelioid hemangioendothelioma of the liver. Cancer 1996:78 (11):2318-2327.

78. Lee JH, Yang HM, Bak UB, Rim HJ. Promoting role of Clonorchis sinensis infection on induction of cholangiocarcinoma during two-step carcinogenesis. Korean J Parasitol 1994; 32:13-18.

79. Lencioni R, Pinto F, Armillotta N, Bartolozzi C. Assessment of tumor vascularity in hepatocellular carcinoma: comparison of power Doppler US and color Doppler US. Radiology 1996; 201:353-358.

80. Levin B. Gallbladder carcinoma. Ann Oncol 1999; 10 129-130.

81. Lewis KH, Chezmar JL. Hepatic metastases. Magn Reson Imaging Clin North Am 1997; 5:319-330.

82. Lim JH, Cho JM, Kim EY, Park CK. Dysplastic nodules in liver cirrhosis: evaluation of hemodynamics with CT during arterial portography and CT hepatic arteriography. Radiology 2000; 214:869-874.

83. Lim JH, Choi D, Cho SK, Kim SH, Lee WJ, Lim HK, Park CK, Paik SW, Kim YI. Conspicuity if hepatocellular nodular lesions in cirrhotic livers at ferumoxides-enhanced MR imaging: importance of Kupffer cell number. Radiology 2001; 220:669-676.

84. Linstedt-Hilden M, Brambs HJ. Two different manifestations of botryoid sarcoma (embryonal rhabdomyosarcoma) of the biliary tree. Bildgebung 1994; 61:40-43.
85. Locker GY, Doroshow JH, Zwelling LA, Chabner BA. The clinical features of hepatic angiosarcoma: a report of four cases and a review of the English literature. Medicine (Baltimore) 1979; 58:48-64.
86. Manfredi R, Maresca G, Baron RL, Cotroneo AR, De Gaetano AM, De Franco A, Pirovano G, Spinazzi A, Marano P. Manfredi R., Maresca G., Baron R.L., et al.: Delayed MR imaging of hepatocellular carcinoma enhanced by gadobenate dimeglumine (Gd-BOPTA). J Magn Reson Imaging 1999; 9:704-710.
87. Marcos-Alvarez A, Jenkins RL. Cholangiocarcinoma. Surg Oncol Clin North Am 1996; 5:301-316.
88. McLarney JK, Rucker PT, Bender GN, Goodman ZD, Kashitani N, Ros PR. Fibrolamellar carcinoma of the liver: radiologic-pathologic correlation. Radiographics 1999; 19:453-471.
89. Mihara S, Matsumoto H, Tokunaga F, Yano H, Ota M, Yamashita S. Botryoid rhabdomyosarcoma of the gallbladder in a child. Cancer 1982; 49:812-818.
90. Miller JH, Greenspan BS. Integrated imaging of hepatic tumors in childhood. Part. I: Malignant lesions (primary and metastatic). Radiology 1985; 154:83-90.
91. Miller WJ, Dodd GD 3rd, Federle MP, Baron RL. Epithelioid hemangioendothelioma of the liver: findings with pathologic correlation. AJR 1992: 159:53-57.
92. Moon WK, Kim WS, Kim IO, Yeon KM, Yu IK, Choi BI, Han MC. Undifferentiated embryonal sarcoma of the liver: US and CT findings. Pediatr Radiol 1994; 24:500-503.
93. Murakami T, Baron RL, Peterson MS, Oliver JH 3rd, Davis PL, Confer SR, Federle MP. Hepatocellular carcinoma: MR imaging with mangoafodipir trisodium (Mn-DPDP). Radiology 1996; 200:69-77.
94. Murakami T, Kim T, Nakamura H. Hepatitis, cirrhosis, and hepatoma. J.Magn Reson Imaging 1998; 8:346-358.
95. Murakami T, Kim T, Takamura M, Hori M, Takahashi S, Federle MP, Tsuda K, Osuga K, Kawata S, Nakamura H, Kudo M. Hypervascular hepatocellular carcinoma: detection with double arterial phase multidetector row helical CT. Radiology 2001; 218:763-767.
96. Nakashima T, Kojiro M. Hepatocellular carcinoma: An Atlas of Its Pathology. Tokyo: Springer-Verlag, 1987.
97. Nerlich AG, Majewski S, Hunzelmann N, Brenner RE, Wiebecke B, Muller PK, Kreig T, Remberger K... Excessive collagen formation in fibrolamellar carcinoma of the liver: a morphological and biochemical study. Mod Pathol. 1992; 5:580-585.
98. Newton WA Jr, Gehan EA, Webber BL, Marsden HB, van Unnik AJ, Hamoudi AB, Tsokos MG, Shimada H, Harms D, Schmidt D, et al. Classification of rhabdomyosarcoma and related sarcomas. Cancer 1995; 76:1073-1085.
99. Noguchi S, Yamamoto R, Tatsuta M, Kasugai H, Okuda S, Wada A, Tamura H. Cell features and patterns in fine-needle aspirates of hepatocellular carcinoma. Cancer 1986; 58:321-328.
100. Nzeako UC, Goodman ZD, Ishak KG. Hepatocellular carcinoma in cirrhotic and noncirrhotic livers: a clinico-histopathologic study of 804 North American patients. Am J Clin Pathol 1996; 105:65-75.
101. Ohsawa M, Aozasa K, Horiuchi K, Kataoka M, Hida J, Shimada H, Oka K, Wakata Y. Malignant lymphoma of the liver. Dig Dis Sci 1992; 37:1105-1109.
102. Oliver JH 3rd, Baron RL, Federle MP, Rockette HE Jr. Detecting hepatocellular carcinoma: value of unenhanced or arterial phase CT imaging or both used in conjunction with conventional portal venous phase contrast-enhanced CT imaging. AJR 1996; 167:71-77.
103. Orsatti G, Hytiroglou P, Thung SN, Ishak KG, Paronetto F. Lamellar fibrosis in the fibrolamellar variant of hepatocellular carcinoma: a role for transforming growth factor beta. Liver 1997; 12:152-156.
104. Parker SL, Tong T, Bolden S, Wingo PA. Cancer statistics. CA Cancer J Clin 1997; 47:5-13.
105. Patil KK, Omojola MF, Khurana P, Iyengar JK. Embryonal rhabdomyosarcoma within a choledochal cyst. Can Assoc Radiol J 1992; 43:145-148.
106. Paulson E.K. Evaluation of the liver for metastatic disease. Semin in Liver Disease 2001; 21 (2):225-235.
107. Peterson MS, Murakami T, Baron RL. MR imaging patterns of gadolinium retention within liver neoplasms. Abdom Imaging 1998; 23:592-599.
108. Peterson MS, Baron RL, Rankin SC. Hepatic angiosarcoma: findings on multiphasic contrast-enhanced helical CT do not mimic hepatic hemangioma. Am J Roentgenol 2000; 175:165-170.
109. Peterson MS, Baron RL, Marsh JW Jr, Oliver JH 3rd, Confer SR, Hunt LE. Pretransplantation surveillance for possible hepatocellular carcinoma in patients with cirrhosis: epidemiology and CT-based tumor detection rate in 430 cases with surgical pathologic correlation. Radiology; 2000; 217:743-749.
110. Pobiel RS, Bisset III GS. Pictorial essay: imaging of liver tumors in the infant and child. Pediatr Radiol 1995; 25:495-506.
111. Polk HC. Carcinoma and the calcified gallbladder. Gastroenterology 1966; 50:582-585.
112. Roebuck DJ, Yang WT, Lam WW, Stanley P. Hepatobiliary rhabdomyosarcoma in children: diagnostic radiology. Pediatr Radiol 1998; 28:101-108.
113. Rofsky NM, Earls JP. Mangafodipir trisodium injection (Mn-DPDP). A contrast agent for abdominal MR imaging. Magn Reson Imaging Clin N Am 1996; 4:73-85

114. Ros PR, Taylor HM. Malignant Tumors of the liver. Textbook of gastrointenstinal radiology, Vol II, second edition. Copyright 2000:1523-1568.
115. Ros PR, Olmsted WW, Dachman AH, Goodman ZD, Ishak KG, Hartman DS. Undifferentiated (embryonal) sarcoma of the liver: radiologic pathologic correlation. Radiology 1986; 160:141-145.
116. Ros PR, Murphy BJ, Buck JL, Olmedilla G, Goodman Z. Encapsulated hepatocellular carcinoma: radiologic findings and pathologic correlation. Gastrointest Radiol 1990; 15:233-237.
117. Runge VM, Lee C, Williams NM. Detectability of small liver metastases with gadolinium BOPTA. Invest Radiol 1997; 32:557-565.
118. Ruymann FB, Raney RB Jr, Crist WM, Lawrence W Jr, Lindberg RD, Soule EH. for the Intergroup Rhabdomyosarcoma Study of CCSG and POG. Rabdomyosarcoma of the biliary tree in childhood: a report from the Intergroup Rhabdomyosarcoma Study. Cancer 1985; 56:575-581.
119. Ryan J, Straus DJ, Lange C. Primary lymphoma of the liver. Cancer 1988; 61:370-375.
120. Sagoh T, Itoh K, Togashi K, Shibata T, Minami S, Noma S, Yamashita K, Nishimura K, Asato R, Mori K, et al.. Gallbladder carcinoma: evaluation with MR imaging. Radiology 1990; 174:131-136.
121. Sakamoto M, Hirohashi S, Shimosato Y. Early stages of multistep hepatocarcinogenesis: adenomatous hyperplasia and early hepatocellular carcinoma. Hum Pathol 1991; 22:172-178.
122. Sanders LM, Botet JF, Straus DJ, Ryan J, Filippa DA, Newhouse JH. CT of primary lymphoma of the liver. AJR 1989; 152:973-976.
123. Schweizer P, Schweizer M, Wehrmann M. Major resection for embryonal rhabdomyosarcoma of the biliary tree. Pediatr Surg Int 1994; 9:268-273.
124. Seneterre E, Taourel P, Bouvier Y, Pradel J, Van Beers B, Daures JP, Pringot J, Mathieu D, Bruel JM. Detection of hepatic metastases: Ferumoxides-enhanced MR Imaging versus unenhanced MR Imaging and CT during arterial portography. Radiology 1996; 200:785-792.
125. Sherlock S, Dooley J. Diseases of the liver and biliary system (9th ed). Oxford: Blackwell Scientific, 1993, pp 44-61.
126. Shirkhoda A, Ros PR, Farah J, Staab EV. Lymphoma of the solid abdominal viscera. Radiol Clin North Am 1990; 28:785-799.
127. Siegel MJ. Pediatric liver imaging. Seminars in liver disease 2001; 21:251-269.
128. SIOPEL III. International society of pediatric oncology: Liver tumours studies. Hepatoblastoma and Hepatocellular Carcinoma. 1998.
129. Smalley SR, Moertel CG, Hilton JF, Weiland LH, Weiand HS, Adson MA, Melton LJ 3rd, Batts K. Hepatoma in the noncirrhotic liver. Cancer 1988; 62:1414-1424.
130. Sons HU, Borchard F, Joel BS. Carcinoma of the gallbladder: autopsy findings in 287 cases and review of the literature. J Surg Oncol 1985; 28:199-206.
131. Soyer P, Roche A, Levesque M, Legmann P. CT of fibrolamellar hepatocellular carcinoma. J Computed Assist Tomogr. 1991; 14:533-538.
132. Soyer P, Gouhiri M, Boudiaf M, Brocheriou-Spelle I, Kardache M, Fishman EK, Rymer R. Carcinoma of the gallbladder: imaging features with surgical correlation. AJR 1997; 169:781-784.
133. Stevens WR, Johnson CD, Stephens DH, Nagorney DM. Fibrolamellar hepatocellular carcinoma: stage at presentation and results of aggressive surgical management. AJR 1995; 164:1153-1158.
134. Stocker JT, Ishak KG. Undifferentiated (embryonal) sarcoma of the liver. Report of 31 cases. Cancer 1978; 42:336-348.
135. Sussman EB, Nydick J, Gray GF. Hemangioendothelial sarcoma of the liver and hemochromatosis. Arch Pathol Lab Med 1974; 97:39-42.
136. Takano H, Smith WL. Gastrointestinal tumors of childhood. Radiol Clin North Am. 1997; 35:1374.
137. Tamburro CH. Relationship of vinyl monomers and liver cancers: angiosarcoma and hepatocellular carcinoma. Semin Liver Dis 1984; 4:158-169.
138. Thorsen MK, Quiroz F, Lawson TL, Smith DF, Foley WD, Stewart ET. Primary biliary carcinoma: CT evaluation. Radiology 1984; 152:479-483.
139. Tsuchida Y, Ikeda H, Suzuki N, Takahashi A, Kuroiwa M, Sakai M, Shimizu H, Shitara T, Yamanouchi H, Hirato J.. A case of well differentiated, fetal-type hepatoblastoma with very low serum alpha-fetoprotein. J Ped Surg 1999; 34:1762-1764.
140. Van Beers B, Roche A, Mathieu D, Menu Y, Delos M, Otte JB, Lalonde L, Pringot J. Epithelioid hemangioendothelioma of the liver: MR and CT findings. J Comput Assist Tomogr 1992; 16:420-424.
141. Walker NI, Horn MJ, Strong RW, et al. Undifferentiated (embryonal) sarcoma of the liver. Pathologic findings and long-term survival after complete surgical resection. 1992; 69:52-59.
142. Wang C, Ahlstrom H, Ekholm S, Fagertun H, Hellstrom M, Hemmingsson A, Holtas S, Isberg B, Jonnson E, Lonnemark-Magnusson M, McGill S, Wallengren NO, Westman L..: Diagnostic efficacy of Mn-DPDP in MR imaging of the liver. A phase III multicentre study. Acta Radiol 1997; 38:643-649.
143. Weiss SW, Enzinger FM. Epithelioid hemangioendothelioma: a vascular tumor often mistaken for a carcinoma. Cancer 1982; 50:970-981.
144. Wernecke K, Peters PE, Kruger KG. Ultrasonographic patterns of focal hepatic and splenic lesions in Hodgkin's and non-Hodgkin lymphoma. The British Journal of Radiology 1987; 60:655-660.

145. Wilbur AC, Sagireddy PB, Aizenstein RI. Carcinoma of the gallbladder: color Doppler ultrasound and CT findings. Abdom Imaging 1997:22:187-190.
146. Winston CB, Schwartz LH, Fong Y, Blumgart LH, Panicek DM. Hepatocellular carcinoma: MR imaging findings in cirrhotic livers and noncirrhotic livers. Radiology 1999; 210:75-79.
147. Worawattanakul S, Semelka RC, Kelekis NL, Woosley JT. Angiosarcoma of the liver: MR imaging pre- and post chemotherapy. Magn Reson Imaging 1997; 15:613-617.
148. Worawattanakul S, Semelka RC, Noone TC, Calvo BF, Kelekis NL, Woosley JT. Cholangiocarcinoma: specrum of appearances on MR images using current techniques. Magn Reson Imaging 1998; 16:993-1003.
149. Yamanaka N, Okamoto E, Ando T, Oriyama T, Fujimoto J, Furukawa K, Tanaka T, Tanaka W, Nishigami T. Clinicopathologic spectrum of resected extraductal mass-forming intrahepatic cholangio-carcinoma. Cancer 1995; 76:2449-2456.
150. Yamashita Y, Fan ZM, Yamamoto H, Matsukawa T, Yoshimatsu S, Miyazaki T, Sumi M, Harada M, Takahashi M..: Spin-echo and dynamic gadolinium-enhanced FLASH MR imaging of hepatocellular carcinoma: correlation with histopathologic findings. J Magn Reson 1994; 4:83-90.
151. Yeo CJ, Pitt HA, Cameron JL. Cholangiocarcinoma. Surg Clin North Am 1990; 70:1429-1447.
152. Yoon W, Kim JK, Kang HK. Hepatic undifferentiated embryonal sarcoma: MR findings. J Computed Assist Tomogr 1997; 21:100-102.
153. Yoshida Y, Imai Y, Murakami T, Nishikawa M, Kurokawa M, Yonezawa T, Tokunaga K, Fukushima Y, Wakasa K, Kim T, Nakamura H, Sakon M, Monden M. Intrahepatic cholangiocarcinoma with marked hypervascularity. Abdom Imaging 1999; 24:66-68.
154. Yu JS, Kim KW, Kim EK, Lee JT, Yoo HS. Contrast enhancement of small hepatocellular carcinomas: usefulness of three successive early image acquisitions during multiphase dynamic MR imaging. AJR 1999; 173:597-604.

6   Imaging of Diffuse Liver Disease

Contents

6.1 Fatty Liver

Accumulation of fat within hepatocytes is commonly found in patients suffering from diabetes mellitus or obesity and after exposure to ethanol or other chemical toxins. In addition, in patients with advanced malignant neoplasms, fatty changes of the liver may be present due to poor nutrition and the hepatotoxic effects of chemotherapy. In most cases, fatty liver is associated with elevated levels of hepatic transaminases [48, 74].

Fatty changes are distributed either diffusely giving rise to a patchy pattern, or present as focal lesions. Frequently, the deposition of fat in the liver reflects regional differences in perfusion. Regions with a decreased portal flow accumulate less fat than areas that have normal or increased perfusion [2].

Generally, fatty changes of the liver have a characteristic pattern. In cases of entire fatty infiltration of the liver, the medial segment of the left lobe adjacent to the falciform ligament tends to accumulate fat, while the other side of the medial segment adjacent to the portal vein usually does not show any pathological changes [78]. A characteristic wedge-shape in certain regions of the liver is frequently indicative of fatty infiltration. Unfortunately, these findings are not sufficiently specific to enable a definitive diagnosis. With computed tomography (CT) imaging, the absence of a mass effect and the presence of normal vascular structures within

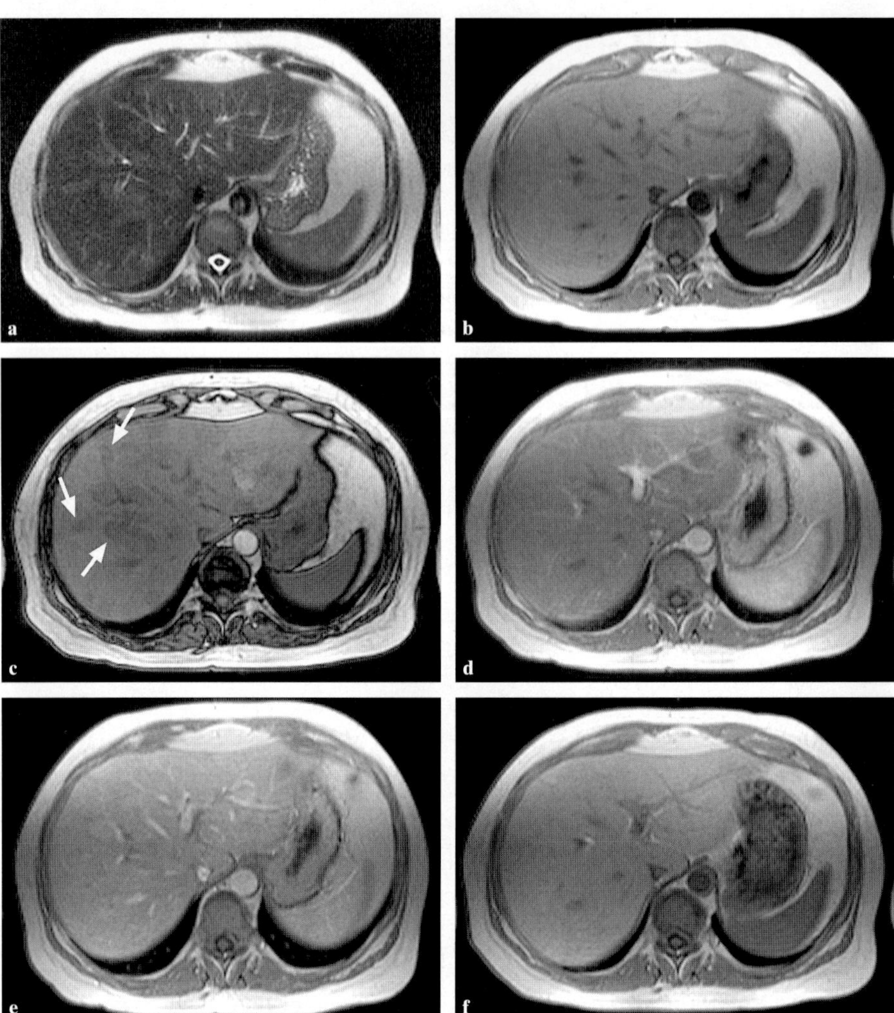

Fig. 1a-f. Diffuse focal fatty infiltration of the liver. A 54-year old female patient six months after high-dose chemotherapy for breast cancer. A follow-up CT study showed multiple hypodense liver lesions suspected to be metastases. Whereas on T2w (**a**) and T1w (**b**) unenhanced images hardly any liver lesions are visible, opposed phase images (**c**) show diffusely distributed hypointense areas (*arrows*). On dynamic and delayed imaging after Gd-BOPTA (0.05 mmol/kg body weight (BW) [(**d**) arterial phase, (**e**) portal venous phase, (**f**) hepatobiliary phase] no regional changes of hepatic blood flow and no differences in Gd-BOPTA uptake can be seen, indicating that no focal liver lesions are present. Overall, MRI allows the diagnosis of diffuse focal fatty infiltration of the liver following high-dose chemotherapy

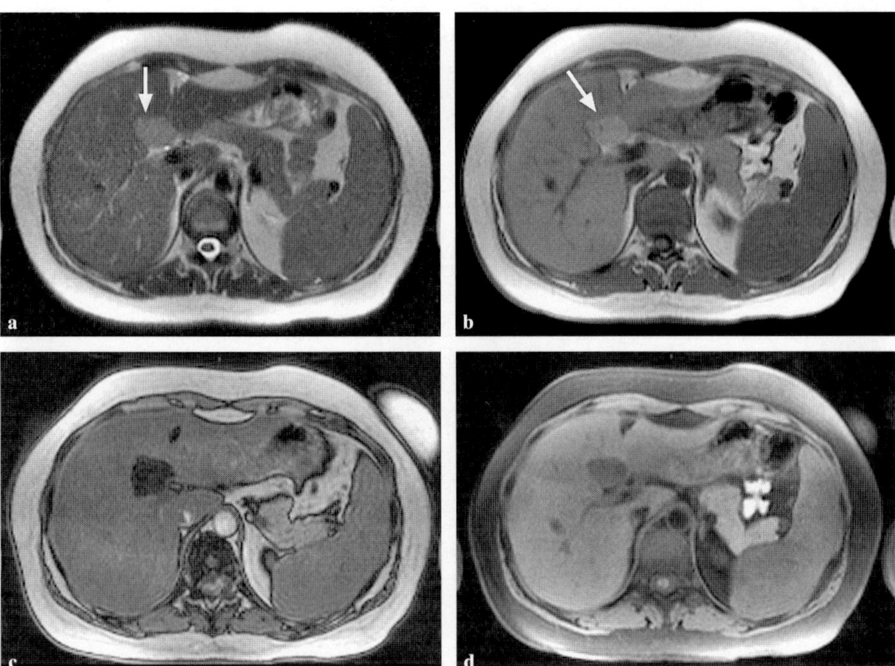

Fig. 2a-d. Focal fatty infiltration of the liver. Typical case of focal fatty infiltration in the area of the portal vein bifurcation. A 62-year old female patient with a history of sigmoid colorectal cancer. Routine follow-up ultrasound detected a focal liver lesion near the liver hilum, indicative of a metastasis of colorectal carcinoma. With MRI both T2w (**a**) and T1w (**b**) images reveal a focal hyperintense liver lesion (*arrows*). The high signal intensity on both T1w and T2w images makes the diagnosis of a liver metastasis of colorectal carcinoma unlikely. Both opposed phase (**c**) and T1w images with fat saturation (fs) (**d**) reveal a significant drop in signal intensity, which allows the accurate diagnosis of focal fatty infiltration of the liver. In this case the high fat content means that even T1w fs images show a significant drop in signal intensity compared to the normal parenchyma

the focal fatty lesions can be considered as helpful to the diagnosis, particularly in very large lesions. With magnetic resonance (MR) imaging, conventional T1-weighted (T1w) spin echo sequences are relatively insensitive to fatty infiltration with differences in signal intensity of only 5-15% between normal liver tissue and tissue containing at least 10% triglycerides.

T2-weighted (T2w) images, moreover, are especially insensitive to fatty infiltration. Thus, the diagnosis of a diffuse or focal fatty infiltration of the liver is based upon the exclusion of a focal or diffuse pathological process. In particular, comparison of CT scans that show regions of decreased attenuation with T2w MR images that show no pathological changes and T1w images that depict a slightly bright lesion may point to the presence of fatty infiltration. With the evolution of chemical shift imaging an accurate differential diagnosis of fatty lesions in the liver is now possible. Thus, fatty infiltration of the liver no longer represents a major diagnostic problem with MRI [32, 77].

In chemical shift imaging, the signal from water and fat is separated on the basis of differences in resonance frequency. This allows an absolute diagnosis of focal or

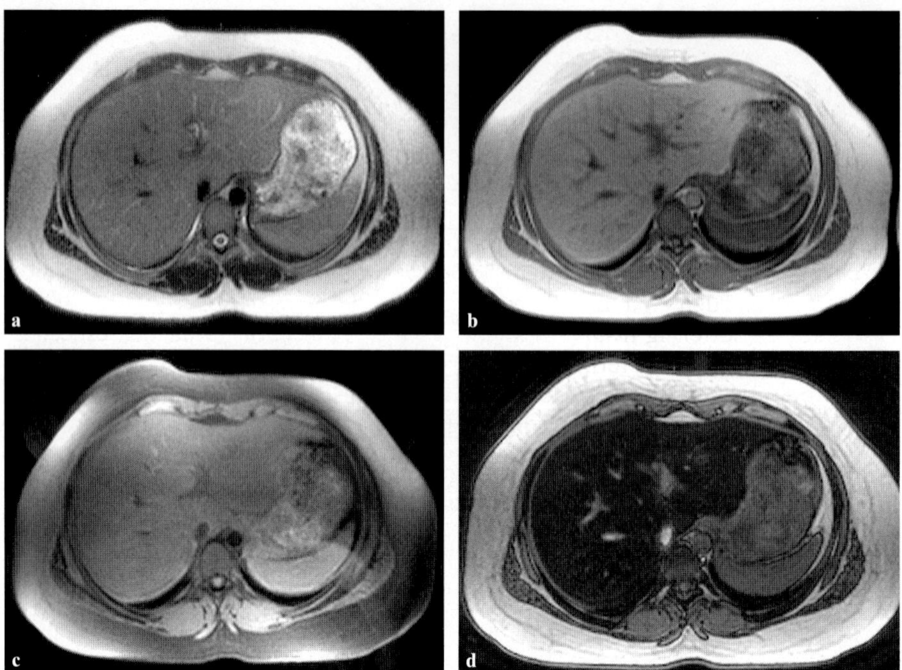

Fig. 3a-d. Diffuse fatty liver. A 26-year old female patient with obesity. Both T2w (**a**) and T1w (**b**) unenhanced images reveal an unusually high signal intensity of the liver parenchyma. In this case T1w fs (**c**) images do not allow the diagnosis of diffuse fatty liver because the signal intensity of the liver is not markedly different from that on T1w images. However, opposed phase images (**d**) easily allow the diagnosis of diffuse fatty liver because of the dramatic reduction of liver parenchyma signal intensity

diffuse fatty infiltration. Apart from the case of lipoma of the liver, opposed phase images are more sensitive for the detection of fatty liver than fat-suppressed images. The intensity in opposed phase images is determined from the absolute value of water intensity minus the fat intensity. Thus, whereas most tissues (including fat) appear similar on in-phase and opposed phase images, fatty liver will be noticeably darker. If, for example, in a given case of focal fatty infiltration fat accounts for 10% of the signal intensity (SI) of the lesion and water accounts for 90% on in-phase images, fat-suppression, assuming that the fat signal is totally suppressed, will lead to an image in which the lesion still has 90% of the signal. However, if opposed phase imaging is applied, using the same repetition time (TR) as on in-phase images, the SI of the lesion will drop to 80% of the in-phase signal (90% water signal minus 10% fat signal) thereby making it easier to detect the signal drop on MR images.

In the case of liver lipoma which contains only fat, the signal of the lesion will not change to any noticeable extent on opposed phase images. On the other hand, on fat-suppressed images the SI of the lesion will drop significantly. (Fig. 1-3)

6.2   Inflammatory Disease

6.2.1   Viral Hepatitis

Acute viral hepatitis is diagnosed primarily by clinical or serological examination; cross sectional imaging is not normally part of the primary diagnostic approach. Typical MR findings in acute viral hepatitis are hepatomegaly combined with edema of the liver capsule. In fulminant forms of acute viral hepatitis diffuse or focal necrosis may be detected on MR images.

In patients suffering from chronic hepatitis, cross sectional imaging, especially MRI, is performed to determine the presence of cirrhosis or ascites and to screen for the presence of hepatocellular carcinoma (HCC). As a frequently occurring, but non-specific sign, a region of high signal intensity surrounding the portal vein branches can be found on T2w images in patients suffering from acute or chronic active hepatitis [38]. In addition, diffuse or regional high signal areas can be identified on T2w images [58, 59].

Typically, in patients with viral hepatitis enlarged lymph nodes can be found at the liver hilum presenting as solitary or confluent. However, in contrast to lymph node metastasis, the portal veins and other structures are not compressed and maintain their shape.

6.2.2   Sclerosing Cholangitis

Sclerosing cholangitis is a disease that affects the intra- and extrahepatic biliary system. Although it may have a variety of pathogenic origins, the histopathological changes are generally comparable. The biliary tracts, in particular, are affected by an intense inflammatory fibrosis [10]. Additionally, enlarged lymphatic nodules localized in the liver hilum may be found. Although the hepatic parenchyma usually presents as normal, a fulminate form of sclerosing cholangitis may occur, leading to liver failure and portal hypertension [80].

Typical findings with MR imaging are diffusely distributed regions of biliary dilatation and areas of periportal inflammation. These features are best distinguished on heavily T2w images when the biliary dilatation presents as areas showing a fluid-equivalent signal localized along branches of the portal veins. On the other hand, periportal inflammation shows a decreased signal intensity on T1w images, while a signal intermediate between that of liver tissue and bile is seen on T2w images. These imaging findings are typically localized in the liver hilum and accompany the intrahepatic portal tracts surrounding the portal vein branches but not the hepatic veins, which are unaffected by this disease. For the differential diagnosis of sclerosing cholangitis, periportal inflammation, biliary obstruction, hepatitis and periportal neoplasm each have to be taken into consideration.

Patients suffering from sclerosing cholangitis frequently develop an occult thrombosis of the main or segmental portal vein as a result of the periportal inflammatory process. This may subsequently lead to a segmental atrophy [9, 28] (Fig. 4).

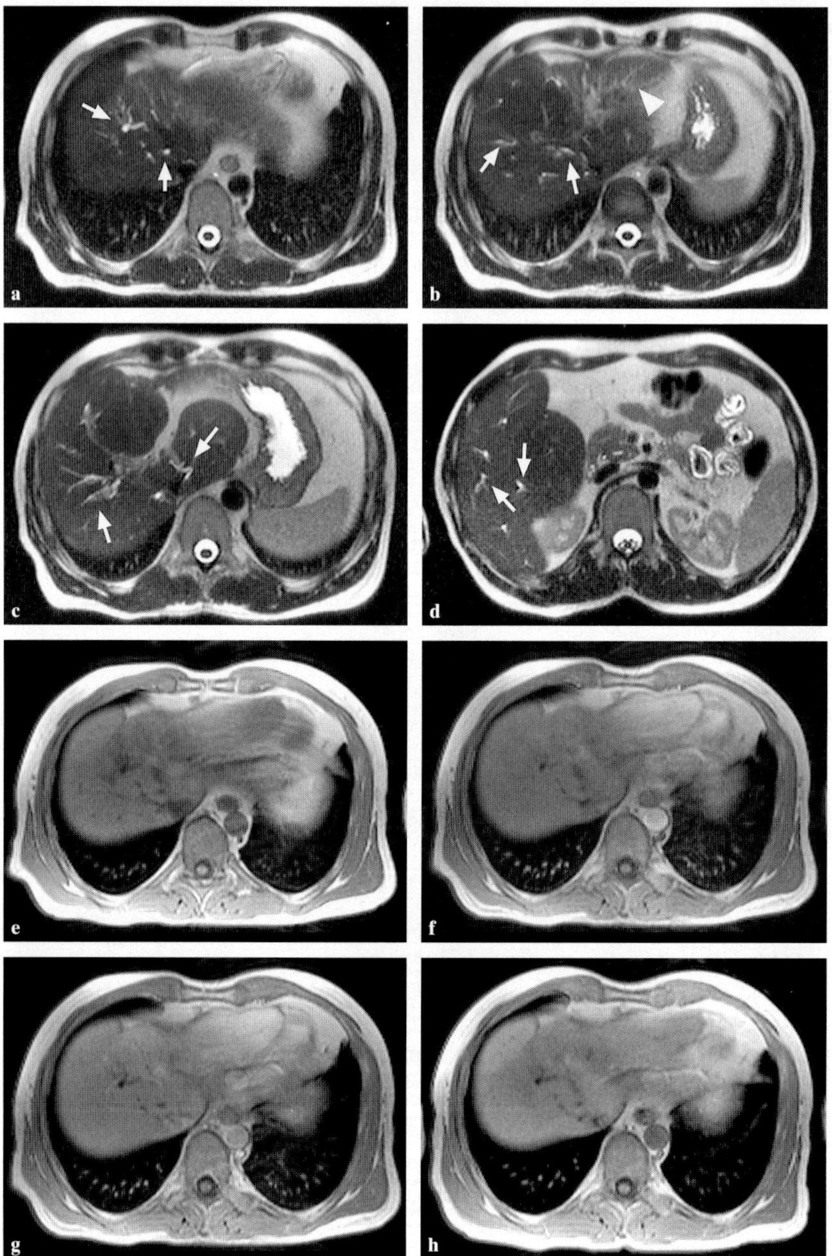

Fig. 4a-h. Primary sclerosing cholangitis. T2w images (**a-d**) show diffusely distributed regions of biliary dilatation (*arrows*) as well as segmental atrophy (*arrowhead in* **b**) of segments 2 and 3 of the liver. Due to the
already advanced stage of the disease, hypertrophy of segment 1 (**c**) can be detected. Unenhanced T1w images (**e**) show a decreased signal intensity of the liver parenchyma. On T1w dynamic imaging [(**f**) arterial phase, (**g**) portal-venous phase] an irregular enhancement due to inflammatory changes can be detected. In the
hepatobiliary phase (**h**), after injection of 0.05 mmol/kg BW Gd-BOPTA, a patchy pattern of the liver can
be detected which corresponds to the affected areas of liver parenchyma in which uneven uptake and excretion of the contrast medium occurs.

6.2.3   Radiation Induced Hepatitis

Due to its size and anatomical location in the abdomen the liver is frequently affected secondarily during radiation therapy of extrahepatic malignancies. Within six months of radiation injury, diffuse edema of the liver can be seen which appears as increased signal intensity on T2w images and decreased signal intensity on T1w images [68].

Portal flow is generally reduced in patients with radiation injured regions of the liver, and, as in the case of patients with concomitant fatty infiltration, the deposition of fat in these areas is usually reduced [22].

6.3   Cirrhosis

Hepatic cirrhosis is a disease that leads to irreversible fibrosis of the parenchyma. It is localized in the spaces between the portal tracts and destroys the normal hepatic architecture. However, the development of cirrhosis in patients suffering from viral hepatitis is frequently inhibited by treatment with interferon [14].

Generally, diagnosis of liver cirrhosis is achieved by histological examination of a liver biopsy, whereas imaging is performed to determine the anatomical distribution of the disease.

Typical features of advanced hepatic cirrhosis in diagnostic imaging are nodular contours and enlargement of the caudate lobe and lateral segment of the left lobe combined with atrophy of the right lobe [26, 59]. However, regional hypertrophy of certain liver segments, such as the caudate lobe, and atrophy of the right lobe are less likely to occur in alcohol induced liver cirrhosis, which is one of the more frequent causes of liver cirrhosis [24].

As liver atrophy seems to be localized around the portal vein and the liver hilum, an empty region in the gallbladder fossa is typically depicted, which contains periportal fat. Although cirrhosis affects the entire organ, the actual volume of fibrous scar tissue is very small compared with the whole liver volume and thus it has little influence on the relaxation times of hepatocellular tissue. For this reason, cirrhosis alone is difficult to depict on MRI [25].

However, as liver cirrhosis is often accompanied by hepatitis or inflammation, cirrhotic livers frequently show prolonged T1 and/or T2 relaxation times [66].

Furthermore, cirrhotic livers tend to accumulate iron, which leads to a decreased hepatic signal intensity. Frequently the distorsion and nodular appearance of intrahepatic vessels is helpful for the diagnosis of cirrhosis on MR images.

Similarly, the decreased caliber of segmental veins compared with the intrahepatic inferior vena cava can be interpreted as a sign of liver cirrhosis [42] (Fig. 5).

6.3.1   Regenerative Nodules

Regenerative nodules frequently arise in cirrhotic livers as a result of heterogeneous regeneration in the grossly distorted liver architecture. These lesions, which are usually less than 5 mm in diameter, show a heterogeneous pattern on MR images. Larger regenerative nodules, measuring more than 5 mm in diameter, can be found in about one third of cirrhotic livers, while nodules larger than 10 mm only occur in about 10% of cases [72].

Regenerative nodules on ultrasound and CT may mimic neoplasms such as HCC, which is a misinterpretation frequently underlined by the fact that intrahepatic vessels are displaced by mass effects. MR imaging is superior for the diagnosis of regenerative nodules because of its better soft tissue contrast. The typical nodular pattern which is due to inflammatory fibrous septa surrounding each regenerative nodule is best depicted on mildly T2w images [49].

An increased deposition of iron compared with surrounding normal liver cells occurs in 25% of regenerative nodules [65]. Hence, their identification as regions with decreased signal intensity on T2w or gradient echo images is improved [64].

Furthermore, the contrast between the fibrous septa and the normal liver parenchyma can be increased by the application of exogenous iron oxide-based contrast agents [18].

As liver cirrhosis with regenerative nodules may also occur in patients suffering from fatty infiltration or presenting with fatty regenerative nodules, opposed-phase T1w imaging is often appropriate to clarify the diagnosis. Since regenerative nodules consist of normal hepatic cells, MRI is the imaging modality of primary choice to exclude HCC, which can usually be differentiated from regenerative nodules due to its increased signal intensity on T2w images. In some cases regenerative nodules may appear as slightly hyperintense on T1w sequences. This is particularly the case when the signal of the surrounding liver parenchyma is reduced due to fibrosis and in cases in which the nodules have accumulated fat [39] (Fig. 6).

Regenerative nodules should be distinguished from the so-called nodular regenerative hyperplasia, which is characterized by multiple hyperplastic nodules occurring in a non-cirrhotic liver. These nodules may sometimes mimic cirrhosis, however, they do not show the tendency to accumulate fat or iron [13].

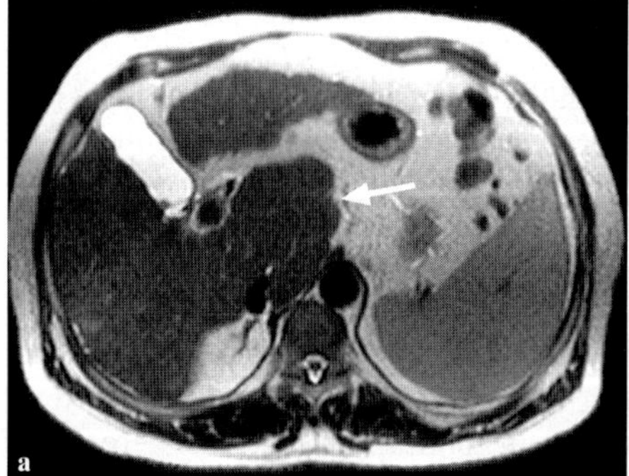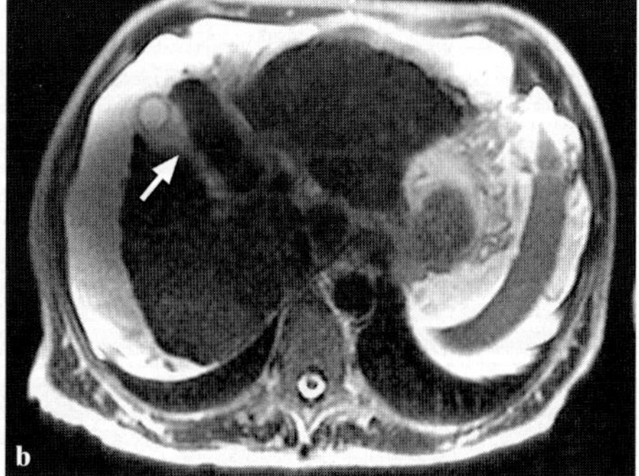

Fig. 5a,b. Typical findings in hepatic cirrhosis. T2w images (**a**, **b**), show nodular contours of the liver surface, enlargement of the caudate lobe (*arrow in* **a**), ascites and atrophy of the right liver lobe with subsequent hypertrophy of the left lobe. Additionally, a typically empty region in the gallbladder fossa (*arrow in* **b**) can be depicted which corresponds to periportal fat

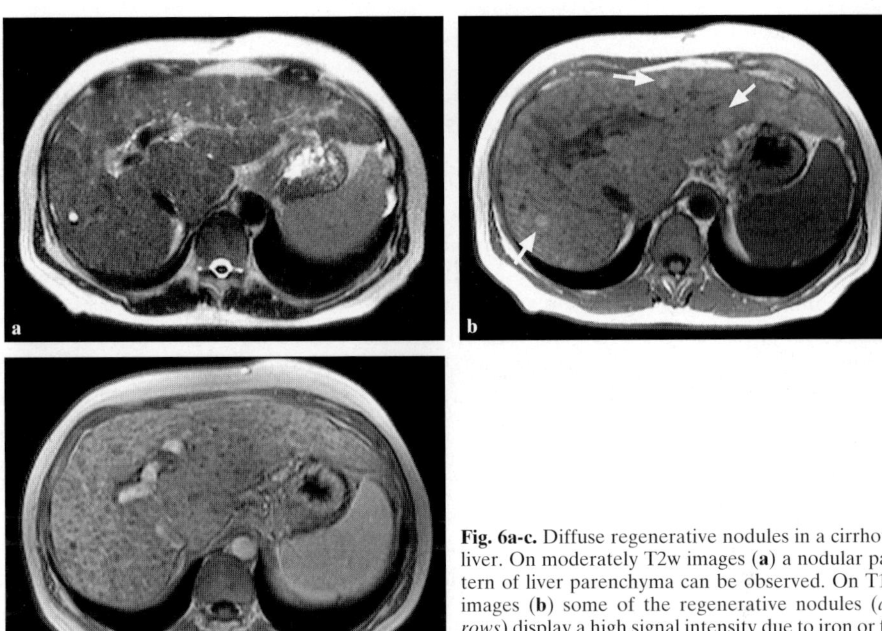

Fig. 6a-c. Diffuse regenerative nodules in a cirrhotic liver. On moderately T2w images (**a**) a nodular pattern of liver parenchyma can be observed. On T1w images (**b**) some of the regenerative nodules (*arrows*) display a high signal intensity due to iron or fat content. On T1w contrast enhanced images (**c**) the diffuse nodular pattern is displayed more clearly

6.3.2 Portal Hypertension

Portal hypertension is frequently a systemic complication of liver cirrhosis and may be caused by an obstruction at the post-sinusoidal (e.g. hepatic vein), sinusoidal (e.g. cirrhosis) or pre-sinusoidal (e.g. portal vein) level [27].

The most common cause of portal hypertension is liver cirrhosis in which there are complications such as variceal bleeding, ascites and splenomegaly. A primary consequence of the increased pressure in the portal tract is the dilatation of vessels. Later, as a result of the development of porto-systemic shunting, the blood flow to the liver diminishes and the size of the portal vessels is reduced again. The increased porto-systemic shunting results in less effective metabolism of absorbed nutrients and the accumulation of toxic metabolites, such as ammonia, in the blood. This may lead to the clinical manifestation of hepatic encephalopathy. As decreased portal flow correlates with the presence of liver atrophy, porto-systemic shunting or portal hypertension contributes to the further regression of liver parenchyma in patients suffering from cirrhosis [35].

An important consequence of portal hypertension is the development of esophageal varices. The rupture of these either spontaneously or as a result of vomiting may lead to life-threatening hemorrhage. Esophageal varices are the result of porto-systemic shunting through the lienal vein, to the left gastric (coronary) veins, which secondarily drain to the thoracic veins such as vena azygos or hemiazygos [79].

Concomitant varices in the spleno-renal venal system and the paraumbical venal net, as well as the presence of anorectal shunts, may reduce the risk of rupture of the esophageal varices, but at the increased risk of hepatic encephalopathy [43].

Therapy of esophageal varices consists of sclerotherapy or surgical intervention to create alternative porto-systemic shunts.

Esophageal varices are usually depicted on T1w or flow sensitive gradient echo images localized anterior to the aorta at the level of the diaphragmatic hiatus [7].

Comparable results to digital subtraction angiography and endoscopy may be achieved by means of flow sensitive MRI. As the neighboring aorta and heart may induce pulsatile artifacts, low flip angles or ECG gating should be used for gradient echo sequences. However, if esophageal varices are not seen, then dilated left gastric veins in the gastro-hepatic ligament may indicate the diagnosis.

Whereas spleno-renal shunts, retroperitoneal shunts and puborectal shunts are difficult to demonstrate on ultrasonography, they are well visualized using MR angiography techniques. Moreover, reversed flow in the central portion of the splenic vein can be considered diagnostic [50].

Paraumbilical shunting may be best diagnosed by following the left portal vein to the superficial veins at the umbilicus through the ligamentum teres hepatis. Dilated veins adjacent to the abdominal wall have a characteristic spider's web appearance, called caput medusae.

In patients with large gastroepiploical veins along the greater curvature of the stomach, esophageal varices induced by a single splenic vein occlusion (e.g. caused by pancreatitis), has to be taken into account as a differential diagnosis.

Enlargements of the gastroepiploic veins can be considered a specific sign of splenic vein occlusion since they are not present in patients with portal hypertension in whom splenic veins are patent. In contrast, occlusion of the splenic vein can be excluded as a primary cause of portal hypertension in patients with paraumbilical varices. However, gastroesophageal and retroperitoneal colaterals may be seen in both conditions [36].

Portal vein velocity and flow volume may be ascertained on MRI using two dimensional phase contrast techniques. With this imaging modality increased portal flow is frequently seen in patients with cirrhosis in cases of recompensation. On the other hand, decreased or even reversed flow within the portal tract has been demonstrated in patients suffering from severe cirrhosis [63].

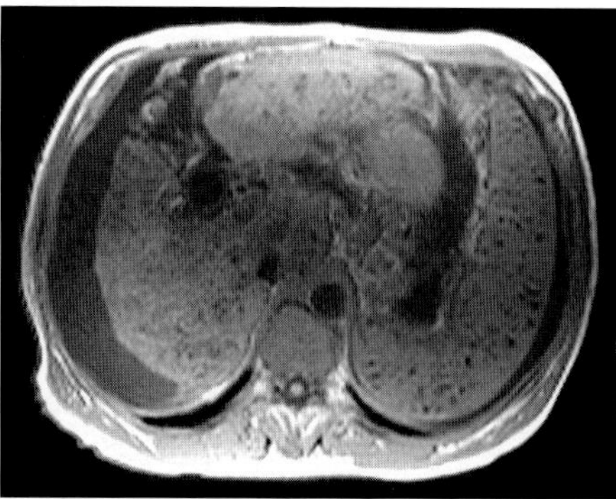

Fig. 7. Gamna-Gandy bodies of the spleen in a patient with portal hypertension due to liver cirrhosis. The T1w image shows diffuse low signal intensity lesions in the spleen which represent siderotic nodules arising due to portal hypertension. Additionally, typical signs of liver cirrhosis including ascites, hypertrophy of the left liver lobe and segment 1 with concomitant hypotrophy of the right liver lobe can be seen

Independent of primary diseases of the gallbladder, a thickened gallbladder wall is frequently found in patients with cirrhosis.

Further clinical manifestations of portal hypertension are ascites and splenomegaly. So-called Gamna-Gandy bodies which represent siderotic nodules within the spleen can arise in patients with portal hypertension and may be detected on T2w or contrast enhanced T1w MRI [54] (Fig.7).

6.4 Iron Overload

Since the liver is a central organ of digestive and reticuloendothelial function, it is heavily involved in the deposition and distribution of iron. Accumulated iron in the liver originates both from intestinally absorbed dietary iron and from particulate iron from damaged erythrocytes. Normally, accumulated iron in the liver is metabolized and delivered to the bone marrow in order to be used for red blood cell production. However, several diseases which increase the uptake of intestinal iron or the liberation of physiologically bound iron may lead to an excessive accumulation of iron in the liver.

Because iron reduces the T2 and T2* relaxation times significantly, MRI is a sensitive and specific imaging modality for the depiction of iron overload and its anatomical distribution. The most frequent diseases that lead to an increased accumulation of iron in the liver are hemochromatosis, siderosis (due to transfusional iron overload), hemolysis and cirrhosis. In addition to an examination of the liver, whole body MRI may be helpful to evaluate the underlying disease by revealing the pattern of increased iron accumulation in extrahepatic tissues.

6.4.1 Hemochromatosis

Hemochromatosis is a disease caused by an increased intestinal absorption of dietary iron, bound as ferritin or hemosiderin, and is characterized by excessive parenchymal iron accumulation [29].

The primary organs affected by hemochromatosis are the liver, pancreas and heart. Thus, liver cirrhosis, diabetes mellitus and cardiomyopathy frequently occur in untreated patients. Patients with longstanding disease and liver cirrhosis are significantly more at risk of developing HCC, thereby worsening the overall prognosis of the disease. Additional clinical manifestations include dermal hyperpigmentation, decreased libido and a slightly increased incidence of extrahepatic malignancies.

In general, menstruating women tend to show a rather moderate development of the disease [47].

Patients with hemochromatosis also demonstrate decreased reticuloendothial function and thus iron storage is mainly limited to the hepatic parenchyma [40]. In contrast, patients without hereditary hemochromatosis who ingest massive amounts of iron demonstrate both parenchymal and reticuloendothial iron overload.

Hemochromatosis has to be differentiated from hemosiderosis, in which increased accumulation of iron arises due to transfusional iron overload, typically in patients with hematological diseases who need regular blood transfusions. In patients with hemosiderosis iron accumulates primarily in the reticuloendothial cells of liver and spleen, while hepatocytes, pancreas and other parenchymal organs are relatively excluded. This difference is of major importance since parenchymal overload has more toxic consequences. However, an accumulation of iron within liver cells may also be seen in certain patients after massive blood transfusions [16, 46].

Since in most cases hemochromatosis is a primary genetic disease, familial screening should be performed in order to detect early liver cirrhosis or HCC. Moreover, the prognosis of patients with hemochromatosis can be improved significantly by reducing serum iron levels by means of repeated phlebotomy [3].

As measurements of serum iron levels and ferritin are not specific and CT findings do not provide satisfactory results, a definitive diagnosis has to be obtained by means of histological examination [58].

Since iron decreases the T2 relaxation time, hemochromatosis is seen as areas of decreased signal intensity on T2w or T2*w MR images [55]. In addition to the liver, the pancreas and heart are other primary affected organs. Therefore, the suspicion of hemochromatosis can be confirmed if each of these organs demonstrates decreased signal intensity on MR images. Parenteral iron accumulation (e.g. in transfusional iron overload), can be excluded as the pathogenic factor in hemochromatosis if the spleen presents with a normal signal intensity (Fig. 8).

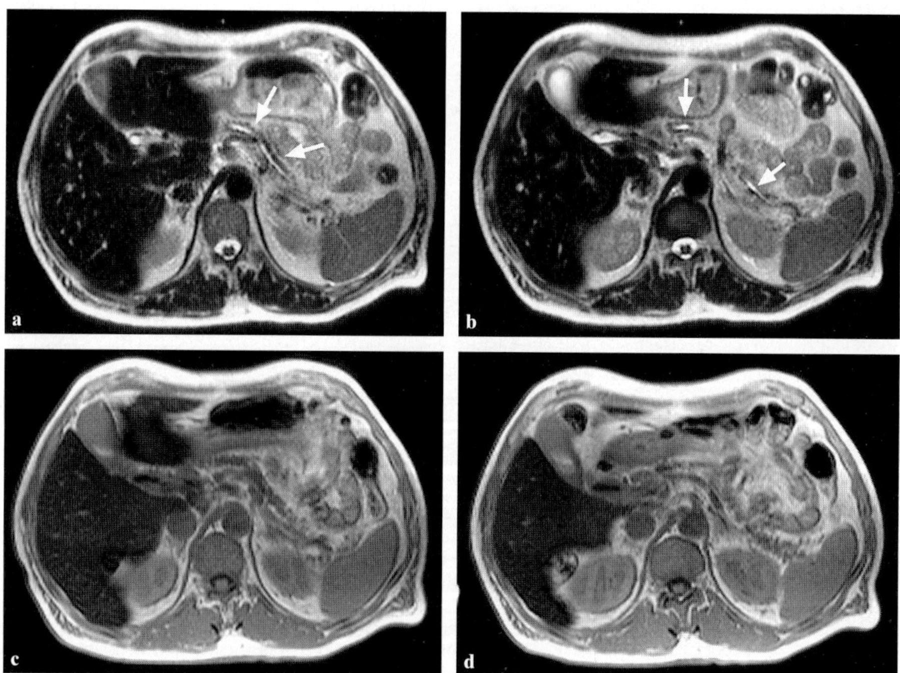

Fig. 8a-d. Hemochromatosis. A typical case of a longstanding hemochromatosis in which the liver and pancreas show decreased signal intensity on T2w (**a**, **b**) and T1w (**c**, **d**) images, while the spleen demonstrates essentially normal signal intensity. Note that the atrophy of the pancreas is displayed best on T2w images (*arrows*). As a result of the atrophy, this patient with longstanding disease developed diabetes mellitus

In normal individuals the liver parenchyma shows an increased signal intensity compared with the skeletal muscles on all sequences. As skeletal muscles are not affected by hemochromatosis they represent a suitable reference tissue to interpret and quantify the decreased signal of affected liver parenchyma [12].

In the early stages of the disease the signal intensity of the pancreas remains normal, particularly in menstruating women. However, as the disease progresses, the signal within the pancreatic tissue decreases. This is particularly evident in symptomatic hemochromatosis. Since MR imaging is able to demonstrate the progression of iron accumulation and the clearing of hepatic iron, it is possible it may serve as a monitoring modality in place of the histological follow-up examinations conducted at present.

Cirrhosis of the liver frequently occurs in patients suffering from untreated hemochromatosis. With MRI it may be detected due to the fact that fibrous septa demonstrate increased signal intensity compared to the low signal intensity

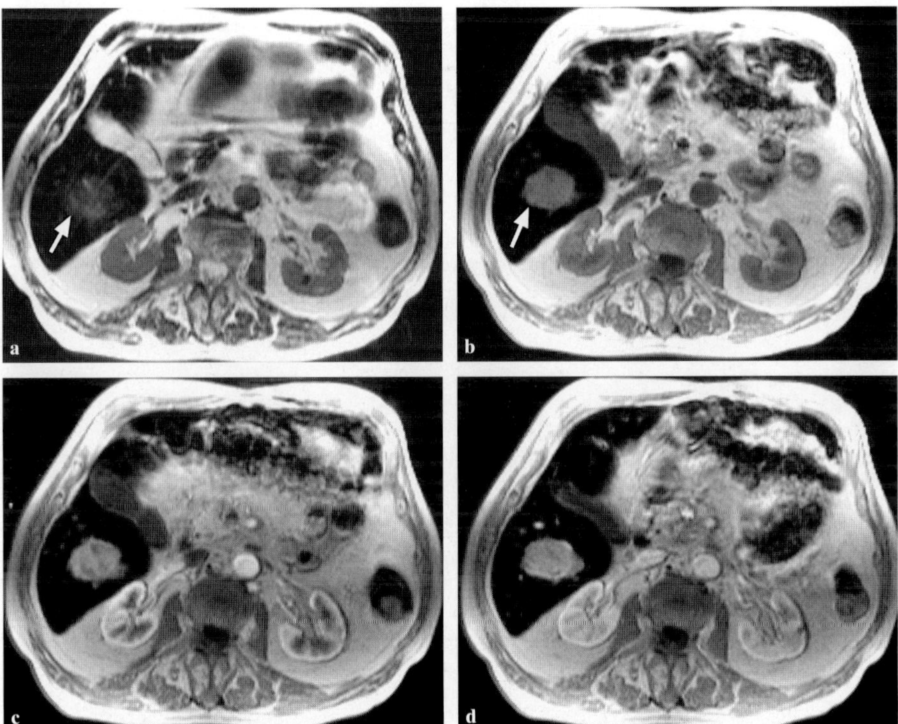

Fig. 9a-d. Hepatocellular carcinoma in a patient with longstanding hemochromatosis. A 74-year old male patient with longstanding hemochromatosis and significantly elevated AFP levels. The unenhanced T2w (**a**) and T1w (**b**) images reveal decreased signal intensity of the liver parenchyma and a hyperintense liver lesion (*arrows*) in the right liver lobe. In this case, iron deposition in the hepatocytes serves as an intrinsic contrast agent enabling the HCC to appear with high signal intensity since iron storage does not take place in the tumor cells. With dynamic imaging [(**c**) arterial phase, (**d**) portal-venous phase] after injection of a gadolinium-based contrast agent, strong hypervascularization of the lesion can be detected which clearly indicates the presence of a hepatocellular carcinoma.

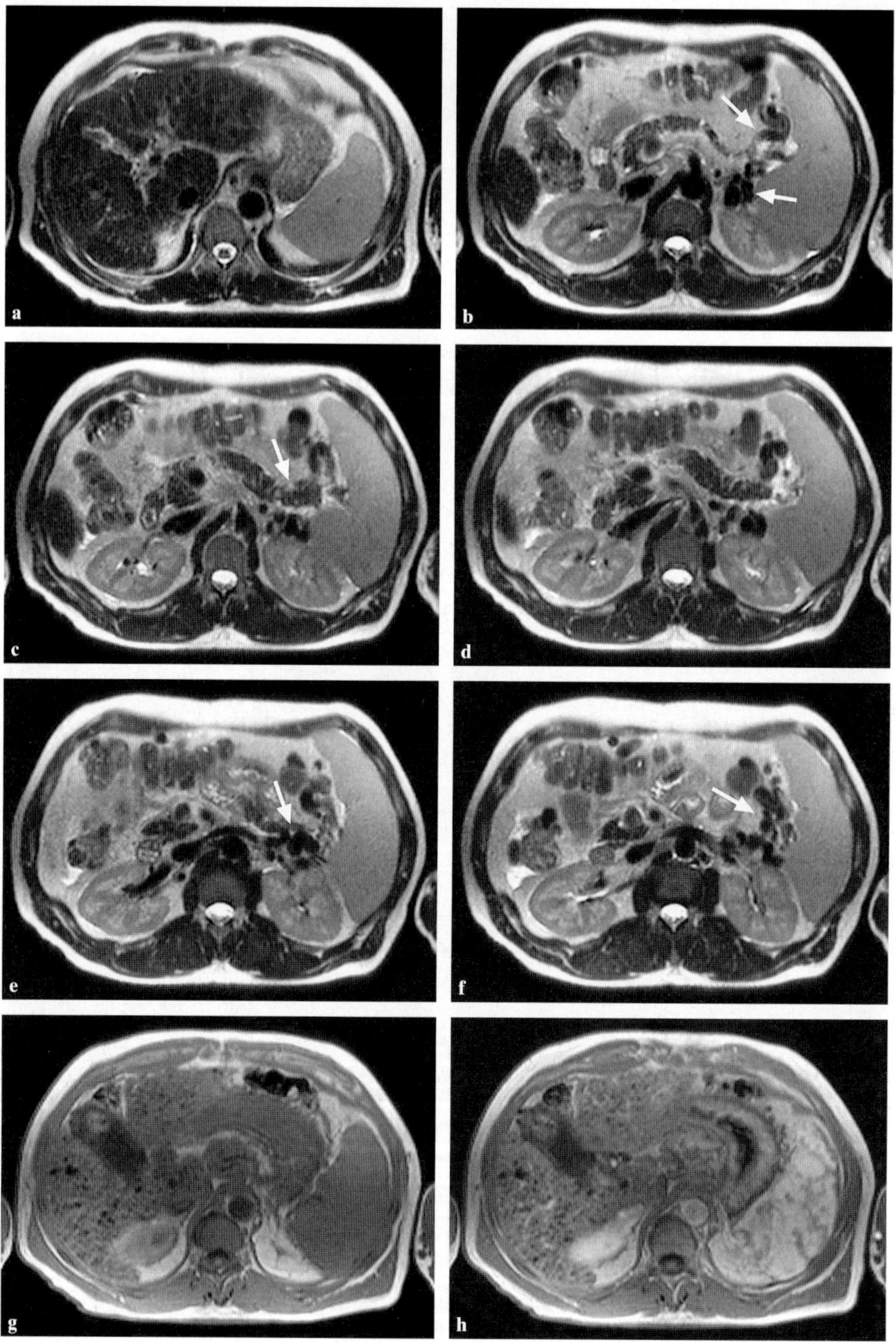

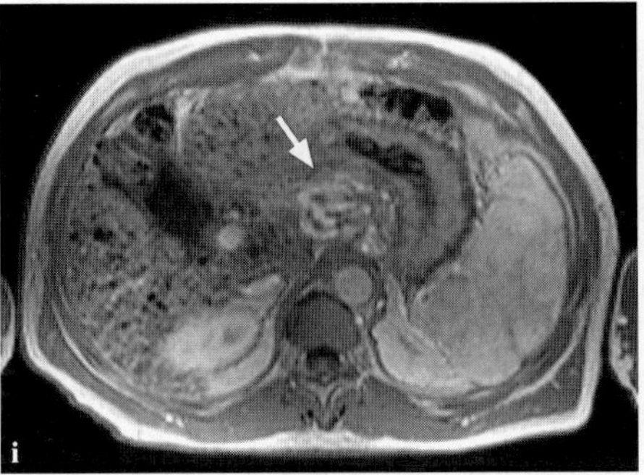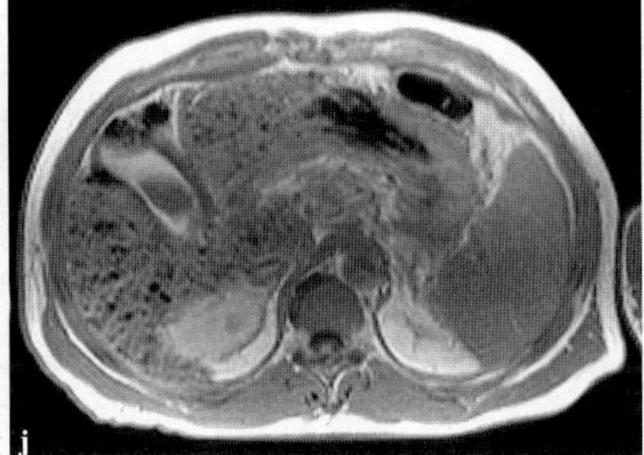

Fig. 10a-j. Patient with longstanding hemochromatosis and subsequent development of liver cirrhosis and portal hypertension. T2w images (**a-f**) show typical signs of liver cirrhosis with hypertrophy of segment 1 and a nodular surface of the liver. Due to the already advanced liver cirrhosis, the signal intensity of the liver parenchyma is not as low as in cases of hemochromatosis without cirrhosis since the inflammatory changes in cirrhosis increase the signal intensity of the liver. However, a decreased signal intensity of the pancreatic tissue (**b-d**) can be noted together with the beginnings of pancreatic atrophy. The spleen is enlarged and multiple collateral vessels in the splenic hilum can be depicted that drain into the left renal vein (**b-f**) (*arrows*). On T1w unenhanced images (**g**) multiple small areas of low signal intensity can be noted that correspond to areas of increased iron storage. The nodular appearance of the cirrhotic liver is much more obvious on dynamic images after Gd-BOPTA [(**h**) arterial phase, (**i**) portal-venous phase]. Additionally, irregular portal-venous collaterals (*arrow*) can be seen near the small curvature of the stomach on the portal-venous phase image (**i**). Only a slight increase of liver parenchyma signal intensity can be noted on the hepatobiliary phase image (**j**), although excretion of Gd-BOPTA into the gall bladder is evident

parenchyma. However, in many cases of hemochromatosis-induced cirrhosis a micronodular pattern is present which is difficult to visualize on MRI [64].

As dysplastic liver cells in HCC do not tend to accumulate iron to the same extent as liver parenchyma in hemochromatosis, HCC usually appear with a high signal intensity compared to the low signal intensity liver tissue. However, similar high signal areas are generally seen on all sequences for most focal liver lesions in cases of hepatic iron overload (Fig. 9)

Liver transplantation is usually indicated for patients with hemochromatosis and advanced liver cirrhosis (Fig. 10). Although the transplanted organ also tends to accumulate iron, the hepatotoxic effect of the accumulation requires a long time to develop and so prognosis is significantly improved. Interestingly, patients suffering from hemochromatosis may serve as donors for liver transplantation because the transplanted liver rapidly clears the accumulated iron [15]

6.4.2 Siderosis

In patients suffering from transfusional siderosis the liver shows a similar decrease of signal intensity to that seen in hemochromatosis. However, transfusional siderosis can easily be distinguished by examination of the signal intensity of the spleen and pancreas. While the spleen demonstrates decreased signal intensity in patients with transfusional siderosis, it usually does not show any signal intensity decrease in cases of hemochromatosis. In contrast, the pancreas usually demonstrates a significant drop of signal intensity in cases of hemochromatosis but remains unchanged in patients with trasfusional siderosis; only in cases of extreme transfusional iron overload (i.e. after transfusion of >100 units of red blood) is the signal intensity of the pancreas affected [55].

Comparable findings are observed with cardiac MR imaging. Whereas no changes in imaging characteristics are seen in the myocardium of patients with transfusional siderosis, in cases of hemochromatosis the myocardium usually demonstrates decreased signal intensity.

Transfusional siderosis frequently occurs in patients suffering from hematological diseases in which erythrocyte transfusion needs to be performed regularly [52].

In addition, parenteral iron overload may occur in patients with rhabdomyolysis in which the bound iron of myoglobin is liberated into the blood and absorbed secondarily by reticuloendothelial cells [53] (Fig. 11, 12).

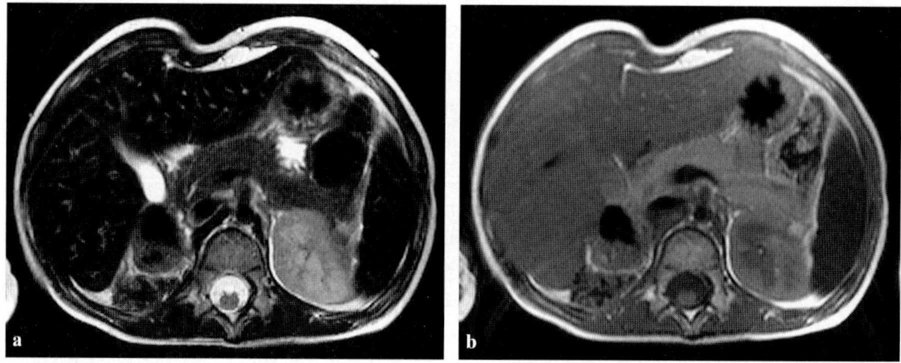

Fig. 11a,b. Transfusional siderosis. 7-year old boy following chemotherapy for right-sided nephroblastoma and multiple blood transfusions. Both T2w (**a**) and T1w (**b**) images reveal decreased signal intensity of the liver and spleen, while the signal intensity of the pancreas is unaffected. This is due to the presence of iron storage in the macrophages of the spleen and liver, rather than in hepatocytes, as occurs in hemochromatosis (Fig. 12).

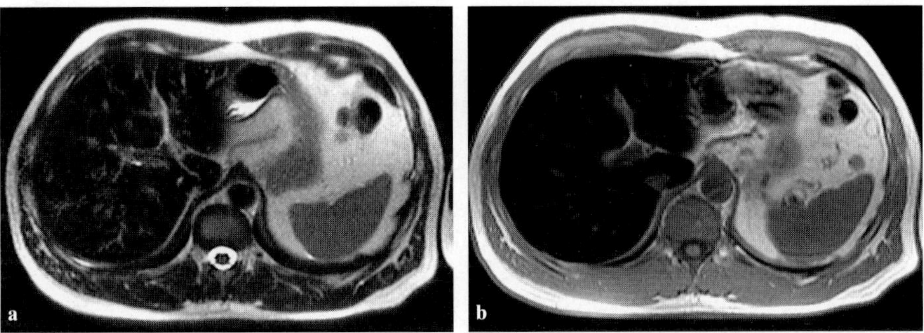

Fig. 12a,b. Hemochromatosis. T2w (**a**) and T1w (**b**) images reveal a dramatically decreased signal intensity of the liver parenchyma while the signal intensity of the spleen remains normal. This permits the differential diagnosis of transfusional siderosis (Fig. 11) to be excluded since in transfusional siderosis the signal intensity of the spleen is also affected

6.4.3 Cirrhosis

A mild accumulation of iron is frequently found in cirrhotic livers, particularly if the cirrhosis is induced by alcohol abuse. However, since the SI of the parenchyma is not greatly reduced in such cases, the misdiagnosis of hemochromatosis, in which the parenchyma demonstrates a massive reduction of SI, can be avoided [4].

6.4.4 Hemolysis

Systemic accumulation of iron may be caused by hemolysis in which hemoglobin is liberated from red blood cells. While extravascular (e.g. splenic) hemolysis leads to a reticuloendothelial deposition of iron, intravascular hemolysis causes a hepato-cellular accumulation, since the released hemoglobin binds to plasma haptoglobin which is taken up by hepatocytes. If the serum hemoglobin level exceeds the transport capacity of haptoglobin, it is filtered through renal glomeruli, reabsorbed and stored within proximal convoluted tubule epithelial cells. For this reason, intravascular hemolysis is characterized by an accumulation of iron in the liver and renal cortex, but not in the spleen. Diseases which lead to intravascular hemolysis and thus show this characteristic imaging pattern, include paroxysmal nocturnal hemoglobinuria and sickle cell disease [61].

6.5 Vascular Pathologies

6.5.1 Portal Vein Thrombosis

The etiology of portal vein thrombosis falls into the Virschow trias comprising reduced blood flow within the vessel, changes in the consistency of blood which affects flow properties, and pathologies of the vessel wall. Thus, etiological factors of portal vein thrombosis are slow flow secondary to cirrhosis, obstruction of the vessel by porto-hepatic lymphadenopathy, direct invasion by cancer, inflammatory changes secondary to pancreatitis, sclerosing cholangitis, abdominal infections, polycytemia vera and benign masses [1, 45, 51, 75].

While portal vein thrombosis often occurs in cases of HCC, it may also be the result of other primary or secondary neoplasms of the liver.

In cases of portal vein occlusion, portal perfusion is maintained due to periportal collateral veins. With progression, the draining collaterals dilate while the thrombosed portal vein retracts to form a so-called "cavernous transformation" which, on ultrasound, may be misinterpreted as patency of the portal vein [44, 76].

MRI is an accurate method to depict portal venous blood flow, intraluminal thrombus and collateral circulation non-invasively and, generally, without the need for contrast medium administration. Moreover, as it is not restricted by body habitus, ascites or abdominal gas, it is superior to duplex sonography [19, 34, 67, 81, 82].

MRI not only aids in the diagnosis of portal vein thrombosis but also in the planning of shunt surgery and hepatic transplantation, and in the monitoring of shunt patency following surgery [5, 17, 60].

Patency of the portal vein can be interpreted on spin echo images by the demonstration of a flow void within the vessel. However, at the confluence of the splenic and the mesenteric veins, an increased signal intensity is frequently seen. In cases of portal vein occlusion, the clot is usually isointense to the liver parenchyma on T1w images, and hyperintense on T2w images [34].

A diagnosis of portal vein thrombosis is likely when the lesion is present on all sequences with comparable size and shape. The suspicion of portal vein thrombosis may be confirmed or excluded following acquisition of flow sensitive gradient echo images [56].

Chronic occlusion of a branch of the portal vein may be accompanied by segmental atrophy and compensatory hypertrophy of other segments [35].

Tumoral obstruction of lobal or segmental portal branches may present on T2w images as wedge shaped regions of increased signal intensity. In such cases the apex usually points to the obstructing tumor, and therefore, MR images should be examined carefully [31].

In livers with preexisting fatty infiltration the area affected by segmental portal vein obstruction shows a decreased accumulation of fat, as fat deliverance correlates with portal flow [2] (Fig. 13).

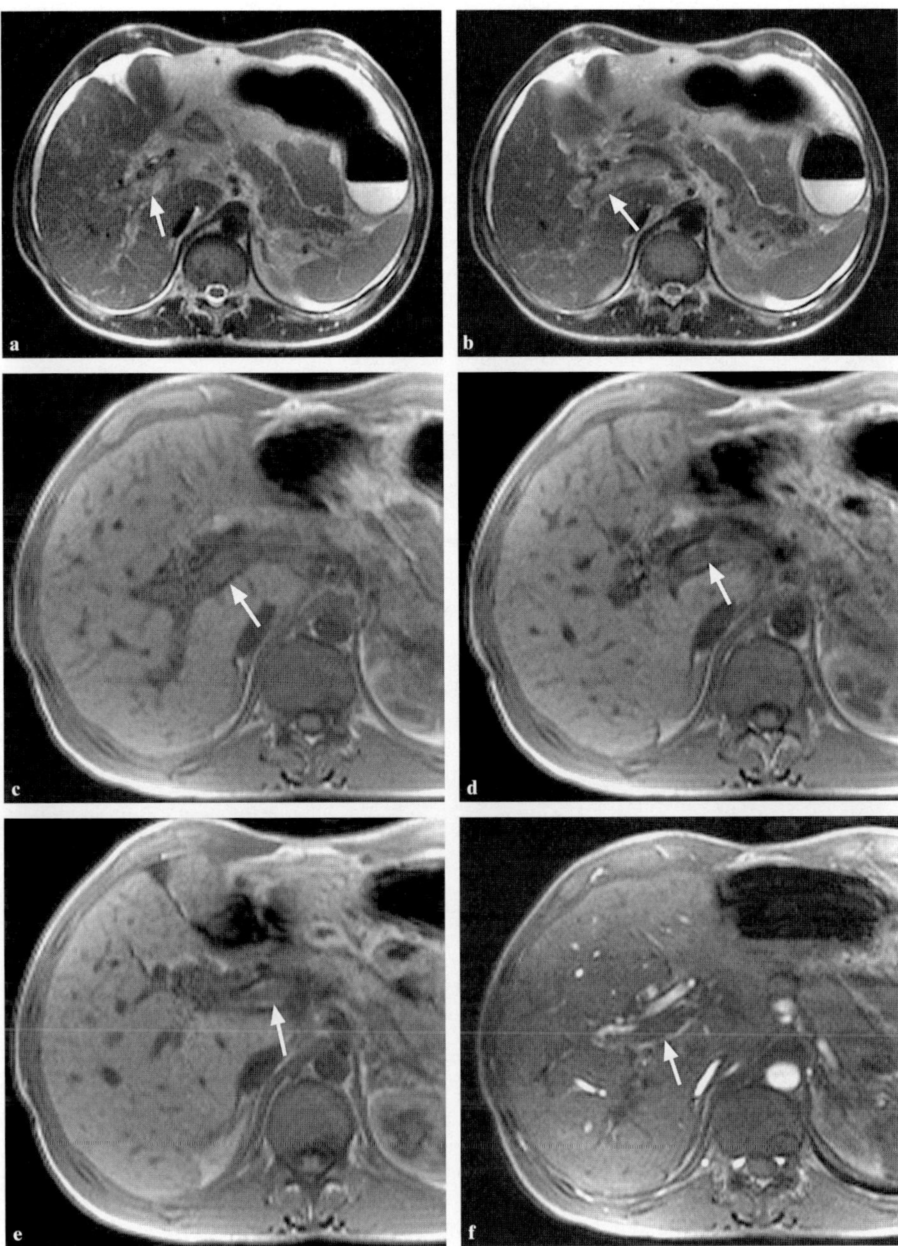

Fig. 13a-r. Subacute portal vein thrombosis. T2w images (**a, b**) reveal intermediate to high signal intensity in the area of the portal vein without any flow void (*arrows*). Additionally, perihepatic and perisplenic ascites can be noted. On T1w images (**c-e**), again, no flow void in the portal vein can be noted although a mass with hypointense and hyperintense areas (*arrows*) does seem to be present in the portal vein. Flow sensitive gradient echo images (**f-k**) clearly depict a thrombus within the portal vein (*arrows*) with some residual peripheral flow indicated by a peripheral high signal intensity rim. The thrombosis can be followed to the confluence of the mesenteric and splenic veins. Irregular enhancement of the liver parenchyma can be noted on arterial phase images after contrast medium injection (**l-n**). On portal-venous phase images (**o-r**), again, the thrombus in the portal vein is clearly depicted and can be followed into the periphery (*arrow*). Note that the mesenteric vein is also occluded (**r**) (*arrow*)

(continued)

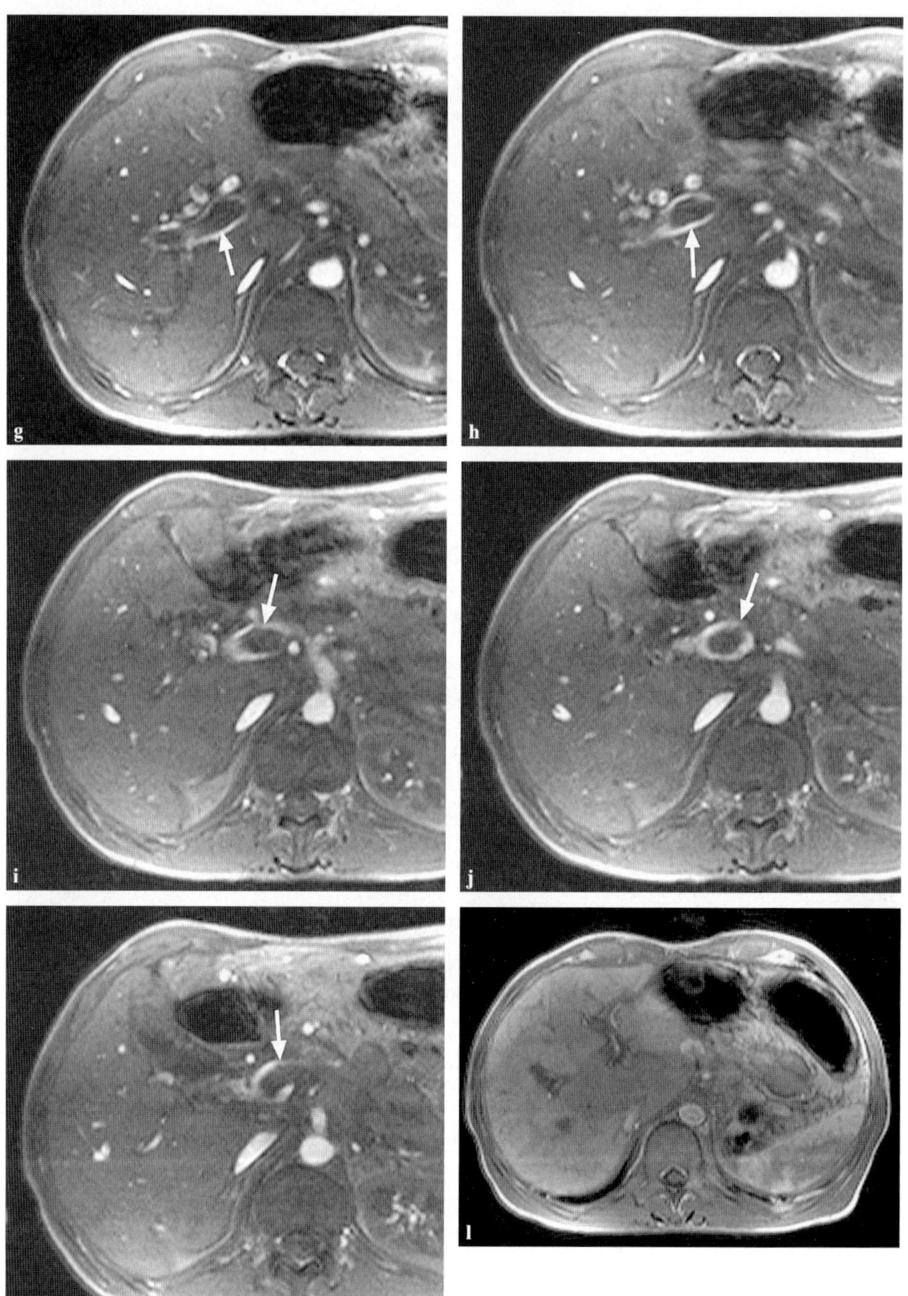

Fig. 13a-r. (*continued*)

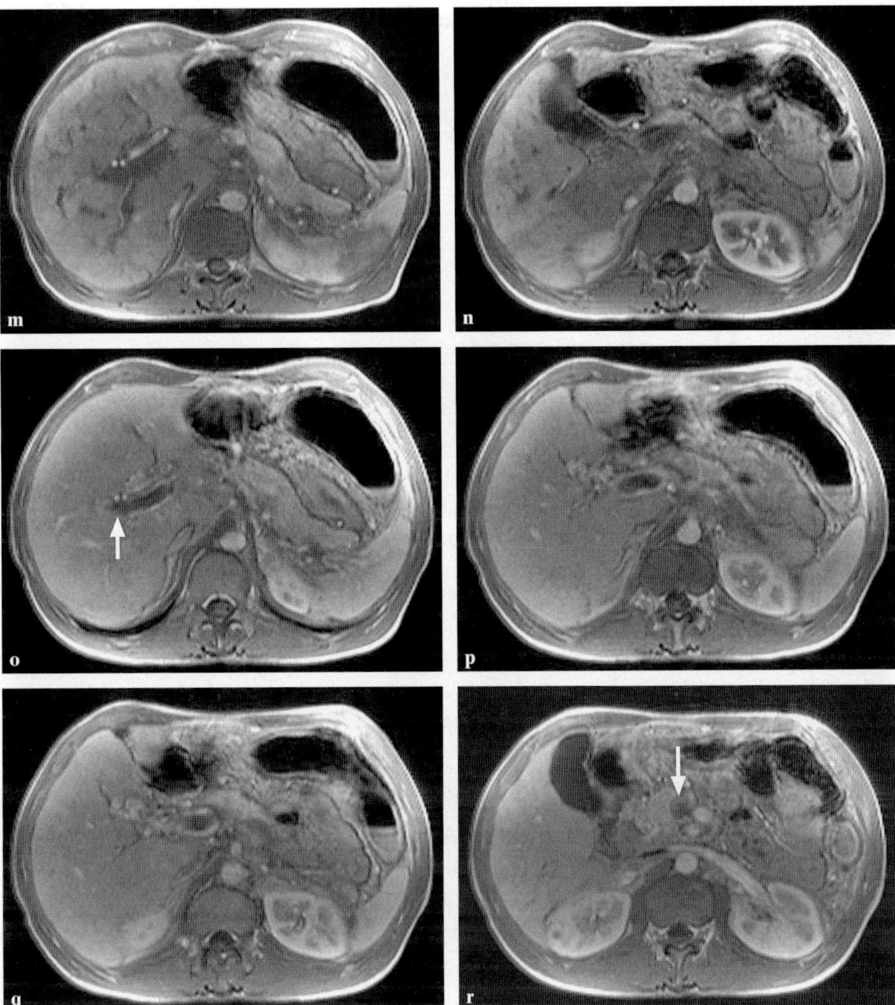

Fig. 13a-r.

6.5.2 Budd-Chiari Syndrome (Acute, Chronic)

Budd-Chiari syndrome is defined as an obstruction of the venous outflow from the sinusoidal bed of the liver. It leads to portal hypertension, ascites and progressive hepatic failure [57].

The treatment of Budd-Chiari syndrome depends on the cause of the obstruction and, hence, careful examination of the hepatic veins, the inferior vena cava (IVC) and the right atrium is necessary [37, 73].

For example, in the Asian population a membranous occlusion of the inferior vena cava is a common cause. In such cases membranectomy should be performed. On the other hand, if a solitary occlusion of the inferior vena cava is present without the hepatic veins being affected, a shunting from the IVC to the right atrium would be the primary treatment of choice.

If only the hepatic veins are obstructed, a shunt between the superior mesenteric vein and the inferior vena cava, a so-called "mesocaval shunt", may be inserted to lower the pressure in the portal-venous system. On the other hand, when both the inferior vena cava and the hepatic veins are occluded the appropriate therapy would be a bypass from the superior mesenteric vein to the right atrium, a so-called "mesoatrial shunting". For patients in whom a neoplasm is the primary cause of a Budd-Chiari syndrome, extensive surgery is often contraindicated.

Given the different therapeutic approaches available, accurate imaging in Budd-Chiari syndrome not only serves for diagnosis but should also indicate the most appropriate therapy for the patient. Ultrasonography may be used to detect hepatic vein occlusion, however, the IVC is not reliably visualized on ultrasonography and ascites in Budd-Chiari syndrome may interfere with the appropriate depiction of the hepatic confluence [41].

In contrast, MRI, which is not affected by the individual constitution of the patient, represents a non-invasive imaging modality for the evaluation of both the intra- and extrahepatic vascular anatomy in Budd-chiari syndrome and the possible intra- or extrahepatic causal pathologies [38].

However, if portocaval shunting is planned, the examination frequently has to be completed by means of venography in order to determine the presence or absence of a significant pressure gradient across the IVC. Even if a patent IVC is demonstrated by non-invasive imaging modalities, a pressure gradient may be present, in most cases due to hypertrophy of the caudate lobe. In such cases, portocaval shunting is contraindicated and shunting has to be performed from the portal venous system to either the right atrium or the left inferior pulmonary vein [5, 60].

Vascular findings. MR imaging is an accurate modality to demonstrate the diverse pattern of vascular changes that are indicative of Budd-Chiari syndrome. Frequently, a significant reduction in caliber or a complete absence of hepatic veins may be found or, alternatively, newly arising intrahepatic collateral veins with a comma-like shape may be seen. Other findings include a constriction of the intrahepatic inferior caval vein or, less commonly, the hepatic veins appear patent but do not show any connection to the inferior caval vein. Since thrombus formation in the hepatic veins may be located some centimeters away from the IVC, patent central hepatic veins and a normal hepatic confluence may be seen.

MRI not only permits the diagnosis of Budd-Chiari syndrome but may also reveal the etiological cause. For example, it is possible to visualize an obstruction of the IVC or the right atrium caused by neoplasms, such as primary sarcomas of the vein, or tumors of the liver, kidney or adrenal gland, and the resulting tumor thrombus formation.

Increased coagulobility of the blood causing thrombosis of the hepatic veins (e.g. in polycytemia vera or paroxysmal nocturnal hemoglobinuria), may be identified by MRI. In patients with polycytemia vera, a diffusely decreased intensity of the bone marrow together with splenomegaly can point to the diagnosis. In patients suffering from paroxysmal nocturnal hemoglobinuria decreased signal intensity in the liver and renal cortex with a normal signal intensity in the spleen is observed [57, 69].

Morphologic features. In most cases of Budd-Chiari syndrome, the hepatic venous outflow is not eliminated completely since a variety of accessory hepatic veins may drain above or below the principal site of obstruction. The most frequent accessory site of venous drainage occurs at the inferior right hepatic vein and the veins of the caudate lobe which drain directly into the inferior portion of the IVC. Additional collaterals draining to other systemic veins may be present, such as the azygos and the vertebral and/or intercostal veins which show characteristic enlargement if present. Reversed flow in some portal vein branches may occur since connections between the portal and the hepatic veins are relatively common [62, 70]. However, the main portal flow usually remains antegrade [30]. Since some hepatic venous drainage is usually preserved for the caudate lobe and for central portions of the right and left liver lobes, a compensatory hypertrophy of the caudate lobe may develop. However, this may lead to a secondary obstruction of the IVC. Although subcapsular hepatic veins may also contribute to collateral blood flow, the resulting venous drainage is usually insufficient to prevent peripheral atrophy of the liver.

In patients with a completely obstructed venous outflow shunting is performed from the hepatic veins and arteries to the portal veins which thereafter demonstrates reversed flow [11].

As a result of collateral venous drainage Budd-Chiari syndrome is typically associated with peripheral hepatic atrophy and, conversely, caudate and central hypertrophy which, together, may lead to a displacement of the porta hepatis towards the anterior portion of the liver [20]. These morphological changes can be visualized on MR imaging, together with a clear depiction of the occluded liver veins. Other findings include regional differences in liver signal intensity due to central lobular necrosis and hepatocellular fat or iron content. Dynamic MR imaging of acute Budd-Chiari syndrome after bolus injection of extracellular contrast agents (Fig. 14) frequently reveals an atypical parenchymal enhancement, which indirectly indicates the presence of increased vascular resistance. Unlike patients with liver cirrhosis, patients with acute Budd-Chiari syndrome demonstrate acute clinical symptoms and a large tender liver without signs of nodular changes. However, in chronic disease, nodular regenerative hyperplasia may develop which may lead to the misdiagnosis of liver cirrhosis [33] (Fig. 15).

Another disease leading to hepatic venous obstruction is the so-called "hepatic veno-occlusive disease". This is often caused by chemotherapy, especially after bone marrow transplantation [8]. In this disease, the post-sinusoidal venules are usually obstructed while the major hepatic veins and IVC do not show pathological changes and remain patent. Since diagnosis by means of MRI is difficult in most

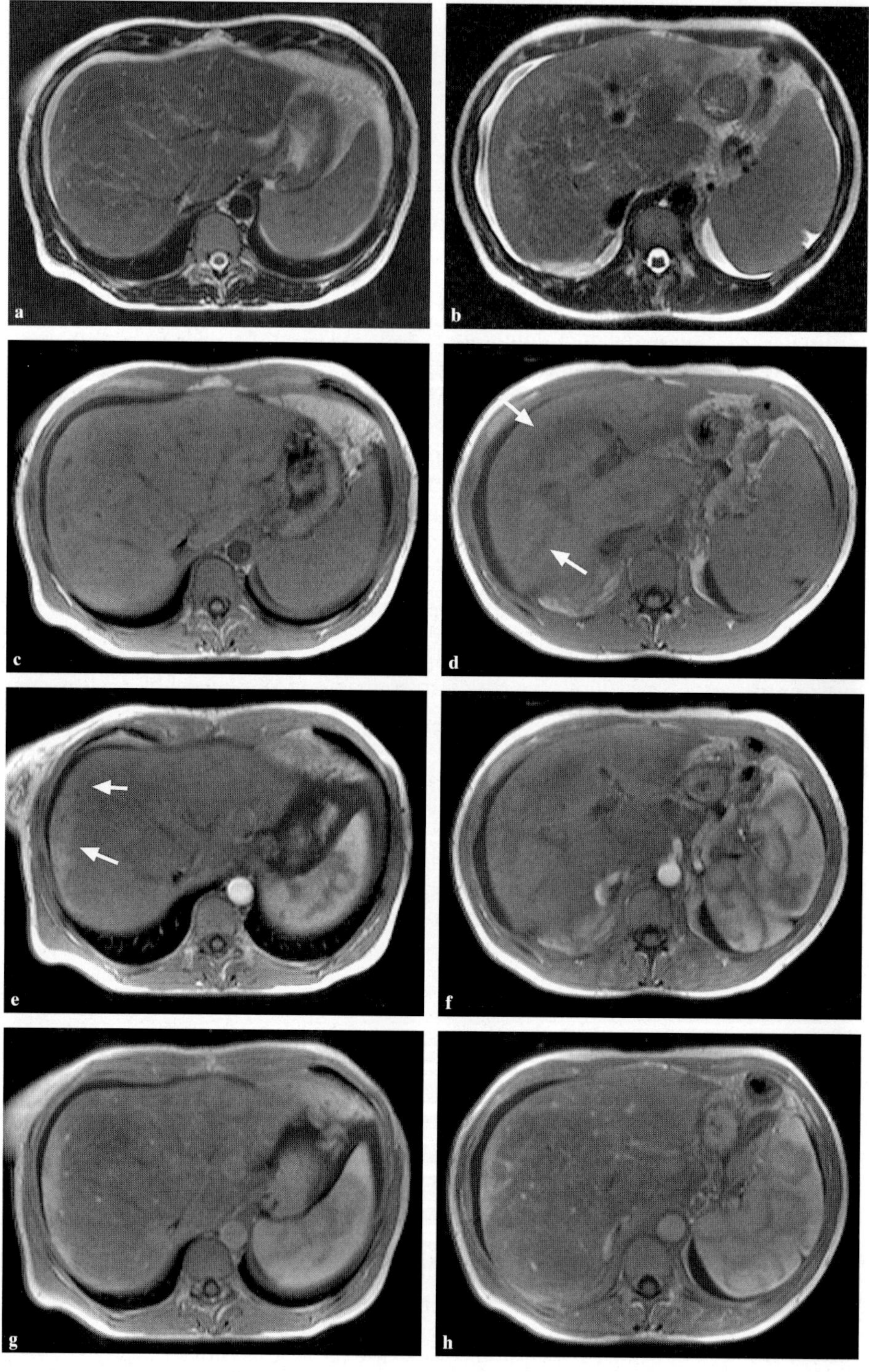

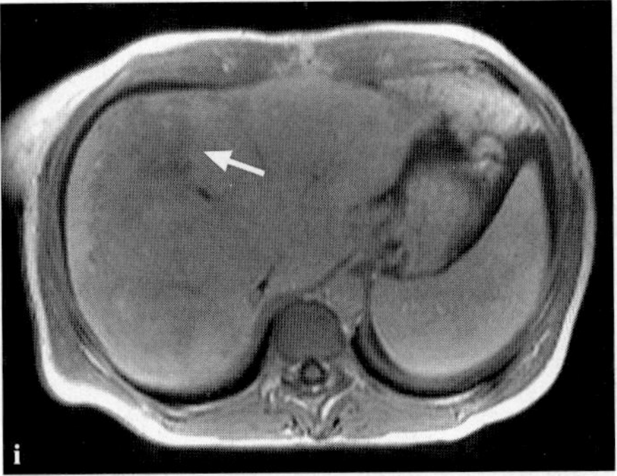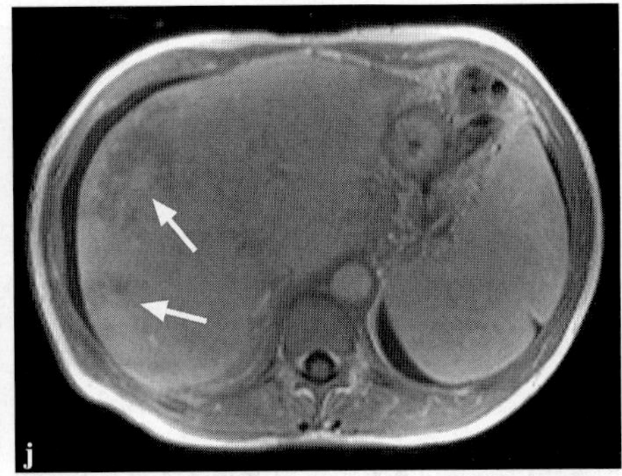

Fig. 14a-j. Acute Budd-Chiari syndrome. T2w images (**a**, **b**) reveal diffuse swelling of the liver and perihepatic and perisplenic ascites. The large intrahepatic liver veins show no signs of flow void and the periphery of the liver parenchyma, especially in the right liver lobe, shows increased signal intensity. On the corresponding T1w images (**c**, **d**), again, the liver veins are depicted only as small hypointense bands and low signal intensity areas in the more caudal parts of the liver can be noted (*arrows*). On contrast enhanced images during the arterial phase (**e**, **f**), only an enhancement of the periphery of the liver can be seen (*arrows*). The more central parts do not show obvious enhancement due to increased vascular resistance. Still no enhancement of portal-venous branches is visible on the portal-venous phase images (**g**, **h**), although enhancement of the central parts of the liver can now be noted. Homogenous enhancement of the left liver lobe and central parts of the right liver lobe is more apparent on equilibrium phase images (**i**, **j**). Peripheral hypointense areas (*arrows*) can still be depicted in the right liver lobe in this phase. These areas correspond to liver necrosis due to acute Budd-Chiari syndrome

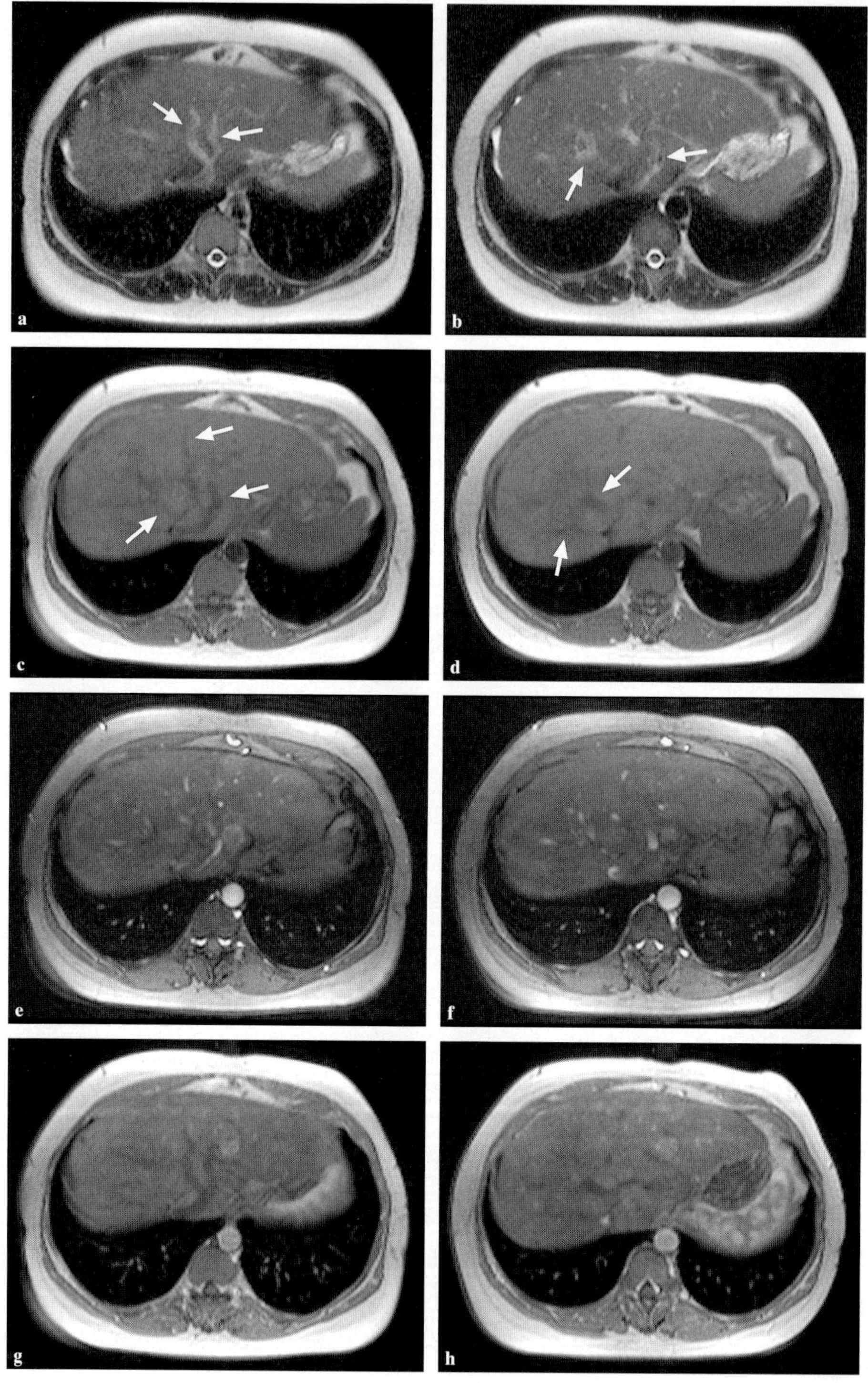

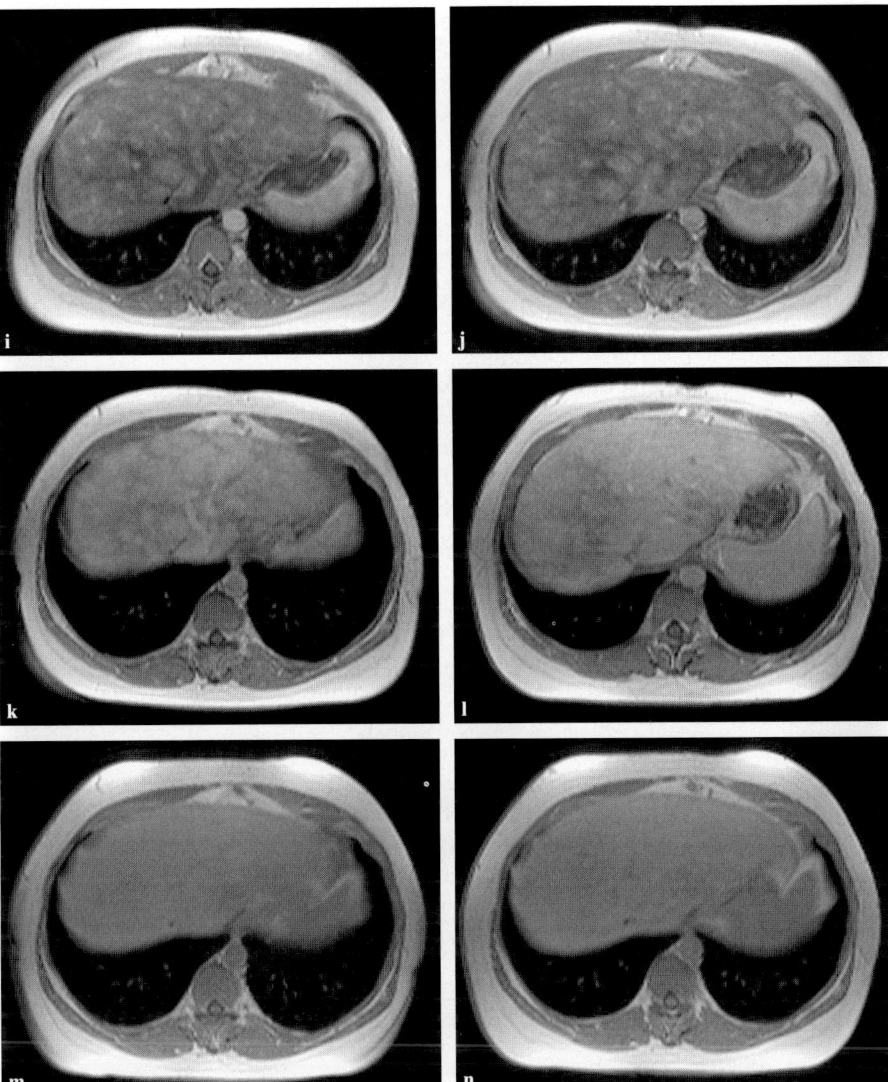

Fig. 15a-n. Longstanding Budd-Chiari syndrome. Unenhanced T2w images (**a**, **b**) reveal a comma-like shape of the intrahepatic collateral veins (*arrows*) that is typical of Budd-Chiari syndrome. These veins (*arrows*) appear with low signal intensity on unenhanced T1w images (**c**, **d**) due to flow void, and show a flow signal on flow sensitive gradient echo sequences (**e**, **f**). As in the case of acute Budd-Chiari syndrome (Fig. 14) delayed enhancement of the liver can be noted on dynamic imaging. Although diffuse enhancement of the liver parenchyma can already be observed on arterial phase images (**g**, **h**), full homogenous enhancement is not yet seen even on portal-venous phase images (**i**, **j**). On the other hand, nodular enhancement due to regenerative processes is visible. Some hypointense areas in the liver parenchyma are still apparent on images acquired 5 min after contrast agent injection (**k**, **l**) indicating decreased blood flow. Isointensity with the surrounding liver tissue is finally observed on images acquired 15 min after contrast agent administration (**m**, **n**)

cases, confirmation needs to be established either by histopathological examination of a biopsy or by wedge hepatic venography. In addition, dynamic MR imaging of the liver in the arterial and portal-venous phases may indicate an increased arterial perfusion of the affected regions and a prolonged liver transit time of the contrast agent [60].

6.5.3 Arterio-Venous Malformations

Arterio-venous (AV-) malformations of the liver are rare and are caused either iatrogenically in liver biopsy and liver surgery, or are distributed diffusely in patients with hereditary hemorrhagic teleangiectasia (HHT; "Osler's disease") [23]. In general, AV-malformations may occur between the hepatic artery and the hepatic vein, as well as between the hepatic artery and the portal-venous system. Typical findings on dynamic MR images of the liver for singular AV-malformations post-biopsy or surgery include a dilatation of the draining hepatic vein and an early enhancement of the hepatic veins (Fig. 16). Shunts between the hepatic artery and the portal-venous system typically lead to increased portal-venous pressure and thus to the usual findings of portal hypertension [21].

In contrast, AV-malformations in Osler's disease are diffusely distributed throughout the liver and may be associated with enlargement of the hepatic artery and increased tortuousity of the vessels in the liver hilum and in the central portions of the liver lobes. In Osler's disease increased arterial perfusion of the liver tissue leads frequently to secondary nodular hypertrophy which may be misinterpreted as a malignant hepatic tumor. These pseudotumors, as in focal nodular hyperplasia, represent a localized overgrowth of hepatocellular tissue and are not real liver tumors. Dynamic MR imaging reveals that these lesions show strong arterial phase enhancement and subsequent isointensity with the surrounding liver tissue in the portal-venous and equilibrium phases. Normal enhancement of the affected tissue in the hepatobiliary phase can be noted with the use of contrast agents with hepatocellular properties such as Gd-BOPTA [71] (Fig. 17).

Severe cases of AV shunting in Osler's disease may lead to right heart failure and, at present, the only curative treatment is liver transplantation [6].

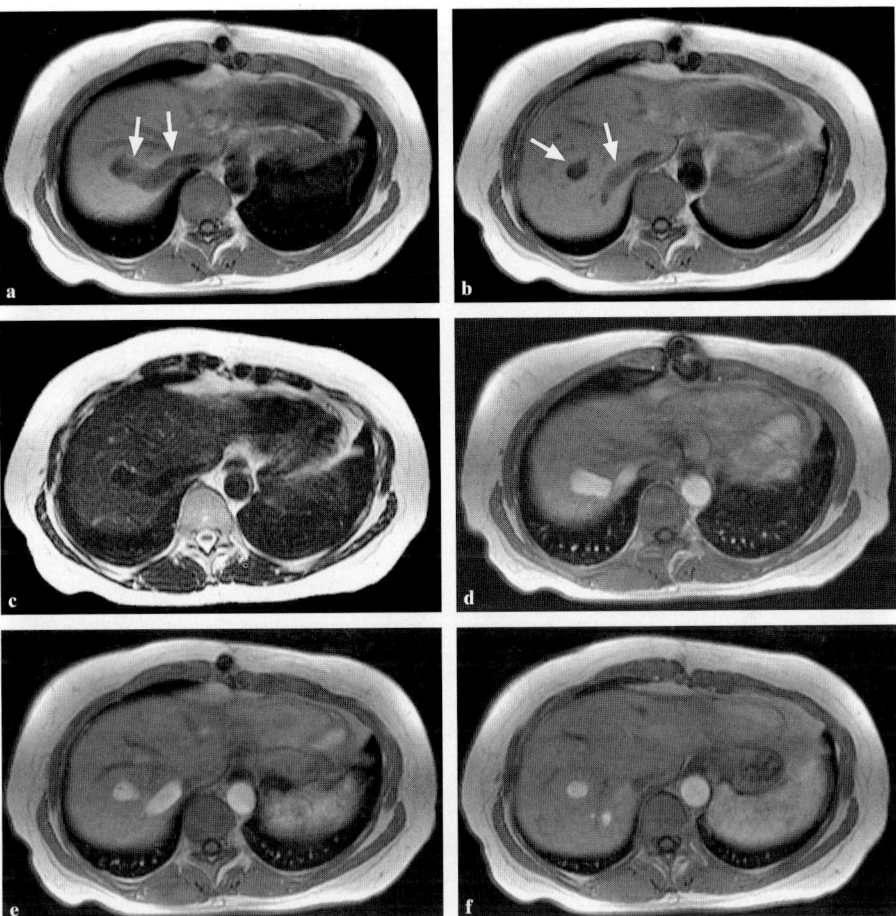

Fig. 16a-f. Iatrogenic AV-shunt post surgery. Unenhanced T1w images (**a**, **b**) reveal dilatation of the draining hepatic veins in AV shunting (*arrows*). The corresponding T2w image (**c**) again reveals flow void in the vessels. Early enhancement of the draining liver veins indicating an AV malformation can be depicted clearly on early arterial phase images (**d-f**) after intravenous injection of paramagnetic contrast agent

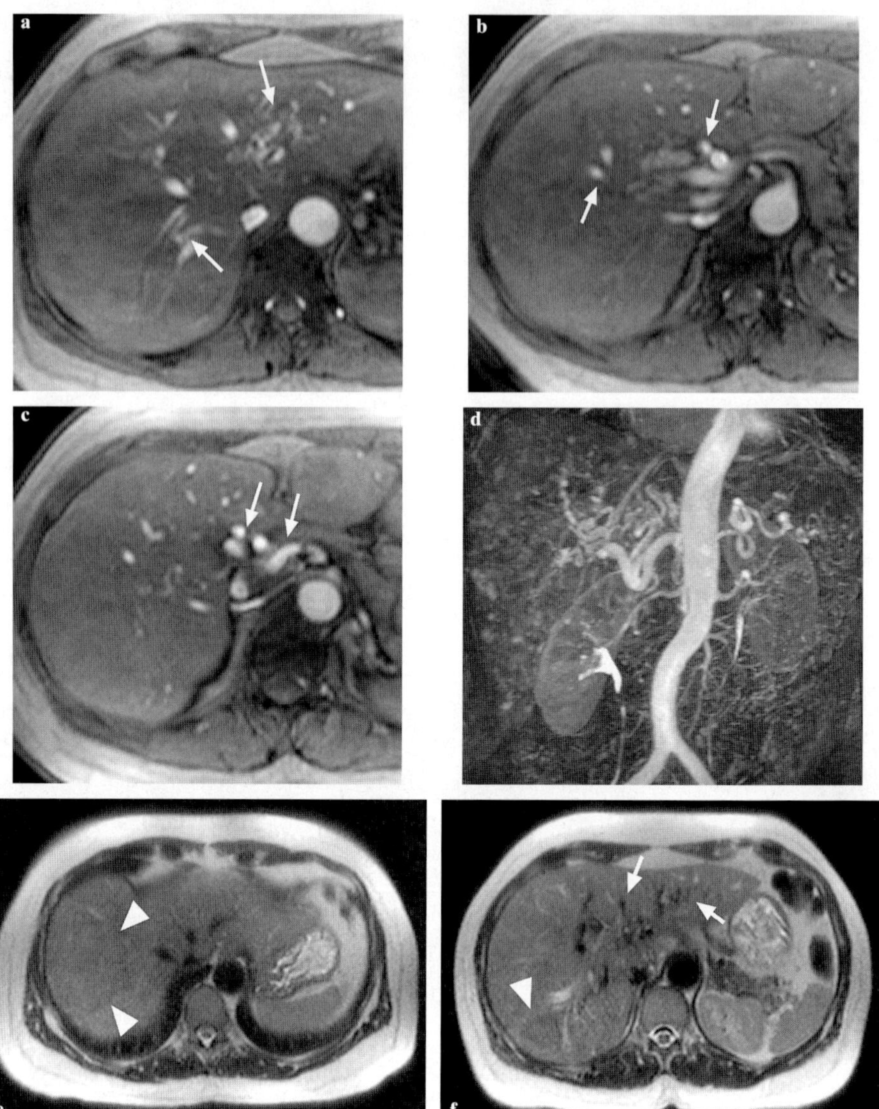

Fig. 17a-r. Diffusely distributed AV-malformations in a patient with Osler's disease. Flow sensitive gradient echo images (**a-c**) reveal enlarged tortuous vessels in the liver hilum and in the more centrally located liver parenchyma (*arrows*), indicating increased flow in the hepatic artery. On contrast enhanced MRA (**d**), the dilatation of the hepatic artery is even more obvious. Again, the tortuous vessels and diffusely distributed small AV malformations in the liver are observed. On T2w images (**e-g**) areas of flow void in the liver can be noted indicating increased flow in branches of the hepatic artery (*arrows*). Additionally, some nodular-appearing liver lesions in the right liver lobe can be depicted (*arrowheads*). On unenhanced T1w images (**h-j**) these liver tumors show an almost isointense signal intensity compared with the surrounding liver tissue. However, in the arterial phase after injection of Gd-BOPTA (**k-m**) these liver lesions are clearly hypervascular (*arrows*). On portal-venous phase images (**n, o**) the lesions are isointense with the surrounding liver tissue. In the hepatobiliary phase one hour after injection of Gd-BOPTA (**p-r**), the lesions appear hyperintense compared to the surrounding liver tissue due to uptake of the contrast agent into hepatocyctes. These liver lesions correspond to a localized overgrowth of hepatocellular tissue similar to that which occurs in FNH. The lesions appear hyperintense in the hepatobiliary phase due to the delayed excretion of the contrast agent into the newly formed bile ductules

(*continued*)

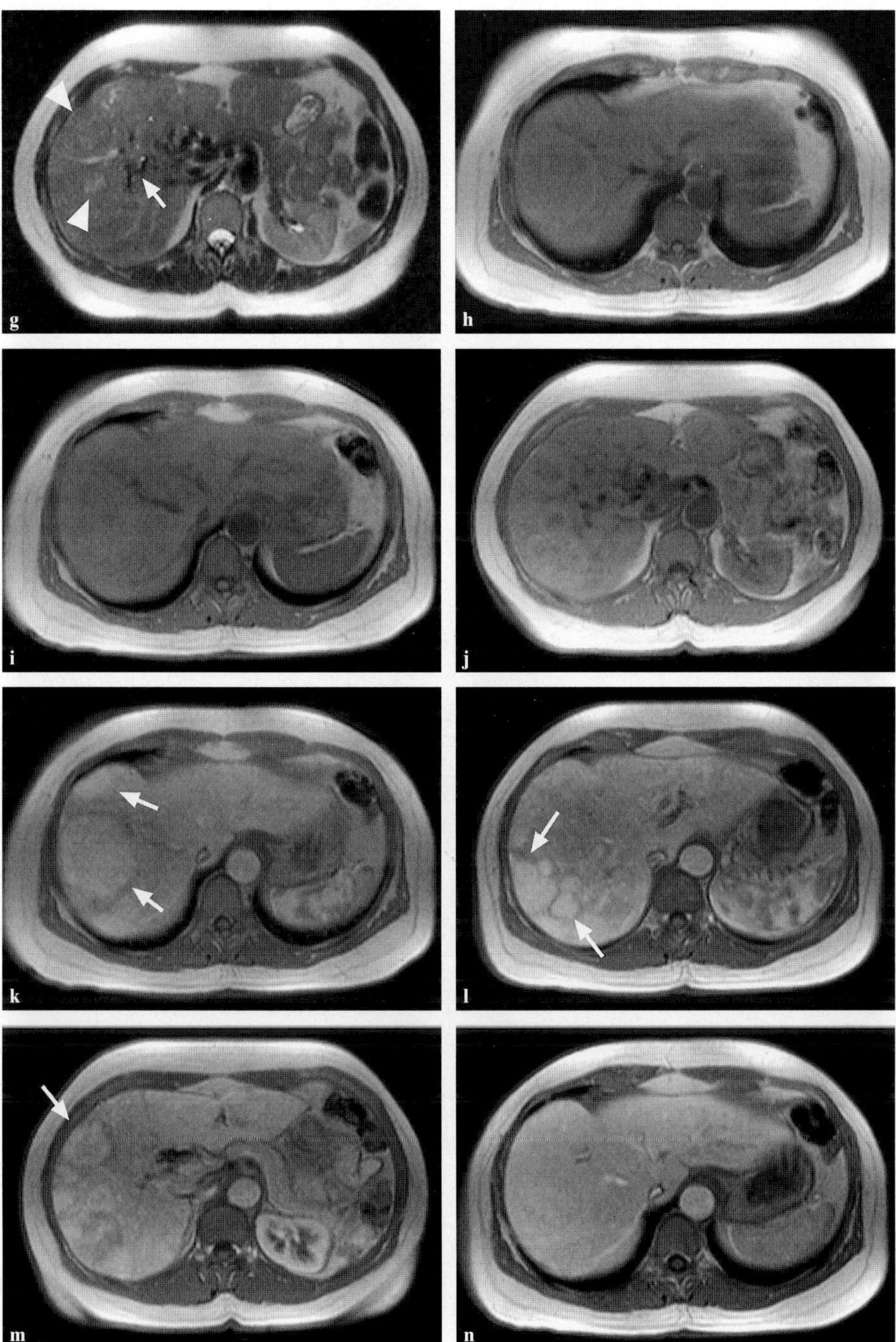

Fig. 17a-r. (*continued*)

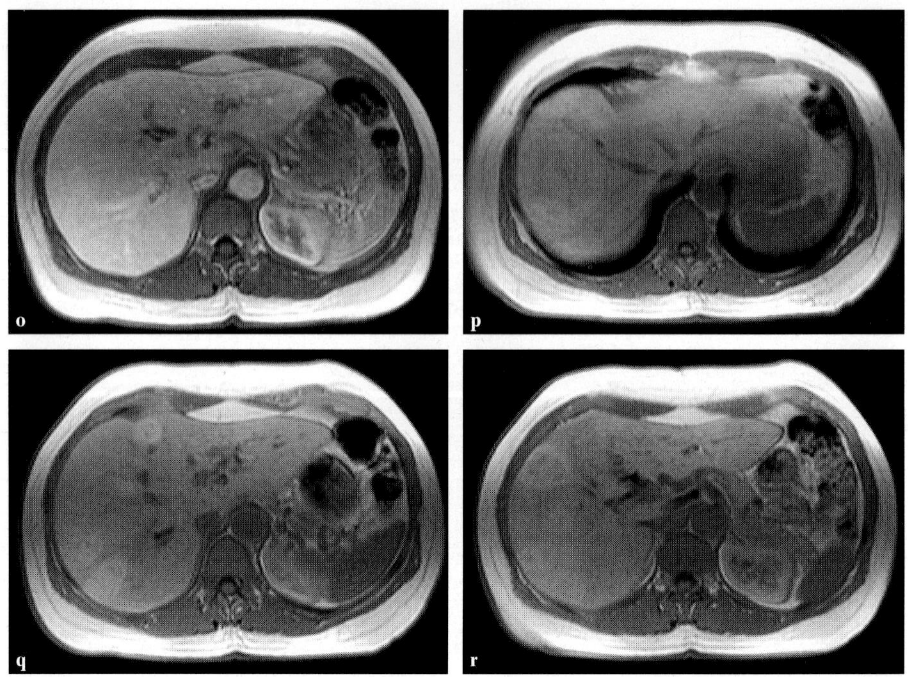

Fig. 17a-r.

References

1. Alpern MB, Rubin JM, Williams DM, Capek P. Porta hepatis: duplex Doppler US with angiographic correlation. Radiology 1987 Jan;162(1 Pt 1):53-6
2. Arai K, Matsui O, Takashima T, Ida M, Nishida Y. Focal spared areas in fatty liver caused by regional decreased portal flow. AJR Am J Roentgenol 1988 Aug;151(2):300-2
3. Bassett ML, Halliday JW, Powell LW. Genetic hemochromatosis. Semin Liver Dis 1984 Aug;4(3):217-27
4. Bassett ML, Halliday JW, Powell LW. Value of hepatic iron measurements in early hemochromatosis and determination of the critical iron level associated with fibrosis. Hepatology 1986 Jan-Feb;6(1):24-9
5. Bernardino ME, Steinberg HV, Pearson TC, Gedgaudas-McClees RK, Torres WE, Henderson JM. Shunts for portal hypertension: MR and angiography for determination of patency. Radiology 1986 Jan;158(1):57-61
6. Boillot O, Bianco F, Viale JP, Mion F, Mechet I, Gille D, Delaye J, Paliard P, Plauchu H. Liver transplantation resolves the hyperdynamic circulation in hereditary hemorrhagic telangiectasia with hepatic involvement. Gastroenterology 1999 Jan;116(1):187-92
7. Brady TM, Gross BH, Glazer GM, Williams DM. Adrenal pseudomasses due to varices: angiographic-CT-MRI-pathologic correlations. AJR Am J Roentgenol 1985 Aug;145(2):301-4
8. Brown BP, Abu-Yousef M, Farner R, LaBrecque D, Gingrich R Doppler sonography: a noninvasive method for evaluation of hepatic venocclusive disease. AJR Am J Roentgenol 1990 Apr;154(4):721-4
9. Caldwell SH, Hespenheide EE, Harris D, de Lange EE. Imaging and clinical characteristics of focal atrophy of segments 2 and 3 in primary sclerosing cholangitis. J Gastroenterol Hepatol 2001 Feb;16(2):220-4
10. Chapman RW, Arborgh BA, Rhodes JM, Summerfield JA, Dick R, Scheuer PJ, Sherlock S. Primary sclerosing cholangitis: a review of its clinical features, cholangiography, and hepatic histology. Gut 1980 Oct;21(10):870-7
11. Chawla Y, Dilawari JB, Mitra SK, Khanna SK. The porta-splenic venous system in the Budd-Chiari syndrome. Trop Gastroenterol 1988 Jan-Mar;9(1):14-7
12. Chezmar JL, Nelson RC, Malko JA, Bernardino ME. Hepatic iron overload: diagnosis and quantification by noninvasive imaging. Gastrointest Radiol 1990 Winter;15(1):27-31
13. Dachman AH, Ros PR, Goodman ZD, Olmsted WW, Ishak KG. Nodular regenerative hyperplasia of the liver: clinical and radiologic observations. AJR Am J Roentgenol 1987 Apr;148(4):717-2
14. Di Bisceglie AM, Martin P, Kassianides C, Lisker-Melman M, Murray L, Waggoner J, Goodman Z, Banks SM, Hoofnagle JH. Recombinant interferon alfa therapy for chronic hepatitis C. A randomized, double-blind, placebo-controlled trial. N Engl J Med 1989 Nov 30;321(22):1506-10
15. Dietze O, Vogel W, Braunsperger B, Margreiter R. Liver transplantation in idiopathic hemochromatosis. Transplant Proc 1990 Aug;22(4):1512-3
16. Dolbey CH. Hemochromatosis: a review. Clin J Oncol Nurs 2001 Nov-Dec;5(6):257-60
17. Edelman RR, Zhao B, Liu C, Wentz KU, Mattle HP, Finn JP, McArdle C. MR angiography and dynamic flow evaluation of the portal venous system. AJR Am J Roentgenol 1989 Oct;153(4):755-60
18. Elizondo G, Weissleder R, Stark DD, Guerra J, Garza J, Fretz CJ, Todd LE, Ferrucci JT. Hepatic cirrhosis and hepatitis: MR imaging enhanced with superparamagnetic iron oxide. Radiology 1990 Mar;174(3 Pt 1):797-801
19. Finn JP, Edelman RR, Jenkins RL, Lewis WD, Longmaid HE, Kane RA, Stokes KR, Mattle HP, Clouse ME. Liver transplantation: MR angiography with surgical validation. Radiology 1991 Apr;179(1):265-9
20. Fisher B, Szuch P, Levine M, Saffer E, Fisher ER. The intestine as a source of a portal blood factor responsible for liver regeneration. Surg Gynecol Obstet 1973 Aug;137(2):210-4
21. Garcia-Tsao G, Korzenik JR, Young L, Henderson KJ, Jain D, Byrd B, Pollak JS, White RI Jr. Liver disease in patients with hereditary hemorrhagic telangiectasia. N Engl J Med 2000 Sep 28;343(13):931-6
22. Garra BS, Shawker TH, Chang R, Kaplan K, White RD. The ultrasound appearance of radiation-induced hepatic injury. Correlation with computed tomography and magnetic resonance imaging. J Ultrasound Med 1988 Nov;7(11):605-9
23. Geisthoff UW, Schneider G, Fischinger J, Plinkert PK. Hereditary hemorrhagic telangiectasia (Osler's disease). An interdisciplinary challenge. HNO 2002 Feb;50(2):114-28
24. Giorgio A, Amoroso P, Lettieri G, Fico P, de Stefano G, Finelli L, Scala V, Tarantino L, Pierri P, Pesce G. Cirrhosis: value of caudate to right lobe ratio in diagnosis with US. Radiology 1986 Nov;161(2):443-5
25. Goldberg HI, Moss AA, Stark DD, McKerrow J, Engelstad B, Brito A. Hepatic cirrhosis: magnetic resonance imaging. Radiology 1984 Dec;153(3):737-9
26. Goyal AK, Pokharna DS, Sharma SK. Ultrasonic diagnosis of cirrhosis: reference to quantitative measurements of hepatic dimensions. Gastrointest Radiol 1990 Winter;15(1):32-4
27. Groszmann RJ, Atterbury CE. The pathophysiology of portal hypertension: a basis for classification. Semin Liver Dis 1982 Aug;2(3):177-86

28. Hadjis NS, Adam A, Blenkharn I, Hatzis G, Benjamin IS, Blumgart LH. Primary sclerosing cholangitis associated with liver atrophy. Am J Surg 1989 Jul;158(1):43-7

29. Holland HK, Spivak JL. Hemochromatosis. Med Clin North Am 1989 Jul;73(4):831-45

30. Hosoki T, Kuroda C, Tokunaga K, Marukawa T, Masuike M, Kozuka T. Hepatic venous outflow obstruction: evaluation with pulsed duplex sonography. Radiology 1989 Mar;170(3 Pt 1):733-7

31. Itai Y, Ohtomo K, Furui S, Minami M, Yoshikawa K, Yashiro N. Lobar intensity differences of the liver on MR imaging. J Comput Assist Tomogr 1986 Mar-Apr;10(2):236-41

32. Itai Y, Ohtomo K, Kokubo T, Makita K, Okada Y, Machida T, Yashiro N. CT and MR imaging of fatty tumors of the liver. J Comput Assist Tomogr 1987 Mar-Apr;11(2):253-7

33. Kane R, Eustace S. Diagnosis of Budd-Chiari syndrome: comparison between sonography and MR angiography. Radiology 1995 Apr;195(1):117-21

34. Levy HM, Newhouse JH. MR imaging of portal vein thrombosis. AJR Am J Roentgenol 1988 Aug;151(2):283-6

35. Lorigan JG, Charnsangavej C, Carrasco CH, Richli WR, Wallace S. Atrophy with compensatory hypertrophy of the liver in hepatic neoplasms: radiographic findings. AJR Am J Roentgenol 1988 Jun;150(6):1291-5

36. Marn CS, Glazer GM, Williams DM, Francis IR. CT-angiographic correlation of collateral venous pathways in isolated splenic vein occlusion: new observations. Radiology 1990 May;175(2):375-80

37. Martin LG, Henderson JM, Millikan WJ Jr, Casarella WJ, Kaufman SL. Angioplasty for long-term treatment of patients with Budd-Chiari syndrome. AJR Am J Roentgenol 1990 May;154(5):1007-10

38. Matsui O, Kadoya M, Takashima T, Kameyama T, Yoshikawa J, Tamura S. Intrahepatic periportal abnormal intensity on MR images: an indication of various hepatobiliary diseases. Radiology 1989 May;171(2):335-8

39. Matsui O, Kadoya M, Kameyama T, Yoshikawa J, Arai K, Gabata T, Takashima T, Nakanuma Y, Terada T, Ida M. Adenomatous hyperplastic nodules in the cirrhotic liver: differentiation from hepatocellular carcinoma with MR imaging. Radiology 1989 Oct;173(1):123-6

40. McLaren GD, Muir WA, Kellermeyer RW. Iron overload disorders: natural history, pathogenesis, diagnosis and therapy. CRC Crtit. Rev. Clin. Lab. Sci. 1984 19:205-266.

41. Menu Y, Alison D, Lorphelin JM, Valla D, Belghiti J, Nahum H. Budd-Chiari syndrome: US evaluation.Radiology 1985 Dec;157(3):761-4

42. Mitchell DG. MR imaging of cirrhosis and its complications. Abdom Imaging 2000 Sep-Oct;25(5):455

43. Mostbeck GH, Wittich GR, Herold C, Vergesslich KA, Walter RM, Frotz S, Sommer G. Hemodynamic significance of the paraumbilical vein in portal hypertension: assessment with duplex US. Radiology 1989 Feb;170(2):339-42

44. Nakao N, Miura K, Takahashi H, Miura T, Ashida H, Ishikawa Y, Utsunomiya J. Hepatic perfusion in cavernous transformation of the portal vein: evaluation by using CT angiography. AJR Am J Roentgenol 1989 May;152(5):985-6

45. Nelson RC, Lovett KE, Chezmar JL, Moyers JH, Torres WE, Murphy FB, Bernardino ME. Comparison of pulsed Doppler sonography and angiography in patients with portal hypertension. AJR Am J Roentgenol 1987 Jul;149(1):77-81

46. Niederau C, Strohmeyer G. Strategies for early diagnosis of haemochromatosis. Eur J Gastroenterol Hepatol 2002 Mar;14(3):217-21

47. Niederau C, Fischer R, Sonnenberg A, Stremmel W, Trampisch HJ, Strohmeyer G. Survival and causes of death in cirrhotic and in noncirrhotic patients with primary hemochromatosis. N Engl J Med 1985 Nov 14;313(20):1256-62

48 .Nomura F, Ohnishi K, Ochiai T, Okuda K. Obesity-related nonalcoholic fatty liver: CT features and follow-up studies after low-calorie diet. Radiology 1987 Mar;162(3):845-7

49. Ohtomo K, Itai Y, Ohtomo Y, Shiga J, Iio M. Regenerating nodules of liver cirrhosis: MR imaging with pathologic correlation. AJR Am J Roentgenol 1990 Mar;154(3):505-7

50. Parvey HR, Eisenberg RL, Giyanani V, Krebs CA. Duplex sonography of the portal venous system: pitfalls and limitations. AJR Am J Roentgenol 1989 Apr;152(4):765-70

51. Patriquin H, Lafortune M, Burns PN, Dauzat M. Duplex Doppler examination in portal hypertension: technique and anatomy. AJR Am J Roentgenol 1987 Jul;149(1):71-6

52. Powell LW, Bassett ML, Halliday JW. Hemochromatosis: 1980 update. Gastroenterology 1980 Feb;78(2):374-81

53. Rupert SA. Pathogenesis and treatment of rhabdomyolysis. J Am Acad Nurse Pract 2002 Feb;14(2):82-87

54. Sagoh T, Itoh K, Togashi K, Shibata T, Nishimura K, Minami S, Asato R, Noma S, Fujisawa I, Yamashita K, et al. Gamna-Gandy bodies of the spleen: evaluation with MR imaging. Radiology 1989 Sep;172(3):685-7

55. Siegelman ES, Mitchell DG, Rubin R, Hann HW, Kaplan KR, Steiner RM, Rao VM, Schuster SJ, Burk DL Jr, Rifkin MD. Parenchymal versus reticuloendothelial iron overload in the liver: distinction with MR imaging. Radiology 1991 May;179(2):361-6

56. Silverman PM, Patt RH, Garra BS, Horii SC, Cooper C, Hayes WS, Zeman RK. MR imaging of the portal venous system: value of gradient-echo imaging as an adjunct to spin-echo imaging. AJR Am J Roentgenol 1991 Aug;157(2):297-302

57. Stanley P. Budd-Chiari syndrome.Radiology 1989 Mar;170(3 Pt 1):625-7

58. Stark DD, Bass NM, Moss AA, Bacon BR, McKerrow JH, Cann CE, Brito A, Goldberg HI. Nuclear magnetic resonance imaging of experimentally induced liver disease. Radiology 1983 Sep;148(3):743-51

59. Stark DD, Goldberg HI, Moss AA, Bass NM. Chronic liver disease: evaluation by magnetic resonance. Radiology 1984 Jan;150(1):149-51

60. Stark DD, Hahn PF, Trey C, Clouse ME, Ferrucci JT Jr. MRI of the Budd-Chiari syndrome. AJR Am J Roentgenol 1986 Jun;146(6):1141-8

61. Tabbara IA. Hemolytic anemias. Diagnosis and management. Med Clin North Am 1992 May;76(3):649-68

62. Takayasu K, Moriyama N, Muramatsu Y, Goto H, Shima Y, Yamada T, Makuuchi M, Yamasaki S, Hasegawa H, Hojo K. Intrahepatic venous collaterals forming via the inferior right hepatic vein in 3 patients with obstruction of the inferior vena cava. Radiology 1985 Feb;154(2):323-8

63. Tamada T, Moriyasu F, Ono S, Shimizu K, Kajimura K, Soh Y, Kawasaki T, Kimura T, Yamashita Y, Someda H, et al. Portal blood flow: measurement with MR imaging. Radiology 1989 Dec;173(3):639-44

64. Terada T, Nakanuma Y. Iron-negative foci in siderotic macroregenerative nodules in human cirrhotic liver. A marker of incipient neoplastic lesions. Arch Pathol Lab Med 1989 Aug;113(8):916-20

65. Terada T, Nakanuma Y. Survey of iron-accumulative macroregenerative nodules in cirrhotic livers. Hepatology 1989 Nov;10(5):851-4

66. The Clinical NMR Group. Magnetic resonance imaging of parenchymal liver disease: a comparison with ultrasound, radionuclide scintigraphy and X-ray computed tomography. Clin Radiol 1987 Sep;38(5):495-502

67. Torres WE, Gaylord GM, Whitmire L, Chuang VP, Bernardino ME. The correlation between MR and angiography in portal hypertension. AJR Am J Roentgenol 1987 Jun;148(6):1109-13

68. Unger EC, Lee JK, Weyman PJ. CT and MR imaging of radiation hepatitis. J Comput Assist Tomogr 1987 Mar-Apr;11(2):264-8

69. Valla DC. Hepatic vein thrombosis (Budd-Chiari syndrome). Semin Liver Dis 2002 Feb;22(1):5-14

70. Van Beers B, Pringot J, Trigaux JP, Dautrebande J, Mathurin P. Hepatic heterogeneity on CT in Budd-Chiari syndrome: correlation with regional disturbances in portal flow. Gastrointest Radiol 1988;13(1):61-6

71. Varma DG, Schoenberger SG, Kumra A, Agrawal N, Robinson AE. Osler-Weber-Rendu disease: MR findings in the liver. J Comput Assist Tomogr 1989 Jan-Feb;13(1):134-5

72. Wada K, Kondo F, Kondo Y. Large regenerative nodules and dysplastic nodules in cirrhotic livers: a histopathologic study. Hepatology 1988 Nov-Dec;8(6):1684-8

73. Wang ZG, Zhu Y, Wang SH, Pu LP, Du YH, Zhang H, Yuan C, Chen Z, Wei ML, Pu LQ, et al. Recognition and management of Budd-Chiari syndrome: report of one hundred cases. J Vasc Surg 1989 Aug;10(2):149-56

74. Wanless IR, Lentz JS. Fatty liver hepatitis (steatohepatitis) and obesity: an autopsy study with analysis of risk factors. Hepatology 1990 Nov;12(5):1106-10

75. Wanless IR, Peterson P, Das A, Boitnott JK, Moore GW, Bernier V. Hepatic vascular disease and portal hypertension in polycythemia vera and agnogenic myeloid metaplasia: a clinicopathological study of 145 patients examined at autopsy. Hepatology 1990 Nov;12(5):1166-74

76. Weltin G, Taylor KJ, Carter AR, Taylor CR. Duplex Doppler: identification of cavernous transformation of the portal vein. AJR Am J Roentgenol 1985 May;144(5):999-1001

77. Wenker JC, Baker MK, Ellis JH, Glant MD. Focal fatty infiltration of the liver: demonstration by magnetic resonance imaging. AJR Am J Roentgenol 1984 Sep;143(3):573-4

78. White EM, Simeone JF, Mueller PR, Grant EG, Choyke PL, Zeman RK. Focal periportal sparing in hepatic fatty infiltration: a cause of hepatic pseudomass on US. Radiology 1987 Jan;162(1 Pt 1):57-9

79. Widrich WC, Srinivasan M, Semine MC, Robbins AH. Collateral pathways of the left gastric vein in portal hypertension. AJR Am J Roentgenol 1984 Feb;142(2):375-82

80. Wiesner RH, LaRusso NF. Clinicopathologic features of the syndrome of primary sclerosing cholangitis. Gastroenterology 1980 Aug;79(2):200-6

81. Williams DM, Cho KJ, Aisen AM, Eckhauser FE. Portal hypertension evaluated by MR imaging. Radiology 1985 Dec;157(3):703-6

82. Zirinsky K, Markisz JA, Rubenstein WA, Cahill PT, Knowles RJ, Auh YH, Morrison H, Kazam E. MR imaging of portal venous thrombosis: correlation with CT and sonography.AJR Am J Roentgenol 1988 Feb;150(2):283-8

7 Imaging of the Liver Post-Surgery and/or Post-Ablative Therapy

Contents

The liver is a common site of metastatic disease following initial spread to the lymph nodes, and, because it is the first major organ reached by venous blood draining from the intestinal tract, it is the most common site of metastatic disease from primary cancer within the abdomen. For patients with systemic spread of metastases, curative treatment is generally not possible and general chemotherapeutic approaches to treatment are indicated. On the other hand, if the liver remains the only site of metastatic disease, surgical resection may represent the only means of cure. Unfortunately, the average survival time of patients with untreated hepatic metastases is between 2 and 8 months [19].

Only about 20% of patients with hepatic metastases are suitable for surgical resection. Thus, there has been growing interest in interstitial approaches to destroying liver metastases *in situ*. As alternatives to major surgery, local ablative therapeutic approaches include thermotherapy and chemotherapy techniques, each of which has the advantage of being repeated in cases of recurrent metastatic lesions [1].

Thermotherapeutic approaches to tumor reduction include the application of physical energy in radio-frequency (RF) ablation, laser-induced interstitial therapy (LITT) and cryotherapy. Chemotherapeutic approaches include the local instillation of drugs, as in alcohol injection, chemotherapeutic drug instillation and regional transarterial chemoembolization (TACE) [22].

7.1   Surgical Resection

The role of surgical resection in the treatment of hepatic metastases of primary colorectal carcinomas is well recognized, and may contribute to the 5-year survival of 25% to 37% of affected patients [9]. However, the approach to the surgical treatment of hepatic metastases from primary tumors other than colorectal cancer is less obvious and appears highly dependent upon the type of primary tumor. Nevertheless, a reported 5-year survival rate of 21% after resection of metastases from non-colorectal carcinomas can be considered comparable to that for metastases from colorectal carcinomas [12]. Whereas outstanding results are obtained for the resection of metastases from neuroendocrine tumors, less favorable results are frequently obtained from the resection of metastases from gastric or breast cancer.

In most cases surgical resection involves the removal of two or more liver segments and post-surgical follow-up imaging does not differ greatly from pre-surgical imaging. However, if the borders of the resected liver lesions have been within two centimeters of the resection margin, special attention to the neighboring areas is needed at follow-up. Using T1-weighted (T1w) imaging, detailed evaluation of the resection margins is sometimes difficult due to susceptibility artifacts caused by surgical clips. Follow-up evaluations are also difficult in cases of atypical resection, and when liver lesions are enucleated with a margin of two to three centimeters. Additionally, signal intensity on unenhanced T1w and T2w images, as well as perfusion with T1w dynamic imaging may be influenced by hemorrhage, seroma formation and ischemia of surrounding liver tissue, particularly during the first one to two months after resection. Thus, follow-up imaging is usually best performed at 3 months or more after resection. In such cases, hyperintense nodular regions on T2w images or irregular vascularization on T1w dynamic images are details that are also seen in untreated liver tissue and are usually indicative of recurrent tumor.

In post-surgical follow-up imaging, special care is needed to detect intrahepatic or intraperitoneal seeding of tumor cells. This is particularly important in instances of atypical resection.

7.2   Radio-Frequency (RF) Ablation

In RF ablation of focal liver lesions an alternating current at frequencies above 250 kHz is used to generate heat and thus destroy tissue without causing stimulation of nerves or muscles. The slow application of electrical energy with low current density, leads to the heating and eventual dehydration of cells and, thereafter, to the degeneration of collagenous structures [6].

Cooled tip RF electrodes with 2–3 cm of exposed metal tip are currently used to deliver the RF energy to the tissue. During lesion ablation a thermocouple measures the local temperature and tissue impedance is monitored continuously while the generator output is increased slowly to 950–1.100 mA. Careful monitoring is necessary to prevent the tissue from boiling. Thus, if the impedance increases by > 10 Ohm, the current needs to be reduced until stable impedance is observed again [5]. The standard RF application generally lasts for 12–25 min and results in typical coagulation necrosis diameters of 2.5–3.7 cm [18].

In cases of complete tumor destruction, T2w magnetic resonance (MR) images acquired post RF ablation typically show an area of low signal intensity, comparable to that of normal liver tissue, surrounded by a hyperintense rim. Conversely, treated lesions typically present as hyperintense on unenhanced T1w images. Following the injection of an extracellular Gd-chelate, T1w images of completely destroyed liver lesions reveal a hypointense, non perfused area, sometimes surrounded by a thin hyperintense rim (Fig. 1). However, if hyperintense nodular foci are detected on T2w images, or if irregular enhancement at the boundaries or within the lesion are observed on post-contrast T1w images, this should be considered as suspicious for residual tumor or local tumor re-growth. The thin rim seen as hyperintense on T2w images and as enhancing on T1w contrast enhanced images reflects a vascularized inflammatory reaction surrounding the central zone of coagulation necrosis [7].

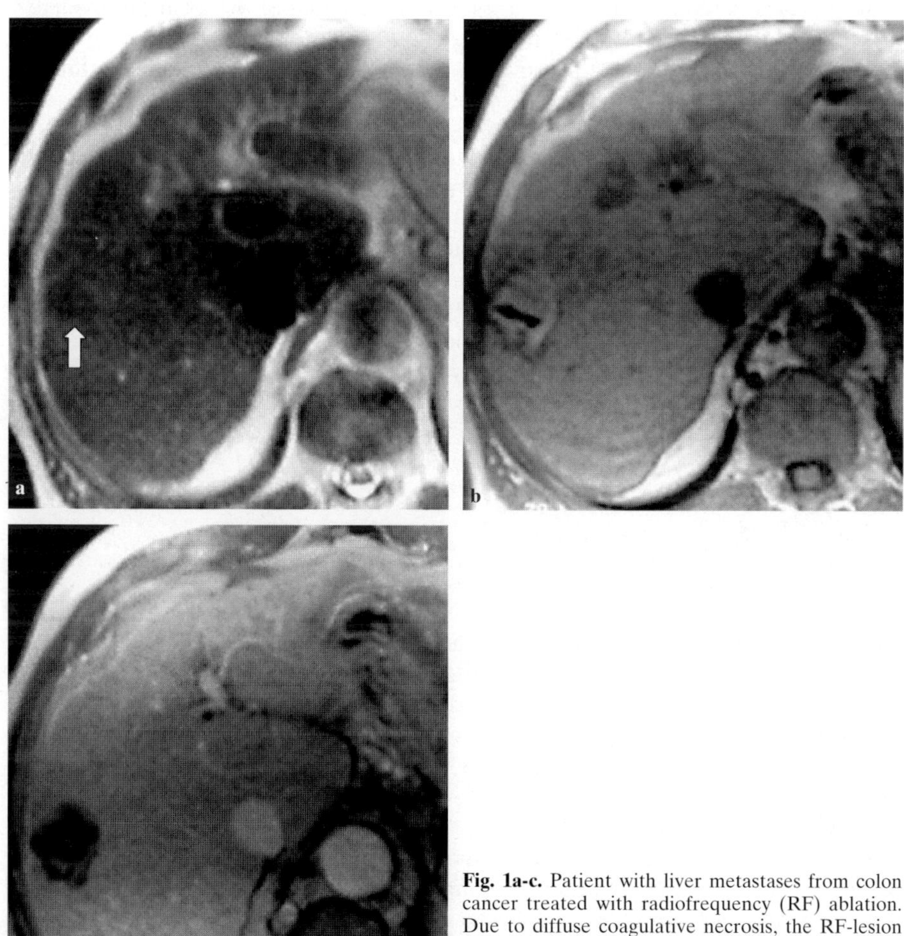

Fig. 1a-c. Patient with liver metastases from colon cancer treated with radiofrequency (RF) ablation. Due to diffuse coagulative necrosis, the RF-lesion (*arrow*) appears slightly hypointense on the T2w image (**a**) and slightly hyperintense on the T1w image (**b**). No enhancement of the RF-lesion is seen during the equilibrium phase after Gd-BOPTA administration (**c**) indicating complete tumor destruction

In RF ablation special attention should be paid not only to complications such as hemorrhage and inflammation, but also to intrahepatic diffusion of the tumor and to seeding along the puncture canal since these areas are not affected by high frequency ablation.

7.3   Laser-Induced Interstitial Therapy (LITT)

Interstitial laser-induced hyperthermia is based on the conversion of laser light into heat. This is typically performed using a Nd:YAG laser at a wavelength of 1064 nm. The technique involves the invasive insertion into the lesion of a laser catheter with a light conducting quartz fiber. The success of the treatment is highly dependent upon the optimal positioning of the laser applicator in the center of the lesion. Hence, precise monitoring during therapy is mandatory. The conversion of laser light into heat in LITT results in cell death followed by coagulative necrosis. Secondary degeneration and atrophy results in tumor shrinkage with minimal damage to surrounding structures.

The size of the heated volume depends on the power of the laser, the irradiation time and the optical and thermal characteristics of the treated tissue. Frequently, lesions with a diameter of 5 cm or more can be treated successfully [21].

T2w MR images acquired approximately 2–3 months after LITT intervention typically reveal a hyperintense lesion surrounded by a hypointense rim. No enhancement of the lesion should be seen on T1w images acquired after injection of a Gd-chelate.

Local tumor recurrence should be considered if T2w images reveal nodular areas of medium to high signal intensity within the treated area or in the hypointense rim surrounding the lesion. The same applies for contrast-enhanced T1w images in which recurrent tumor growth is indicated if enhancement is seen of central areas of the lesion or of peripheral nodular structures [2].

7.4   Cryotherapy

Cryosurgery is defined as local tumor destruction *in situ* caused by the freezing of tumor cells. Cryosurgery is employed mainly in patients with prostatic malignancies and, in some centers, also for the treatment of patients with liver metastases and primary liver tumors such as hepatocellular carcinoma (HCC).

Since cryotherapy does not destroy the walls of large vessels, such as the inferior caval vein, or large liver veins and portal branches, this approach is particularly well-suited to the treatment of unresectable lesions located near these vessels.

Frequently, resection and cryotherapy may be combined during one invasive procedure. Moreover, cryosurgery is appropriate as an adjunct in liver surgery (so-called "Edge Cryotherapy") in cases in which a very close or histologically-positive resection margin is anticipated. During this procedure, flat cryoprobes are held against the resection edge of the remaining liver and adequate freezing is performed to a depth of at least 1.5 cm into the liver.

The mechanism of tumor cell destruction in cryotherapy depends on the location of the tumor tissue in relation to the cryoprobe. In areas close to the cryoprobe temperatures rapidly fall to –190 °C causing ice crystals to form within and around the cells. Subsequent thawing and rehydration results in rupture of the cell membrane and hence tissue death. At distances slightly more removed from the cryoprobe, the temperature drops more slowly and ice forms within the small vessels. Since cell membranes impede intracellular ice crystal formation in this case, the parenchymal cells dehydrate to equilibrate the resulting chemical gradient. This results in expansion of the blood vessels, which, upon thawing, subsequently rupture resulting in tissue hypoxia. Thus, cell death in cryotherapy is a combination of intra- and extracellular ice crystal formation, cellular dehydration, rupture and hypoxia from small vessel destruction [10, 20].

As a result of these changes, lesions after cryotherapy may show signs of hemorrhage on conventional unenhanced T1w and T1w images with fat saturation (FS) and appear hyper- or isointense on T2w images. On contrast-enhanced T1w images, the destroyed tissue is seen as a hypovascular region. In cases of complete tumor destruction, contrast-enhanced T1w images acquired during the equilibrium phase reveal a hypointense region frequently surrounded by a closed hyperintense rim, made up of granulation tissue (Fig. 2, 3). If this rim is interrupted, the site of the interruption can be considered as representing residual tumor, since typically neither a rim nor evidence of edema is seen in tumor tissue.

Often the size of the resulting cryo-lesions remains relatively stable for 3–6 months. Thereafter, they begin to shrink until they are either no longer visible or can be identified only through the presence of a small scar formation (Fig. 4) [2].

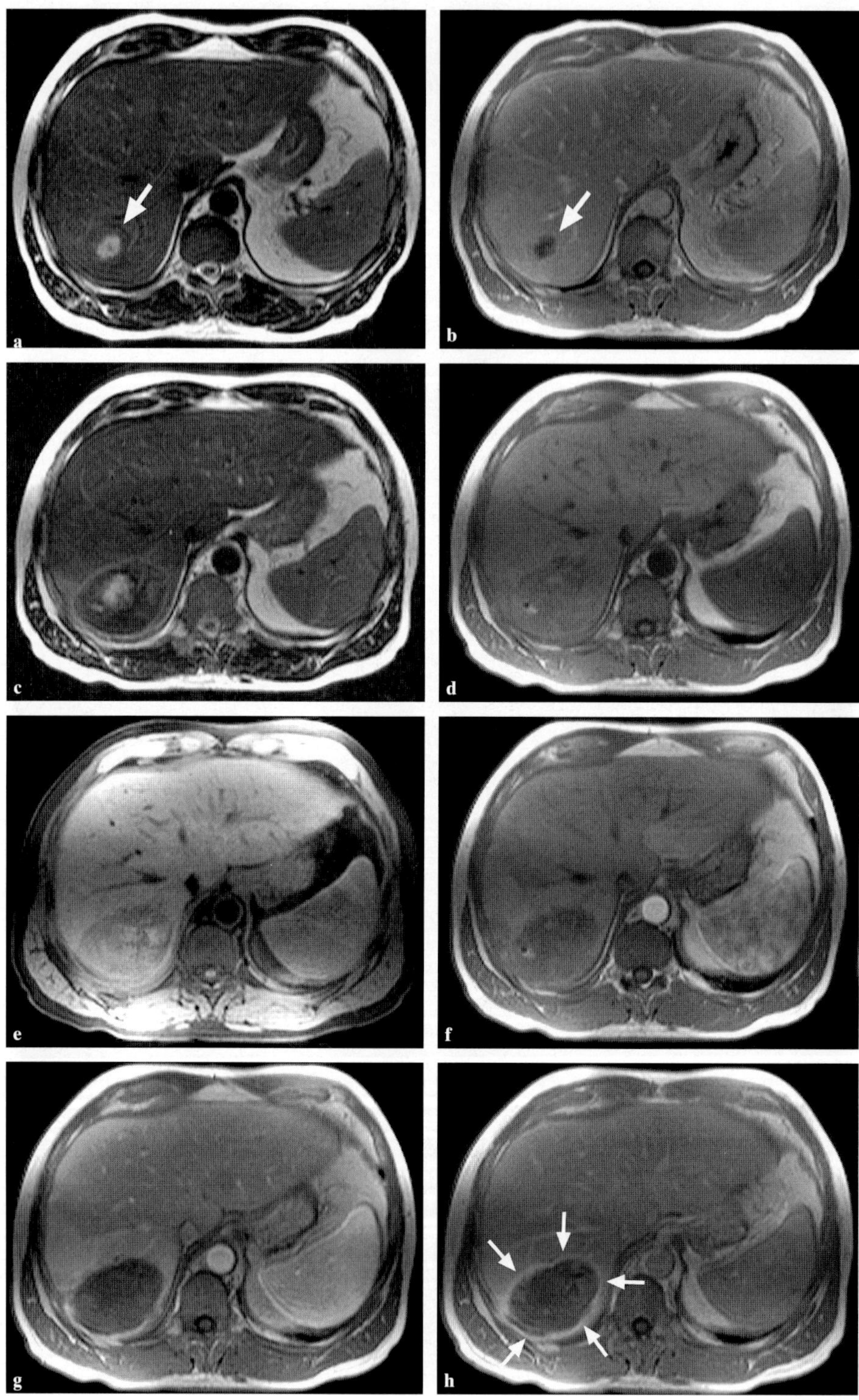

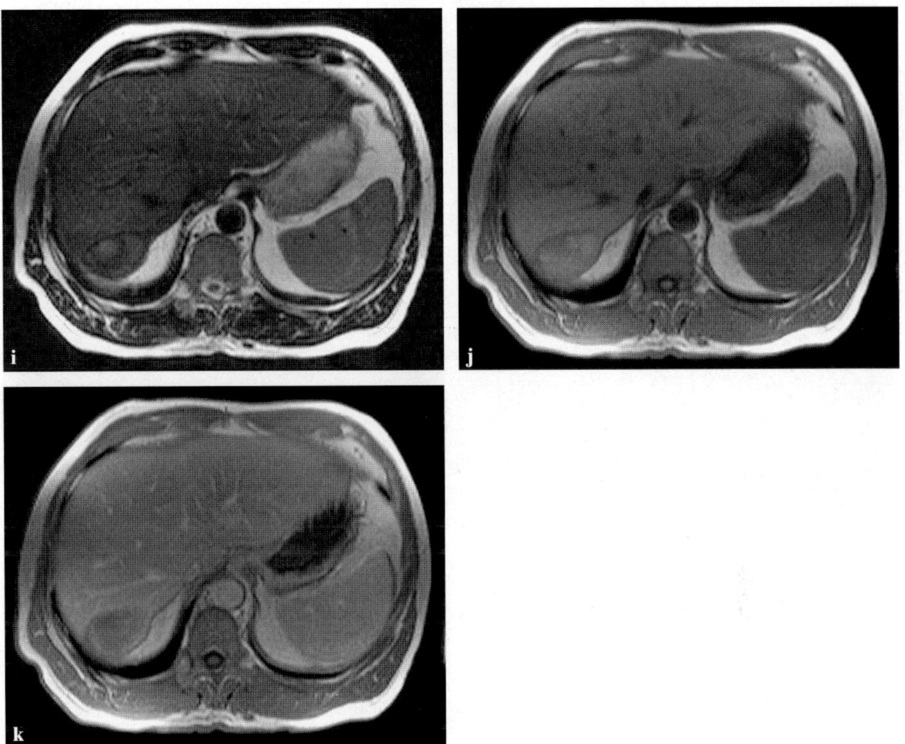

Fig. 2a-k. Liver lesions post-cryotherapy / no residual tumor. Images pre-cryotherapy (**a**: T2w, **b**: T1w contrast enhanced equilibrium phase post-Gd) show a partially necrotic metastasis of colorectal cancer (*arrows*). One week after cryotherapy, the T2w image (**c**) shows a partially hyperintense, partially hypointense region surrounded by a high signal intensity rim. On the corresponding T1w (**d**) and T1w fs (**e**) images, high signal intensity areas within the cryolesion can be detected indicating hemorrhage. Dynamic imaging in the arterial phase (**f**) reveals segmental hypervascularization of the affected liver segment, which is even more obvious in the portal-venous phase (**g**). However, no peripheral enhancement of the cryolesion is detected, indicating no residual tumor. In the equilibrium phase (**h**) a closed hyperintense rim (*arrows*) surrounding the lesion is observed without any enhancement of central areas. This indicates complete destruction of the tumor tissue.
A T2w image acquired six months after cryotherapy (**i**) still shows the cryolesion with non-homogeneous, partially high signal intensity. On the corresponding T1w image (**j**), inhomogeneous high signal intensity can be observed. On contrast enhanced images in the equilibrium phase (**k**), still no enhancement of the central areas of the lesion is visible and a closed hyperintense rim surrounding the lesion can still be seen

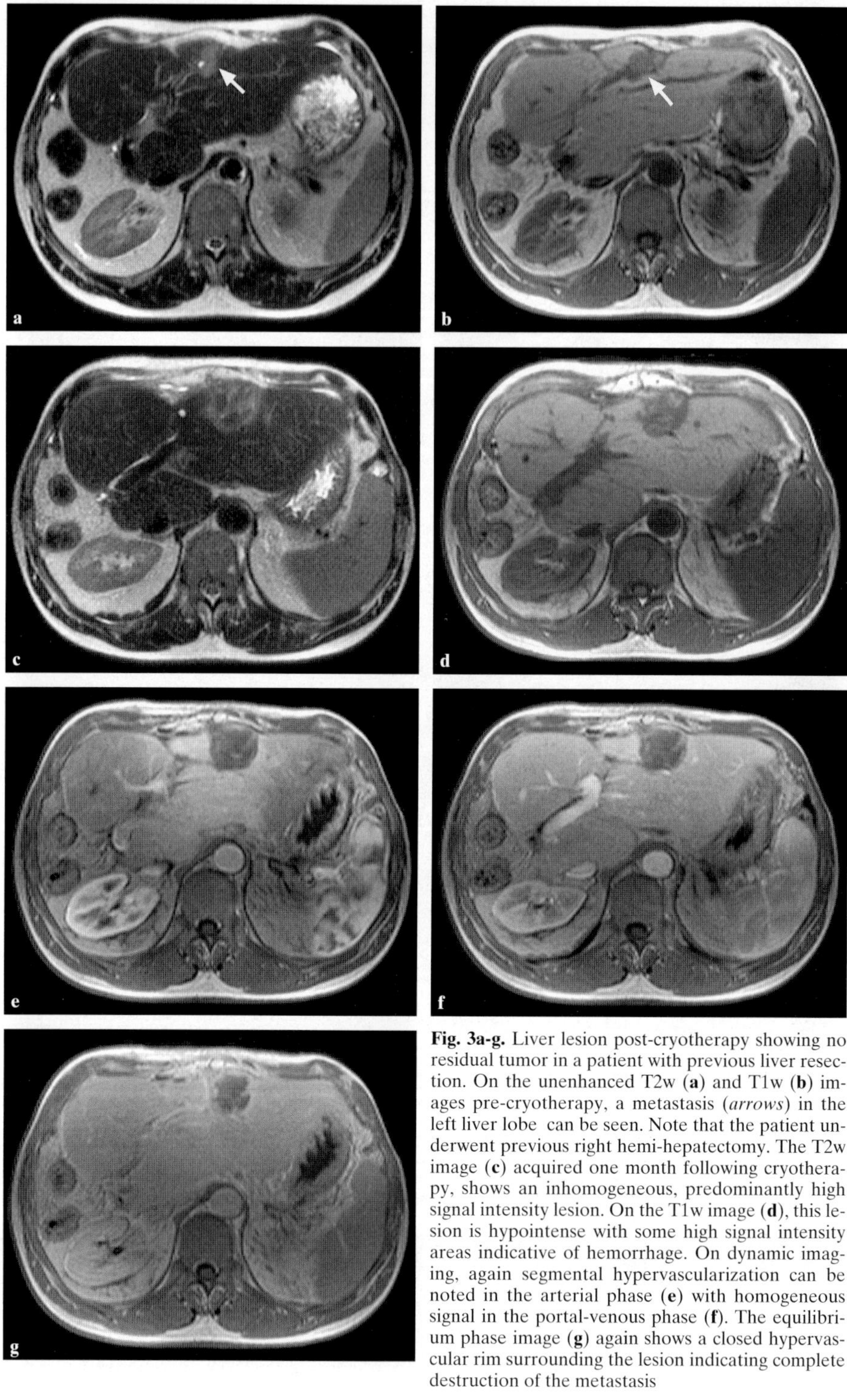

Fig. 3a-g. Liver lesion post-cryotherapy showing no residual tumor in a patient with previous liver resection. On the unenhanced T2w (**a**) and T1w (**b**) images pre-cryotherapy, a metastasis (*arrows*) in the left liver lobe can be seen. Note that the patient underwent previous right hemi-hepatectomy. The T2w image (**c**) acquired one month following cryotherapy, shows an inhomogeneous, predominantly high signal intensity lesion. On the T1w image (**d**), this lesion is hypointense with some high signal intensity areas indicative of hemorrhage. On dynamic imaging, again segmental hypervascularization can be noted in the arterial phase (**e**) with homogeneous signal in the portal-venous phase (**f**). The equilibrium phase image (**g**) again shows a closed hypervascular rim surrounding the lesion indicating complete destruction of the metastasis

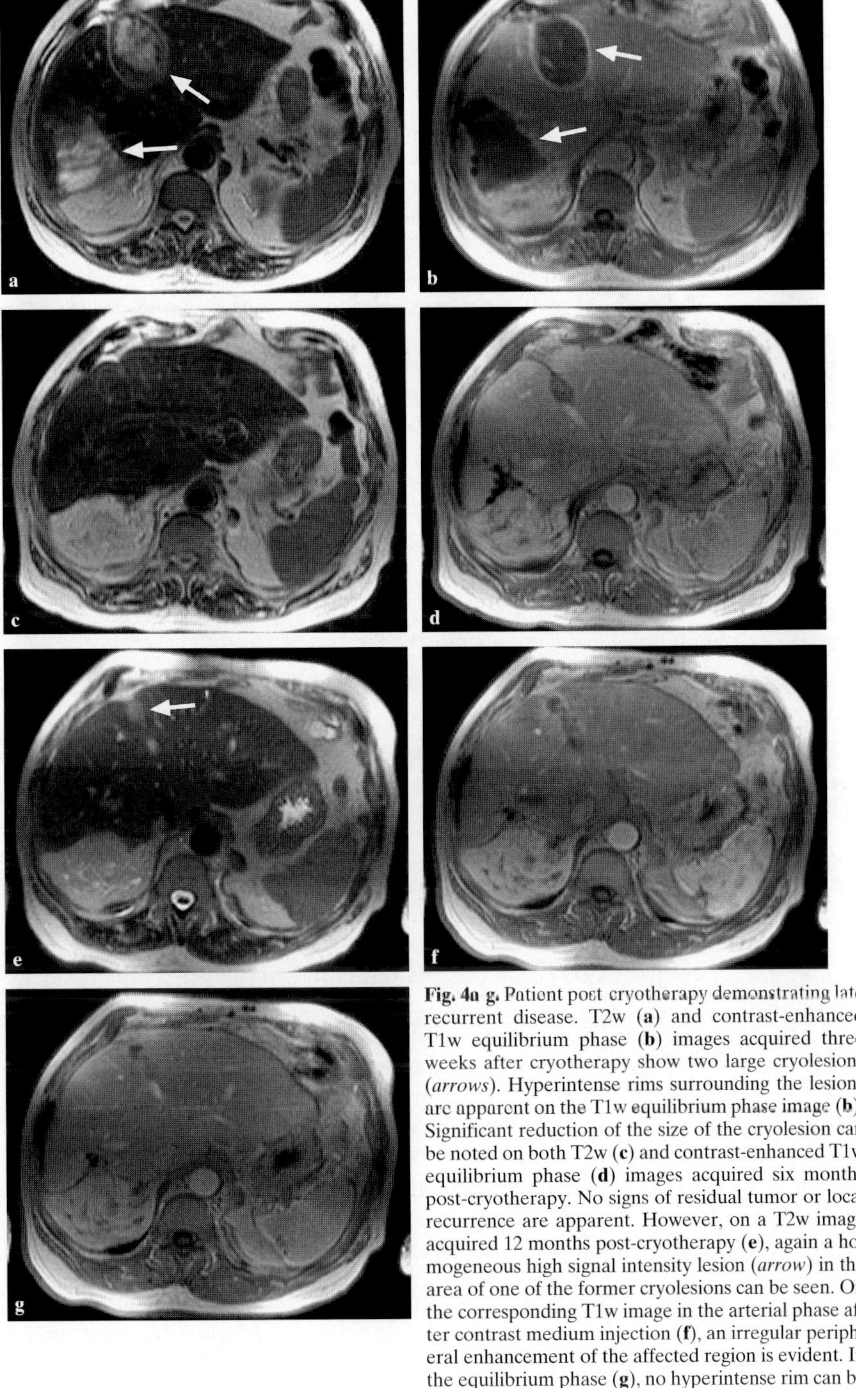

Fig. 4a-g. Patient post cryotherapy demonstrating late recurrent disease. T2w (**a**) and contrast-enhanced T1w equilibrium phase (**b**) images acquired three weeks after cryotherapy show two large cryolesions (*arrows*). Hyperintense rims surrounding the lesions are apparent on the T1w equilibrium phase image (**b**). Significant reduction of the size of the cryolesion can be noted on both T2w (**c**) and contrast-enhanced T1w equilibrium phase (**d**) images acquired six months post-cryotherapy. No signs of residual tumor or local recurrence are apparent. However, on a T2w image acquired 12 months post-cryotherapy (**e**), again a homogeneous high signal intensity lesion (*arrow*) in the area of one of the former cryolesions can be seen. On the corresponding T1w image in the arterial phase after contrast medium injection (**f**), an irregular peripheral enhancement of the affected region is evident. In the equilibrium phase (**g**), no hyperintense rim can be observed. Taken together, these observations indicate local recurrent disease

7.5 Loco-Regional Drug Application

7.5.1 Percutaneous Ethanol Injection

Several studies have shown that percutaneous ethanol injection (PEI) is an effective alternative to surgery in cases of small HCC. Tumor cell destruction is achieved by alcohol-induced immediate coagulative necrosis of the affected tissue as a consequence of protein denaturation and cellular dehydration [16].

The maximum diameter of HCC lesions that can be treated successfully by PEI is approximately 3 cm. Larger lesions are less amenable to treatment with this technique because the ethanol distributes less homogeneously, resulting in incomplete necrosis of the lesion. This equally applies for the treatment of liver metastases for which PEI is of limited effectiveness for local tumor control [8].

T2w MR images acquired post-PEI reveal areas of markedly decreased signal intensity, which correspond to regions of ethanol induced coagulative necrosis. Tumor recurrence should be considered if an area of increased signal intensity is observed within the lesion. However, in rare cases, necrosis with high signal intensity may be observed in the centre of the lesion. This is typically indicative of liquefactive necrosis and should be borne in mind for differential diagnosis. Contrast-enhanced T1w images reveal a hypovascular area similar to that seen in computed tomography (CT) studies. However, recurrent or residual tumor should be considered if enhancement is detected within the first 3–6 months post-therapy (Fig. 5) [11, 17].

7.5.2 Regional Transarterial Chemoembolization (TACE)

Neither systemic or local chemotherapy nor chemoembolization are particularly effective techniques for the treatment of liver metastases. They are mainly considered as a second line of treatment in patients with metastases of colorectal carcinoma or HCC. Nevertheless, TACE is frequently used for curative treatment of HCC, especially in Asia.

TACE therapy is based on the differential blood supply of normal liver tissue and hepatic tumors. Whereas arterial perfusion accounts for about 25% of the blood supply in normal liver parenchyma, it may be as much as 95% in hepatic neoplasms, depending on the histology of the tumor. Thus, solid liver tumors are frequently accessible to arterial embolization and/or intra-arterially applied chemotherapy, while surrounding liver tissue is not affected to the same extent due to its mainly portal venous blood supply. In addition, direct application of chemotherapeutics leads to an increased level of the chemotherapeutic drug within the lesion with a concomitant reduction of systemic side effects [3].

Typically, chemoembolization involves the injection of an emulsion of iodized oil, followed by a chemotherapeutic drug and embolization particles through an arterial catheter advanced into the segmental or subsegmental arteries feeding the tumor.

Chemoembolization may reduce the total tumor volume, which may secondarily allow surgical resection or interventional ablation of inaccessible tumors. In ad-

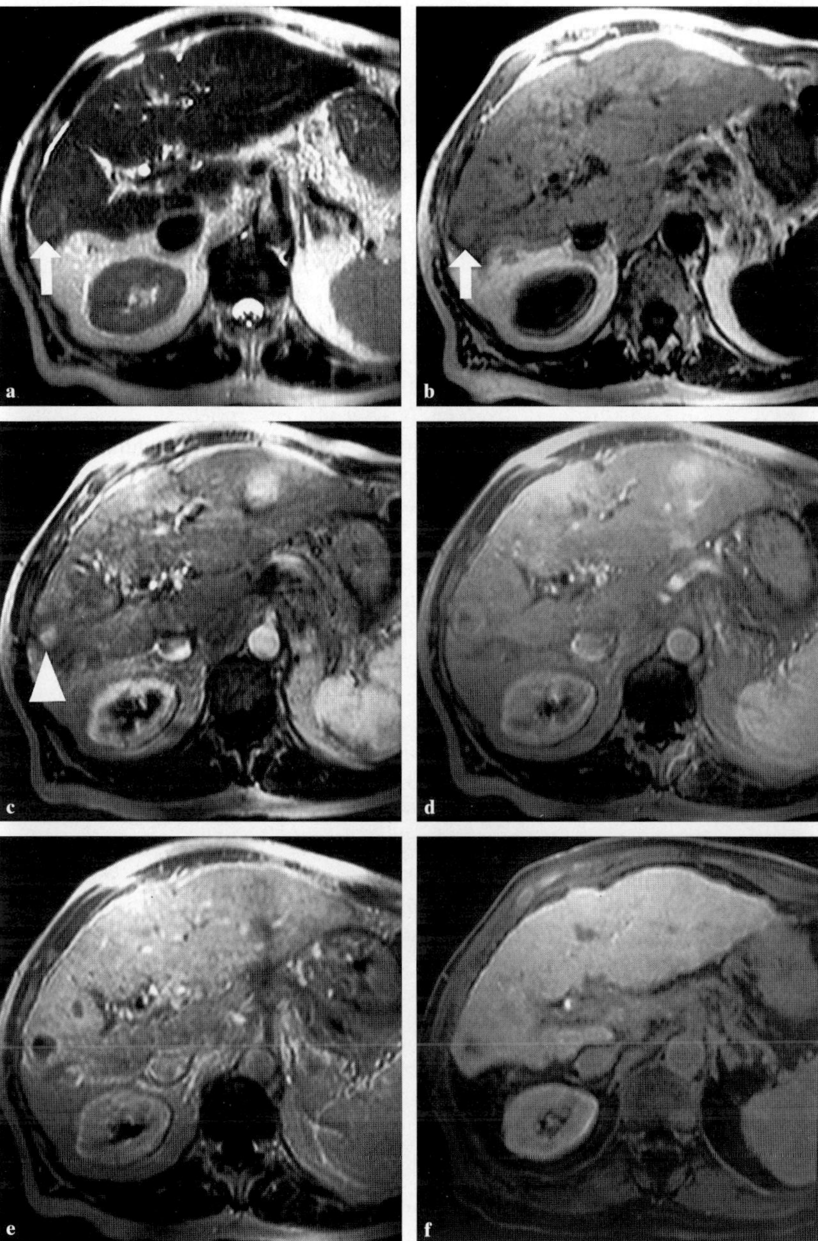

Fig. 5. HCC post-percutaneous ethanol injection (PEI) / residual tumor. The nodule (*arrow*) appears hypointense with slightly hyperintense peripheral areas on T2w images (**a**) and hyperintense on T1w images (**b**) after PEI treatment. A focal hypervascular area (*arrowhead*), representing focal residual tumor, is seen during the arterial phase after the bolus injection of Gd-BOPTA (**c**). The portal-venous and equilibrium phase images (**d** and **e**, respectively) reveal contrast agent washout from the residual tumor and an overall hypointense appearance. The delayed hepatobiliary phase image (**f**) indicates that the residual tumor does not significantly take up Gd-BOPTA. This case is typical of residual tumor in a case of HCC treated by percutaneous ethanol injection. The arterial phase image is the most sensitive phase after contrast medium injection for the detection of residual or recurrent tumor

dition it is performed in cases of ineffective systemic chemotherapy and in cases of therapy-resistant pain arising from dilatation of the liver capsule.

TACE is generally contra-indicated in a number of situations: when significant reduction of synthetic liver function is apparent; when 75% or more of the liver tissue is affected by the neoplasm; in cases of ascites, when the Karnowski Index is < 50%; and in cirrhotic livers when the liver parenchyma has an increased arterial supply. Additionally, TACE may only be performed in cases of portal-venous obstruction if sufficient collaterals are present [14].

MR imaging is increasingly being used in patients after injection of iodized oil (lipiodol). In this regard, MRI is generally preferred to CT for post-TACE imaging since the high concentration of lipiodol within the tumor can make it very difficult to recognize possible disease recurrence on CT [13].

Follow-up imaging after TACE is necessary between the first week and approximately 2–3 months after the procedure. If T1w MR dynamic imaging is performed within the first week after TACE, the increased signal intensity seen in tumor nodules that accumulate lipiodol can sometimes make it difficult to detect residual hypervascular tumor tissue. Decreased signal intensity on T2w images may also be observed within the first week after treatment. However, remaining areas of higher signal intensity on T2w images may not necessarily indicate residual tumor tissue, since the T2 relaxation time is also influenced by early concomitant modifications, such as ischemia, hemorrhage, edema and initial colliquative necrosis [4].

Whereas early follow-up after TACE is often inconclusive for the detection of recurrent tumor, follow-up T1w and T2w MR imaging performed at 2 to 3 months after therapy is very sensitive. Typically, a reduction of the T2 relaxation time, resulting in a decrease of signal intensity, can be observed in completely destroyed tumors on T2w images acquired at 2 to 3 months post TACE. At this time-point, the decreased T2w signal intensity is more likely to be a result of coagulative necrosis induced by TACE than an effect of lipiodol [15].

Completely destroyed tumors are similarly revealed as areas of low signal intensity on T1w images. Thus, dynamic imaging after the injection of Gd-based contrast agents is very sensitive for the detection of tumor recurrence, especially of hypervascular lesions such as HCC. Typically, areas of high signal intensity on T2w images and contrast-enhanced T1w dynamic phase images, acquired at 2 to 3 months after treatment, can be considered as indicative of tumor recurrence [4].

References

1. Bown SG. Phototherapy in tumors. World J Surg 1983 Nov;7(6):700-9
2. Braga L, Semelka RC, Pedro MS, de Barros N. Post-treatment malignant liver lesions. MR imaging. Magn Reson Imaging Clin N Am 2002 Feb;10(1):53-73
3. Chen HS, Gross JF. Intra-arterial infusion of anticancer drugs: theoretic aspects of drug delivery and review of responses. Cancer Treat Rep 1980 Jan;64(1):31-40
4. De Santis M, Torricelli P, Cristani A, Cioni G, Montanari N, Sardini C, Ventura E, Romagnoli R. MRI of hepatocellular carcinoma before and after transcatheter chemoembolization. J Comput Assist Tomogr 1993 Nov-Dec;17(6):901-8
5. De Santis M, Alborino S, Tartoni PL, Torricelli P, Casolo A, Romagnoli R. Effects of lipiodol retention on MRI signal intensity from hepatocellular carcinoma and surrounding liver treated by chemoembolization. Eur Radiol 1997;7(1):10-6
6. Desinger K, Stein T, Tschepe J, Müller G. Investigation on radio-frequency current application in bipolar technique for interstitial thermotherapy (RF-ITT). Minim Invasive Med 1996;7:92-97
7. Dromain C, de Baere T, Elias D, Kuoch V, Ducreux M, Boige V, Petrow P, Roche A, Sigal R. Hepatic tumors treated with percutaneous radio-frequency ablation: CT and MR imaging follow-up. Radiology 2002 Apr;223(1):255-62
8. Ebara M, Ohto M, Sugiura N, Kita K, Yoshikawa M, Okuda K, Kondo F, Kondo Y. Percutaneous ethanol injection for the treatment of small hepatocellular carcinoma. Study of 95 patients. J Gastroenterol Hepatol 1990 Nov-Dec;5(6):616-26
9. Gayowski TJ, Iwatsuki S, Madariaga JR, Selby R, Todo S, Irish W, Starzl TE. Experience in hepatic resection for metastatic colorectal cancer: analysis of clinical and pathologic risk factors. Surgery 1994 Oct;116(4):703-10; discussion 710-1
10. Lee F, Bahn DK, McHugh TA, Onik GM, Lee FT Jr. US-guided percutaneous cryoablation of prostate cancer.Radiology 1994 Sep;192(3):769-76
11. Lencioni R, Bartolozzi C, Caramella D, Di Coscio G. Management of adenomatous hyperplastic nodules in the cirrhotic liver: US follow-up or percutaneous alcohol ablation? Abdom Imaging 1993;18(1):50-5
12. McCarter MD, Fong Y. Metastatic liver tumors. Semin Surg Oncol 2000 Sep Oct;19(2):177-88
13. Murakami T, Nakamura H, Tsuda K, Nakanishi K, Hori S, Tomoda K, Mitani T, Kozuka T, Monden M, Wakasa K. Treatment of hepatocellular carcinoma by chemoembolization: evaluation with 3DFT MR imaging. AJR Am J Roentgenol 1993 Feb;160(2):295-9
14. Pentecost MJ. Transcatheter treatment of hepatic metastases. AJR Am J Roentgenol 1993 Jun;160(6):1171-5
15. Sakurai M, Okamura J, Kuroda C. Transcatheter chemo-embolization effective for treating hepatocellular carcinoma. A histopathologic study. Cancer 1984 Aug 1;54(3):387-92
16. Shiina S, Tagawa K, Niwa Y, Unuma T, Komatsu Y, Yoshiura K, Hamada E, Takahashi M, Shiratori Y, Terano A, et al. Percutaneous ethanol injection therapy for hepatocellular carcinoma: results in 146 patients. AJR Am J Roentgenol 1993 May;160(5):1023-8
17. Sironi S, De Cobelli F, Livraghi T, Villa G, Zanello A, Taccagni G, DelMaschio A. Small hepatocellular carcinoma treated with percutaneous ethanol injection: unenhanced and gadolinium-enhanced MR imaging follow-up. Radiology 1994 Aug;192(2):407-12
18. Solbiati L, Goldberg SN, Ierace T, Livraghi T, Meloni F, Dellanoce M, Sironi S, Gazelle GS. Hepatic metastases: percutaneous radio-frequency ablation with cooled-tip electrodes. Radiology 1997 Nov;205(2):367-73
19. Stangl R, Altendorf-Hofmann A, Charnley RM, Scheele J. Factors influencing the natural history of colorectal liver metastases. Lancet 1994 Jun 4;343(8910):1405-10
20. Steele G Jr. Cryoablation in hepatic surgery. Semin Liver Dis 1994 May;14(2):120-5
21. Vogl TJ, Muller PK, Mack MG, Straub R, Engelmann K, Neuhaus P. Liver metastases: interventional therapeutic techniques and results, state of the art. Eur Radiol 1999;9(4):675-84
22. Vogl TJ, Mack MG, Muller PK, Straub R, Engelmann K, Eichler K. Interventional MR: interstitial therapy. Eur Radiol 1999;9(8):1479-87

Subject Index